Any nurse who takes seriouson
should know about this imp.tri-
bution to our profession. In ...u, an understanding of values and belief. ...may differ from our own
world view, is more importan. ...u. According to many polls, the USA
is a religious country and every religion is practiced by its citizens. However,
nursing has done little to address or incorporate these facts in nursing education and practice. This well-written, informative book can change that. If you
strive to be a better student, clinician, researcher, teacher, or administrator,
you will greatly benefit from reading this book. I highly recommend it.

Anne J. Davis, RN, PhD, DSc (hon), FAAN
Professor Emerita
University of California, San Francisco
Nagano College of Nursing, Japan
International Consultant, Nursing Ethics

Marsha Fowler and her colleagues are making a new and very important
appeal to nursing to see religion not as an extra or external element, but as
something inherent in life. By writing not *about* religion, but *from* within
religious traditions, they show the strengths of all religions to argue and act
in socially appropriate ways by holistic and just means, based on the intrinsic
sacredness of life. They show how religions and religious ethics underscore
the completeness of coherent nursing care and theory. The more I read of
this book, the more I realized how different its message is from other books
and how this message is significant. Other recent international texts on issues
of social ethics have also pointed in the direction of a deeper morality than
has been current. Together these texts make a convincing case, and this book
has the potential to blaze the way for new understandings of the need for
and the delivery of care, in particular nursing care. I hope the book will catch
the imagination of nurses everywhere and that people run with its message.

Verena Tschudin, RN, PhD
Visiting Senior Fellow
University of Surrey
Guildford, United Kingdom

The reader of this exceptionally well-written book will find that classical
dialogues, as well as a more contemporary exposé of philosophies and theories, that have shaped and continue to shape nursing practice, are expertly
discussed. The editor and the authors are some of the top thinkers in the field,
providing a level of intellectual stimulation that will enhance new heights in
critical thinking about the epistemological origins of ideas in nursing. It is a
book of a coherent set of chapters written to raise as many profound questions as it answers. I expect that nursing science and its theoretical basis will

be profoundly influenced by the analyses provided in this volume and the promise that it holds. Kudos to Dr. Marsha Fowler!

Afaf Ibrahim Meleis, PhD, DrPS (hon), FAAN
Margaret Bond Simon Dean of Nursing
University of Pennsylvania School of Nursing
Professor of Nursing and Sociology
Director of the School's WHO Collaborating Center for Nursing
and Midwifery Leadership
University of Pennsylvania

Religion, Religious Ethics, and Nursing finally gives voice to a thoroughly thoughtful and important scholarship that will transform our collective capacity for meaningful dialogue and robust theoretical development. This articulate and scholarly anthology reclaims the middle ground that has been missing from the spirituality discourse in modern nursing literature. Recognizing the centrality of sacred text and tradition as foundational to the human experience of cultures and communities across history and place, it invites an integrative and authentic respect for world religions and for the powerful role they play in shaping the health and illness experience. In their delightful polyvocality, the authors illuminate a profoundly shared moral core, one of reverence for the kinds of questions that all religions confront about the meaning of life and death, the purpose of human suffering, and the value of compassionate engagement.

Sally Thorne, RN, PhD, FCAHS
Professor, School of Nursing
University of British Columbia

To provide a broad and comprehensive view of world religions with a special emphasis on their relevance to health, illness, death, and dying is not a task for the faint-hearted. It is an undertaking that must be approached with great caution lest it fall into the marshes of essentialism and meaningless generalities. So it was not without trepidation that I approached this 19-chapter tome. To my great relief I discovered a sophisticated and highly pertinent analysis of the state of contemporary religion, a critique of the deafening silence in nursing on religion, and a meaningful sweeping look at the world's major religions. There is no cookbook presented here, nor are there trite excursions into transculturalism. Rather, this text teaches about religion and religious beliefs, makes a sustained argument for religion as a positive and as yet untapped force for nurses and nursing, and refreshingly looks the counter arguments straight in the eye and takes them on.

Sioban Nelson, Dean and Professor
Lawrence S. Bloomberg Faculty of Nursing
University of Toronto

Religion, Religious Ethics, AND Nursing

Marsha D. Fowler, PhD, MDiv, MS, RN, FAAN, teaches in Southern California, United States, where she is a professor of Ethics and Spirituality. She is a past chairperson of both the California Nurses Association and American Nurses Association ethics committees and was a member of the Task Force for the Revision of the Code of Ethics for the American Nurses Association. She has numerous publications: peer-reviewed journal articles, book chapters, and books on ethics, bioethics, religion, and spirituality in nursing. Her educational background includes a PhD in Religion & Social Ethics, a Master of Divinity degree, a Master of Science degree (Nursing), and a diploma in Spiritual Direction. She has been a Joseph P. Kennedy, Jr. Fellow in Bioethics at Harvard University and a WK Kellogg Foundation National Leadership Fellow. In 1992, she received the American Nurses Association Honorary Human Rights Award. In 1996, she was the recipient of the Friends World Committee for Consultation Bogert Fund Award for the Study and Practice of Christian Mysticism. She is a fellow of the American Academy of Nursing and currently serves as the Chair of the Academy's Expert Panel on Global Nursing and Health. She is a clergy member of the Presbyterian Church (USA). She has lectured extensively both nationally and internationally, including Russia, the United Kingdom, Jordan, Colombia, Canada, Japan, and South Korea. Her areas of research include ethics in nursing, suffering, religion in nursing, health disparities, and health policy in global health.

Sheryl Reimer-Kirkham, PhD, RN, is a professor in the School of Nursing at Trinity Western University, Langley, British Columbia, Canada. She is the Director of the graduate nursing (MSN) program and teaches Health Care Ethics, Health Policy, and Qualitative Research. Her research program focuses on social justice and pluralism in health care and nursing education. A current funded research project examines religion, spirituality, culture, gender, and place in home health care. She is a founding member of Trinity Western University's Religion in Canada Institute and Institute of Gender Studies, and the Critical Research in Health and Health Inequities Unit at the University of British Columbia. She has recently been awarded a 2010 Award of Excellence in Nursing Research by the College of Registered Nurses of British Columbia.

Richard Sawatzky, PhD, RN, is an Associate Professor of Nursing at Trinity Western University, Canada. His research focuses on methods of patient-reported outcomes and quality of life measurement, and the intersections of spirituality, religion, culture, and other sources of diversity in various health care contexts. He has a particular methodological interest in the use of latent variable mixture modeling for examining sample heterogeneity with respect to individuals' self-reports about their health status and quality of life. He is a member of the International Society for Quality of Life Research and the International Society for Quality of Life Studies.

Elizabeth Johnston Taylor, PhD, RN, is an associate professor, Loma Linda University School of Nursing, Loma Linda, California, United States. Her experiences as an oncology nurse led to an interest in the relationship between illness and spirituality. She pursued this interest in her doctoral program at the University of Pennsylvania, and a postdoctoral fellowship at UCLA. She has also completed two units of Clinical Pastoral Education and Training in spiritual direction. She has received funding for her research and training from several sources, including the National Cancer Institute, the Agency for Health Care Policy and Research, and John Templeton Foundation. She has numerous publications on nursing spiritual care and patient spiritual and religious responses to illness. Her books include *Spiritual Care: Nursing Theory, Research, and Practice* (Prentice Hall, 2002) and *What Do I Say? Talking with Patients about Spirituality* (Templeton Press, 2007). She is authoring the clinical companion book *Religion: A Clinical Guide for Nurses* (Springer Publishing Company, 2012).

Religion, Religious Ethics, AND Nursing

Marsha D. Fowler, PhD, MDiv, MS, RN, FAAN
Sheryl Reimer-Kirkham, PhD, RN
Richard Sawatzky, PhD, RN
Elizabeth Johnston Taylor, PhD, RN

EDITORS

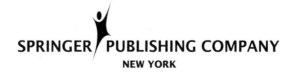

SPRINGER PUBLISHING COMPANY
NEW YORK

Springer Publishing Company, LLC
11 West 42nd Street
New York, NY 10036
www.springerpub.com

Acquisitions Editor: Margaret Zuccarini
Composition: S4Carlisle Publishing Services

ISBN: 978-0-8261-0663-6
E-book ISBN: 978-0-8261-0664-3

11 12 13/ 5 4 3 2 1

The author and the publisher of this Work have made every effort to use sources believed to be reliable to provide information that is accurate and compatible with the standards generally accepted at the time of publication. The author and publisher shall not be liable for any special, consequential, or exemplary damages resulting, in whole or in part, from the readers' use of, or reliance on, the information contained in this book. The publisher has no responsibility for the persistence or accuracy of URLs for external or third-party Internet Web sites referred to in this publication and does not guarantee that any content on such Web sites is, or will remain, accurate or appropriate.

Library of Congress Cataloging-in-Publication Data

Religion, religion ethics, and nursing / Marsha Fowler ... [et al.].
  p. ; cm.
Includes bibliographical references and index.
ISBN 978-0-8261-0663-6 (alk. paper) – ISBN 978-0-8261-0664-3 (e-book) 1. Nursing–Religious aspects.
2. Nursing ethics. 3. Religious ethics. I. Fowler, Marsha Diane Mary.
[DNLM: 1. Nurse's Role. 2. Religion and Medicine. 3. Ethics, Nursing. 4. Spirituality. WY 87]
RT85.2.R45 2012
201'.661073–dc23
                    2011027642

Printed in the United States of America by Bang Printing

Dim heddwch heb gyfiawnder.

Without justice there is no peace.

Contents

Contributors

Rowaida Al Maaitah, DrPh, MPh, RN President of the Hashemite University in Jordan, Consultant for Her Royal Highness Princess Muna Al-Hussein for Health and Social Development, Zarqa, Jordan

Melania Calestani, PhD, MSc Research Fellow, Middlesex University, London, UK

Janice Clarke, PhD, RGN Senior Lecturer at the Institute of Health and Society, University of Worcester, Worcester, UK

Muntaha K. Gharaibeh, PhD, MSC, RN Dean and Professor of Nursing, Jordan University of Science and Technology, Irbid, Jordan

Chaya Greenberger, PhD, MSN, FNP, RN Head of the Department of Nursing, Jerusalem College of Technology/Machon Tal, Jerusalem, Israel

Sonya Grypma, PhD, MN, RN Associate Professor, School of Nursing, Trinity Western University, Langley, BC, Canada

Auntie Joan Hendricks Aboriginal elder of the Ngugi people from Moreton Island; Deputy Chair, Council for Australian Catholic Women Brisbane, QLD, Australia

Harjit Kaur, MSoc Sc Program Manager, Ending Violence Association of British Columbia, Vancouver, BC, Canada

Anita Noble, DNSc, CNM, CTN-A, IBCLC Senior Faculty, Henrietta Szold/Hadassah-Hebrew University School of Nursing, Faculty of Medicine, Jerusalem, Israel

Barbara Pesut, PhD, MSN, RN Canada Research Chair in Health Ethics and Diversity, University of British Columbia, Kelowna, BC, Canada

Donna Scemons, PhD, RN, FNP-C, CNS   Family Nurse Practitioner Healthcare Systems, Inc., Castaic, CA, USA

Sonya Sharma, PhD, MAMRes   Research Associate, Department of Theology and Religion, Durham University, Durham, UK

Savitri W. Singh-Carlson, PhD, MSN, RN   Assistant Professor in Nursing, California State University at Long Beach, Long Beach, CA, USA

Bhartendu Srivastava, PhD, MScTech   Past President, Hindu Cultural Society and Hindu Prarthana Samaj, Toronto, ON, Canada

Raman Srivastava, BMSc (Honors)   Research Associate, Toronto, ON, Canada

Rani Srivastava, PhD, MScN, RN   Chief of Nursing and Professional Practice, Center for Addiction and Mental Health, Toronto, ON, Canada

Landa Terblanche, PhD, M. Art et Scien, RN   Dean and Associate Professor, School of Nursing, Trinity Western University, Langley, BC, Canada

Barbra Mann Wall, PhD, RN, FAAN   Associate Professor of Nursing, Associate Director of the Barbara Bates Center for the Study of the History of Nursing, University of Pennsylvania, Philadelphia, PA, USA

Nereda White, PhD   Professor and Director, Centre for Indigenous Education and Research, Australian Catholic University, Banyo, QLD, Australia

Foreword

The Reverend Dr. Marsha Fowler and her colleagues have written a landmark book that will change and enlighten the discourse on religion and spirituality in nursing. The authors address the awkward silence on religion in nursing theory and education and with insightful scholarship move beyond the current level of knowledge and limited discourse on religion in nursing theory, education, and practice. This book is path-breaking in that it delivers new ways to think about the relationships among ethics, health, caregiving, moral imagination, religion, and spirituality. They trace and defend the roots of secular or nonsectarian nursing education while holding onto the influence of religion and spirituality for nurses, patients, and all health care.

The authors wisely note that the nurses cannot effectively compartmentalize their own religious faith because much of the impetus and moral imagination for nursing come from religious or spiritual understanding. They encourage respect and a better knowledge of religion in health and health care practices and against abusing the nurse–patient relationship by focusing on "converting" or proselytizing the ill person. Starting with Nightingale's injunction against proselytizing, the authors show that using the nurse–patient relationship to gain converts to one's own religion violates the caregiving practices and moral stance of most religions.

Religion, Religious Ethics, and Nursing articulates diverse religious moral sources of caring for family, strangers, neighbors, and the marginalized poor and vulnerable. Fowler and her coauthors astutely avoid a superficial cookbook account of the health care implications of various religious rituals and practices, and call for understanding the moral sources and various religious understandings that guide our understanding and conduct in relation to one another as fellow human beings who are all embodied, vulnerable, and in need of care by others. The authors describe their rationale for presenting different religious knowledge of health and health care: "Understanding what a tradition means by health and concepts more central to health provides a stronger foundation for nurses to engage with religious patients, and may broaden how nursing understands its own theory and practice." For example, in chapter 12 on Islam, Muntaha Gharaibeh and Rowaida Al Maaitah note:

> Jurists and scholars in Islam agree that the aim of Islamic Shari'a is to safeguard the five objectives of life, namely: faith, body, offspring, property and mind. The scholars of Islam express these five sublime objectives in terms of the five essentials. They mean by the word 'essentials' the fundamentals, without which life may not be possible. When any of these fundamentals is undermined, life will be compromised and may become chaotic.

Understanding these five Islamic essentials can guide nurses in their support of the repair of a damaged or disordered Islamic lifeworld that may occur as a result of loss, injury, or suffering. Fowler and her colleagues make it clear that the internal diverse moral sources for caring for the vulnerable and promoting health and well-being stem from the religious understandings of what health, caregiving, and well-being mean within various religious traditions.

Social justice and religious moral sources are presented in chapter 2 in ways that link community health nursing, health promotion, and public health. For example, Fowler and Reimer-Kirkham describe how diverse religious groups organize and engage in many effective endeavors to increase social justice and provide humanitarian aid during times of disaster, breakdown in civility or war, in community development, service, and social advocacy. All of these aims clearly fit within the scope of public health, health promotion, and community health nursing.

A more comprehensive view of spirituality and religious traditions in the current secular and postmodern age demands that antireligious positions such as ultimate faith in science, human will, and intelligence be considered as yet another spiritual and belief-laden stance. In this view, the antireligious may assert equally strong claims about ultimate reality and goals as religious believers and thinkers. Likewise the broad syncretic New Age beliefs and spiritual practices are viewed as evolving religious stances, with many assertions and assumptions about health, caregiving, and sickness or disease, all calling for understanding, study, and respect.

This work is current and forward-looking in a postmodern secularized and global world where people mingle and create new religious practices and beliefs. While calling for respect for religious traditions based upon knowledge and understanding, the authors agree that we live in what Taylor has called *A Secular Age.*[1] However, this secularism is pluralistic with much blending of religious traditions within families and even within congregations.

Religion, Religious Ethics, and Nursing is central to humanities and social science studies in nursing education. The authors have written a wonderfully accessible, scholarly book on the role of religion in health care and caring practices. I think readers of the future will look back on this work as a beginning of a new level of discourse on religion, health care, nursing, and healing practices. Current readers will find new insights to help them through the maze of rich and diverse moral visions for health and well-being rooted in diverse religious traditions.

Patricia Benner, PhD, RN, FAAN
Professor Emerita of Nursing
Department of Social and Behavioral Sciences and Nursing
University of California, San Francisco

NOTE

1. Taylor, Charles. *A Secular Age*. Cambridge, MA: Harvard University Press, 2007.

Preface

The title *Religion, Religious Ethics, and Nursing* may conjure expectations for a "world religions" approach to the subject matter of this book. Readers may thus be startled to find that this work contains no charts about what Catholics, Protestants, Jews, and Buddhists believe—the stuff of "introduction to nursing" textbooks. The intent of this book is, instead, to lay the foundation for a deeper exploration of religion and religious ethics as they intersect with nursing theory, education, research, and practice. This work is intended for the classroom, clinicians, and nurse researchers and nurse ethicists who require a theoretical basis for a consideration of religious diversity, religious ethics, religious social ethics, and nursing. While this book points toward practice, it is not a practice-oriented guide. That task is left to the companion volume *Religion: A Clinical Guide for Nurses* (2012, Springer Publishing Company) written by our colleague Elizabeth Johnston Taylor. So what might the reader encounter in this book?

The first section examines theoretical questions. Chapter 1, "Religion and Nursing," explores nursing's neglect of religion in the light of the deep religious faith of Florence Nightingale and her desire for nursing education to be non-sectarian, and in the light of the secularization of society. This chapter also tackles the perspective that *religion* is a Western construct, a Western invention, that does not reflect the reality of the non-Western world. The chapter concludes with a discussion of how *religion* is defined.

Chapter 2, "Religious Ethics, Religious Social Ethics, and Nursing," begins with a series of caveats in the study, understanding, and exercise of religion. These caveats then inform a discussion of four sources of religious-moral authority that religious traditions and their followers utilize in moral analysis and decision making: sacred writings and sacred stories, tradition, reason, and religious experience. While religions are concerned for the inner life or the spiritual journey, they are also concerned for the shape of the world, with issues of justice and peace. The chapter concludes with an examination of religious social ethics and its involvement in "repairing the world."

Some clarification must be offered at this point. It is customary in religious studies circles to number years as *BCE* (Before the Common Era) and *CE* (in the Common Era) instead of the Christian designations *BC* and *AD*. That practice has been adopted in this book. As a further note, we have chosen to retain some technical or specialized religious terminology commonly found in theological or religious works so that the reader may become acquainted with the more common terms used in religious studies and theology. Additionally, it is common in religious literature written within and for its faith community to employ several devotional conventions. For example, in some Jewish texts, "God" is spelled "G-d," omitting the "o" so as to show reverence for the divine name. In Islam, "peace be upon him" or "PBUH" is written after the name of the Prophet. These are devotional conventions used within the community and are not customarily used in a broader academic literature outside of the community of faith it represents.

Chapter 3, "Religion and Theoretical Thinking in Nursing," discusses how religion has influenced nursing's theoretical thinking and addresses some of the ethical implications of the use of religious ideas in a diverse society. It begins with a brief discussion of the influences of religion on early nursing theory, including nursing models, meta-paradigm development, and nursing diagnosis. It then discusses current trends in religion and spirituality in the broader social context and their influence on nursing theory. The ethical issues of proposing theoretical views in nursing that do not adequately encompass the religious views of patients are then outlined. The chapter concludes with a proposed approach to incorporating religion into nursing theoretical thinking that allows for both the diverse experience of religious individuals and the scientific basis of the nursing discipline.

Chapter 4, "Feminist and Religious Ethics in Nursing," explores the complex relationships between nursing, religion, and feminism with particular emphasis on ethics. Although nursing has strong and continuing roots in institutional religion, feminist critiques of institutional religion have profoundly influenced the construction of religion in current nursing discourse. This chapter will illustrate some of the contributions that feminist ethics can make to religious ethics in nursing and reveal how each provides a lens to understanding what is good and right to do within the discipline. Following the lead of feminist developments in the sociology of religion, this chapter will propose a broader vision for the contributions of feminist ethics to religion and religious ethics in nursing.

Chapter 5, "A Critical Reading Across Religion and Spirituality: Contributions of Postcolonial Theory to Nursing Ethics," provides an overview of postcolonial theory as one form of critical inquiry particularly salient for the study of religion and spirituality, and highlights several methodological and practice implications for nursing ethics. The chapter examines the contributions of postcolonial theory, arguing that critical perspectives offer invaluable analytic tools in the critical analysis of religion, spirituality, and health/

nursing. In so doing, it urges a re-thinking of nursing's typical de-emphasis of creedal religions in the quest for a universal spiritual experience.

Chapter 6, "Intersectional Analyses of Religion, Culture, Ethics, and Nursing," asserts that in the presence of unprecedented global migration and societal diversity, religion and spirituality need to be understood as intertwined with other social categories such as gender, ethnicity, and class. Referred to as intersectionality, these interrelationships shape how identities are lived out and how social disadvantage and oppression operate in collective ways. The intersectionality of religion/spirituality with other social classifications has, as the chapter suggests, not been adequately accounted for in the fields of nursing and nursing ethics. At the level of social ethics, religion/spirituality are implicated in the intersecting social determinants of health and health inequities. In the realm of clinical nursing ethics, a lens of intersectionality gives insight into the complexities of moral agency, ethical decision making, and relational practice.

The succeeding section on historical research on religious nursing provides two examples of research by nurse-historians. This section is intended to show the promise that such historical research holds for understanding both nursing and religious nursing, how religion has influenced the development of nursing, and how religious nursing has influenced both nursing and health care worldwide. These two chapters constitute an implicit call for additional historical research internationally.

The third section of the book includes seven religious-tradition specific chapters on Hinduism, Judaism, Christianity, Islam, Sikhism, Religions of Native Peoples, and emergent non-religious spiritualities, sometimes termed New Age spiritualities. The intent of these chapters is *not* to provide an "essentials" approach or overview of the beliefs of the tradition, nor to examine the health-related implications of certain religious prescriptions and proscriptions. Rather, the aim of these chapters is to explore how these traditions conceptualize various concepts that are pivotal to nursing, including health, well-being, compassion, nursing, care of the stranger, or community. While the impulse might be to start with the particulars of what a religious tradition says about, for example, diet or infertility or family structure, knowing this will not assist the nurse to actually understand what lies behind these norms. Understanding what a tradition means by *health* and concepts more central to health provides a stronger foundation for nurses to engage with religious patients, and may broaden nursing's understanding of its own theory and practice. Additional religious traditions are utilized as examples throughout the text. The limited number of traditions that we examine in greater depth serves as an implicit invitation to nursing to research the religion-nursing intersections of other traditions as well.

The two chapters of the fourth section, "Religion and Nursing Practice," review the research on religion and provide illustrative clinical vignettes pertaining both to patients and to nurses who are religious. Chapter 16,

"Religion and Patient Care," explores how patient or family religious beliefs and practices affect responses to illness challenges and health care. After considering how religion may be associated with health, the chapter illustrates how religiosity colors the interpretation of illness and health behaviors. Because the existent empirical evidence provides considerable insight into how religious coping influences response to illness and how religion has an impact on health care decision making, these areas are examined as well. The chapter reviews not only the impact of these religious beliefs, but also the interplay of religious practices and health, and the religious care that patients want and get. The chapter concludes by identifying implications this evidence provides for clinical nursing practice.

Chapter 17 reviews the literature that suggests the ways in which the religiosity of nurses influences their practice of nursing. It explores ways in which personal religiosity may or may not be appropriately brought to the bedside, and directly addresses the ethical issue of proselytizing in the clinical setting.

The 18th chapter, "The Measurement of Religious Concepts in Nursing," is specifically intended for the nurse researcher or consumer of nursing research. It addresses problems in the measurement of religious concepts for nursing theory and practice based on individuals' self-reports, including the concepts of religious affiliation, religious attendance (participation in religious services or activities), religious orientation, private religiousness, religious coping, and religious beliefs, values, and experiences. The results of studies that answer these questions vary and must be interpreted in light of the characteristics of the measurement instruments that were used and the populations and purposes for which they were developed. This chapter explores the processes and assumptions underlying the measurement validation of religious concepts and the corresponding inferences that may be warranted.

The book concludes with a brief epilogue, "Looking Back and Looking Ahead: A Concluding Postscript." The intent of this brief section is to draw together both the problems and promise that an exploration of religion by nursing might hold. It takes a critical look backward, and an anticipatory look forward to where nursing might go in its study of religion, religious ethics, and nursing theory and practice.

This work is, then, anything but a world-religions approach to religions and nursing. It is our hope that its readers will find it provocative, challenging, and enriching and that it will spur further interest in a topic that has, to nursing's disadvantage, lain fallow.

Marsha D. Fowler
Easter 2011
6th day of Passover 5771
4th day of Chol Hamoed 5771

Acknowledgments

Unlike Athena, who sprang forth full grown from the head of Zeus, no book comes to life quite so precipitously or unassisted. This book emerged from a small gathering of nursing faculty brought together by a networking grant, written by Barb Pesut, which underwrote the travel that allowed us to meet together. We shared a concern for the direction of the nursing literature toward a spirituality that excluded concerns for religion, even while it tended to utilize quasi-religious measures to evaluate spirituality. Over the course of two years we gathered in Vancouver, British Columbia, Canada, and in Loma Linda and Pasadena, California, USA, to collaborate on a series of journal articles and responses to our articles. At the completion of the small grant, we retained an interest in continuing to work together in the domain of religion, ethics, and nursing. This book is the product of that continued collaboration.

Yet, work on religion in nursing remains at the fringes of nursing's interests. Despite nursing's claims to whole-person, holistic care, and despite its incorporation into some codes of ethics, religion receives little more than token mention here and there in the nursing literature. It is mentioned as one of many aspects of "coping mechanisms," it is alluded to when nursing wishes to say that spirituality is not religion, and it receives mention when exceptions to blood transfusions are discussed. At no point does the nursing literature discuss the ways in which religions might view person, health, nursing, society, or environment and how religious faith might condition a patient or a nurse's perspective on the aims of nursing care. Furthermore, the nursing literature is blind to the millennia of religious ethical discourse on every aspect of human life and community, the thousands of years of wisdom literature that richly addresses the human condition and suffering, and the social impetus found in many religions toward the amelioration of the poverty and misery that give rise to disease. Nursing has ignored and shunned religion to its own detriment.

This work seeks to be a beginning remedy to that neglect. Yet it remained to find a publisher who would risk a book on a taboo topic. Years ago,

probably sometime in the 1970s, a friend and nursing colleague was looking, rather desperately, for a publisher. She had a book proposal, a genius
proposal, but it was out of the ordinary and no one was interested in even
looking the proposal, despite its obvious exceptional quality. Then one day
she and I were at a nursing conference, roaming around the exhibits, and we
stopped by the Springer booth. There was a charming older woman, well-
spoken in English with a German accent. She was alone in the booth—a
small booth compared with others. She sat and spoke at great, great length
with my friend and told her that Springer would publish her book. We were
astounded and asked how this could be. She said that this was exactly the
kind of book that Springer looked for. We pressed harder and she said that
she was a member of the Springer family and knew what they looked for.
What I remember so vividly is Ursula Springer's response that gave my
friend such hope after terrible discouragement and has given me a long-
standing fondness for Springer. Over the years, I came to know Springer as
a publisher of exceptional quality and prescience. Ursula Springer was subsequently made an honorary fellow of the American Academy of Nursing
for her commitment to publishing in nursing. I was, thus, delighted when
Springer took on this book and Margaret Zuccarini became our editor. We
are greatly indebted to Margaret and Springer for their support of this project and to Ursula Springer for taking Springer so deeply and well into nursing publishing.

There are many persons who have helped us along the way. We are
grateful for the labors of our contributors in Australia, Canada, Israel,
Jordan, the United Kingdom, and the United States who have made this
a multinational endeavor. We owe a debt of gratitude to Verena Tschudin,
of London, who generously lent us her wise counsel and enormous talents
at review and editing. There are many others, too numerous to name, who
have supported this work, tolerated our neglect of relationships, covered
our bases while we labored, and provided words of encouragement or
impulsion as the occasion demanded. We are grateful for their perseverance
and steadfast commitment to us, even if and whenever we muttered and
grumbled.

The focus of this book is on religion as a resource for nurses, patients,
and the nursing community as it engages in patient care, conceptualizes
fundamental nursing concepts, grapples with both the new and enduring issues that confront nursing, and participates in addressing health disparities
and the social determinants of illness worldwide. We do not deny that religion, both historically and in the present, can be put to toxic, self-serving,
patriarchal, and imperialist and colonialist uses. We do not dismiss the harm
that has been done in the name of religion, but to some extent we temporarily set it aside in order to focus on the irenic, life-giving, healing, wise, and
just uses of religion. We "acknowledge" that harm while at the same time we

acknowledge the heroes of many faiths whose impetus has been to heal and repair the world, respond to human need, and to make it more just.

Over the months that we have been preparing this work, there seems to have been a quiet and as yet tentative expression of interest in religion at nursing conferences, particularly ethics conferences. We hope that this work will further that interest and place it in a broad critical, global, and theoretical footing for nursing education and research. Further, our intent is for this book to serve as a theoretical backdrop for Elizabeth Johnston Taylor's book *Religion: A Clinical Guide for Nurses* that is written to assist nurses in direct clinical practice. But nursing's ethics has never been solely a "bedside" ethics. It has always been, at the same time, a social ethics. In recent years, globalizing forces have brought population ethics, health policy, health politics and diplomacy, and the global politics of religion more acutely into nursing's awareness. It is our hope that the critical–theoretical aspects of this volume will help to address those globalizing forces as they interact with both nursing and religion.

1

Religion and Nursing

Marsha D. Fowler

The year 2010 marked the hundredth anniversary of the death of the greatest American humorist of the late 1800s and early 1900s, Samuel Langhorne Clemens, better known by his pen name Mark Twain. Twice there had been premature reports of his death. A man of incisive and acerbic wit, on the occasion of the first announcement of his death, Mr. Twain responded that ". . . the report of my death is an exaggeration."[1] On the second occasion, May 4, 1907, *The New York Times* published a premature obituary reporting that Twain and the yacht on which he was traveling were lost at sea.[2] Upon his return to land, his arrival having been delayed by a deep fog, Mr. Twain promised

> . . . that I will make an exhaustive investigation of this report that I have been lost at sea. If there is any foundation for the report, I will at once apprise the anxious public. I sincerely hope that there is no foundation for the report, and I also hope that judgment will be suspended until I ascertain the true state of affairs.[3]

When it comes to premature obituaries, Twain is in good company. Pope John Paul II's death was announced prematurely on three occasions. Queen Elizabeth, the Queen Mother; Alfred Nobel of Nobel Prize fame; Lucien Bouchard, former premier of Quebec; actor Sean Connery; and Aden Abdulle Osman Daar, first President of Somalia, were all prematurely bid farewell.

On April 8, 1966, the cover of *Time Magazine*, in black with bright red letters, asked "Is God Dead?"[4] Indeed, over the years there have been numerous reports that God is in fact dead. We believe that these reports are "an exaggeration" and we hope ". . . that judgment will be suspended until

[we] ascertain the true state of affairs." For many years it had been predicted that religion would, in time, become less and less important and eventually disappear as societies modernize. Had these prognoses been accurate there would be no need for a book on religion and religious ethics, as they interact with nursing theory and practice. Instead, God and religion seem to have defied the dire prognosis and made a miraculous recovery. Now, the study of religion is more important to nursing than ever, as will be shown in the chapters that follow, and the reasons for nursing to study religion now go well beyond considerations for direct patient care.

Nursing has largely, if not entirely, neglected religion; thus it is important to look at a number of issues, including the social context and aspirations of nursing that might have fostered such neglect. Specifically, the secularization theories of sociology have become important to explore. Then we turn to the person called Nightingale and her faith as it influenced nursing. Nursing has customarily been cast as having deep roots in religion. These references are often to nursing in the middle ages and the case for a specifically *religious* motivation in that era, as opposed to a military objective, a desire to secure an education not otherwise available to a woman, as a place for the widow, or the "lovelorn," needs to be explored more fully by our nursing historians. Nonetheless, it is surely the case that Florence Nightingale was a woman of deep and enduring religious faith, yet she chose to advance a nursing education that was secular in nature. We must see why this is the case. It will be important, thereafter, to examine nursing's claim to whole-person, holistic care in the face of its silence on religion. We will conclude this chapter with an examination of a perspective in the field of religious studies that *religion* is a Western construct, and with the problems of defining *religion*.

SECULARIZATION, SCIENCE, RELIGION, AND NURSING'S ASPIRATIONS

Friedrich Nietzsche's philosophical novel, *Thus Spake Zarathustra*, is largely responsible for popularizing the phrase "God is dead." The phrase also appears in Nietzsche's earlier work, *The Gay Science*. The concept appears thrice, each with a different narrative. Sections 125 and 108, respectively, state

> God is dead. God remains dead. And we have killed him. How shall we comfort ourselves, the murderers of all murderers? What was holiest and mightiest of all that the world has yet owned has bled to death under our knives: who will wipe this blood off us? What water is there for us to clean ourselves? What festivals of atonement, what sacred games shall we have to invent? Is not the greatness of this deed too great for us? Must we ourselves not become gods simply to appear worthy of it?[5]

After Buddha was dead people showed his shadow for centuries afterwards in a cave—an immense frightful shadow. God is dead: but as the human race is constituted, there will perhaps be caves for millenniums yet, in which people will show his shadow—And we—we have still to overcome his shadow![6]

Nietzsche (1844–1900) did not maintain in a literal sense that there once was a God who had now died. Rather, his view pointed toward the increasing secularization of Europe and the rise of modern science that "killed" a need for a Christian God. Yet, in Zarathustra, the protagonist proclaims that "Dead are all the gods"[7] so that it is all gods who are killed in Nietzsche's thought, not the God of Christianity alone. For Nietzsche, with the death of God came the death of the religiously based and embedded Western European social meaning and value structures and their attendant ethics; universal moral norms; and objective truth by which lives might be oriented. Into this vacuum created by the death of God steps Nietzsche's *übermensch* (*über-*, superior, transcendent; *mencsh*, member of humanity); as the goal that humanity sets for itself.[8] The *übermensch* is the creator of new values motivated by and rooted in a regard for this world and this life, not in religion. Nietzsche proposes a *perspectivism* that rejects the notion of objective ethical or philosophical truths with the claim that what is judged to be true reflects cultural understandings, social location, and individual circumstance. For Nietzsche, truth is now intersubjective in nature. Secularization was leading to the death of God, that is, to an inability of the Christian faith adequately to address the compelling moral and social questions of the day. Our interest here is not in the ethical system that Nietzsche formulates to replace that which is lost when religion dies, but rather our interest is in the Western notion that science is tied to secularization and the interaction that premiss might have with the development of nursing knowledge in the 20th and 21st centuries.

THE SECULARIZATION THESIS

The brief "God is Dead" movement of the 1960s was distinctly a theological movement in Europe and America that was part of a broader "secularization" thesis that began much earlier. Its chief proponents were Protestant Christian theologians Gabriel Vahanian, Paul Van Buren, William Hamilton, Harvey Cox, and Thomas J. J. Altizer and Jewish Rabbi Richard Rubenstein, collectively referred to as the Radical Theologians.[9–12] In *The Death of God*, Vahanian argues that the experience of the sacred, of deity, had ebbed and the secular modern mind had lost any sense of the meaningfulness it had once held, as well as its place in contemporary thought and discourse.[13] Both Van Buren and Hamilton held with Vahanian that there was a loss of meaningfulness of the transcendent and, thus, God was in fact dead in modern thought. They would replace this loss with Jesus as an exemplar of human action-in-love. Altizer[14] and Altizer and Hamilton,[15] however, went further. They rejected the possibility of a belief in a transcendent God. They held that God had imparted God's spirit in Jesus and that spirit remained in the world, but Jesus was dead. For Altizer, God had truly died. Rubenstein is situated among those theologians and writers who wrestled with the meaning of the Holocaust. He argued that the Holocaust had shattered any possibility of continued belief in the God of the covenant of Abraham and Israel as God had been traditionally understood. More specifically, he maintained that belief in God's election (chosenness) of the people of Israel and in God's omnipotence (all-powerfulness) was no longer possible. Unlike Altizer, he did not reject belief in God or in faith or religion, but rather that the Holocaust had forever changed the way in which God could be conceived and hereinafter a new way had to be found.[16]

As a theological perspective, the Death of God movement breathed heavily for about 10 years and then died before God did. The diversity, however, of the meaning of the "Death of God" is similar to the diversity of meaning surrounding the concept of *secularization*. Shiner traces the history of the term secularization with its first instance of usage that corresponds to contemporary historical usage found in the negotiations for the Peace of Westphalia.[17]

The Holy Roman Empire of central Europe was a collection of kingdoms ruled over by "princes" who sought to increase their own power and territories at the expense of the emperor and empire. The emperor did not govern autonomously, but found his powers restricted by the power of the princes. When the Protestant Reformation ensued in the 1500s and 1600s, the religious unity of the Empire was sundered. War broke out between Catholics and Protestants, notably the Thirty Years War, which was largely fought on German soil but eventually involved almost all European nations. This would to be the last great religious war fought on the European continent. That war ended with the Peace of Westphalia, a series of treaties signed in 1648 in Germany.[18] The French portion of the treaties introduced the term *secularization*. In addition to establishing national borders and sovereign nation-states, Westphalia also effected secularization, that is, a transfer of lands and possessions from ecclesiastical (church) control to civil control. In addition, the princes could now choose the religion of their own states, whether Protestant or Roman Catholic, and impose that religion on their people. The people were now entirely subject to their own ruler and the laws of their nation.

This remained the meaning of the term in English from the 1700s to the late 1800s.[19,20]

The early 1900s saw the rise of the social sciences, with their interest in giving an account of modernity. This account included a concern for modernization, industrialization, urbanization, bureaucratization, rationalization, and secularization and their interrelationships. The social sciences sought to formulate theories of society that would have a predictive capability, much like other sciences.[21] Specifically modernization of society was linked to secularization as a consequence. It was predicted that as societies modernize, they would also secularize to the point that religion would eventually disappear, a view asserted by such prominent European figures as Auguste Comte, Herbert Spencer, Émile Durkheim, Max Weber, Ernst Troeltsch, Karl Marx and Frederick Engels, and Sigmund Freud.[22–28] The belief that religion would eventually die out was the prevailing wisdom of the social sciences for the late 19th and most of the 20th century and continues to be debated in this century. Hadden observes that

> . . . the founding generation of sociologists were hardly value-free armchair scholars . . . they believed passionately that science was ushering in a new era that would crush the superstitions and oppressive structures that the Church had promoted for so many centuries. Indeed, they were all essentially in agreement that traditional forms of religion would soon be a phenomenon of the past.[29]

In 1905, Max Weber maintained that the rationalization of society, that is, the development of a rational worldview, and the expansion of knowledge through science would ultimately make belief in the supernatural impossible. At the macrolevel, as opposed to the individual level, science would lead to the *disenchantment* of society, that is, to the loss or devaluation of "mystery" and the "supernatural," or the demystification of society.[30] The advance of science and technology was identified as *progress*. Epistemology would shift toward a reliance upon science for the formation and advance of knowledge, and the religious knowledge and ways of understanding the world, along with notions of divine authority, would largely fade away and disappear completely. According to this line of thought, only those more "primitive" thinkers, those who cling to superstition, would continue to embrace religion and find it credible. In 1959, Talcott Parson's perspective on secularization in *The Social System* is summarized by Mills as,

> Once the world was filled with the sacred—in thought, practice, and institutional form. After the Reformation and the Renaissance, the forces of modernization swept across the globe and secularization, a corollary

historical process, loosened the dominance of the sacred. In due course, the sacred shall disappear altogether except, possibly in the private realm.[31]

As secularization theory developed, however, it became clear that there were eventually multiple "secularizations." Shiner divides them into two categories: dialectical and historical. Dialectical secularization theories are those that hold a polarity between sacred and profane and see the sacred as indestructible. Historical versions of secularization theory focus on the loss of Christianity as the central force of Western society and culture, and hold the loss of the *sacral*, which is a sense of the sacred in society and culture, as irreversible. Shiner writes that

> Those who take a dialectical view are apt to believe that a revival of the "sense of the sacred" or the "cosmic dimension" is essential to a renewal of Christian faith and life; those of an historical bent envisage the possibility of both a non-religious world and a non-religious Christian faith.[32]

It should be noted that theories of secularization arose in Europe and the United States and largely had as their object of scrutiny Christianity and "historically Christian" societies, hence the limitation to Christianity in these works cited. It has been argued that secularization theories are not so much theories as amalgamations of theses that form a *secularization paradigm* more than a secularization theory.[33] However, it must be further noted that none of the early secularization theorists claimed that secularism was universal, that is, that it would also apply to, for example, largely Buddhist, Muslim, or Jewish nations. Weber went so far as to postulate that the potential for secularization is a feature of Protestant Christian societies.[34] Bruce, in his assessment of Western societies, asserts that

> ". . . individualism, diversity and egalitarianism in the context of liberal democracy undermine the authority of religious beliefs . . . religion diminishes in social significance, becomes increasingly privatized, and loses personal salience except where it finds work to do other than relating individuals to the supernatural."[35]

That "work" is cultural in nature and includes cultural defense (as in ethnic conflicts) and cultural transition (as with immigrant populations). Thus, it would seem that these theorists viewed the West as particularly susceptible to secularization. More recent theorists have widened the reach of secularization theory to all modernized or modernizing societies, including those rooted in non-Christian religions.

The most vigorous view of early secularization theories was that modernization leads to "the disenchantment of the world" and its disillusionment, that is, an ablation of its illusions.[36] Affirmation of supernatural forces, gods, or spirits is little more than nonscientific, even antiscientific, superstition that would give way to reason, science, and the scientific worldview. Society would come to be organized around rational and scientific principles. Of course, there would always remain small pockets of non- or antirational belief, attitudes, and behaviors that would persist in the face of the availability of scientifically promulgated and validated knowledge. But these would be aberrations. Churches would close, be repurposed, or embrace a secular, religionless religion; that is, a religion without a supernatural element.

As secularization theories developed in the late 19th and early- to mid-20th centuries, divergent understandings of *secularization* arose. They included (a) the loss of the authority of religion in the social and cultural life of a nation; (b) the loss of control over social institutions by religious bodies; (c) a decline in belief in superhuman or supernatural forces, gods, and spirits; (d) a decline in religious belief; and (e) a decline in participation in religious institutions.[37,38]

Secularization theories have met with significant opposition. Rodney Stark has been a vigorous opponent of secularization theory. He locates the first appearance of secularization theory in about 1710 in a work by Thomas Woolston. Stark writes "Thus, as far as I am able to discover, it was Thomas Woolston who first set a date by which time modernity would have triumphed over faith. Writing in about 1710, he expressed his confidence that Christianity would be gone by 1900."[39] He then proceeds to detail a number of dire predictions of the death of Christianity that have been profoundly wrong. Stark maintains that social scientists

> . . . have failed to recognize the dynamic character of religious economies. To focus only on secularization is to fail to see how this process is part of a much larger reciprocal structure . . . Western intellectuals have misread the secularization [of a particular set of religious organizations] as the doom of religion in general . . . secularization is only one of three fundamental and interrelated processes that constantly occur in all religious economies. The process of secularization is self-limiting and generates two countervailing processes. One of these is *revival* . . . Secularization also stimulates *religious innovation*.[40]

Thus, for Stark and Bainbridge, secularization, revival, and religious innovation are always going on in any society. They understand secularization as the first of a three-phase process. First the churches or religious groups become "eroded by secularization" and more "worldly," that is, more "secular." This produces, in response, a segment that breaks away in protest, seeking "to restore vigorous otherworldliness to a conventional faith." These breakaway groups are referred to as *sects*. This comprises their second stage, *revival*. Secularization and revival then prompt *religious innovation*, that is, the formation of new religious traditions.[41] They write,

> New religions constantly appear in societies. Whether they make any head-way depends on the vigor of conventional religious organizations. When new faiths that are better adapted to current market demand spring up, older faiths are eclipsed. Thus did Christianity, Islam, Buddhism, and other great world faiths wrest dominant market positions from older faiths.[42]

Traditional secularization theory reached its zenith in the 1960s with such proponents as Harvey Cox and Peter Berger.[43,44] Since that time, it has un-dergone considerable challenge as well as refinement. Some of those who originally led the charge for secularization theory have since, by and large, come to reject it. Peter Berger, an Austrian-born American sociologist, is one such person. Well known for his work with Thomas Luckman on *The Social Construction of Reality*, in recent decades he has written extensively on the sociology of religion and economics.[45,46] He had predicted the universal secu-larization of the world, but now holds that such an affirmation runs counter to the available data. By the late 1980s, Berger had come to reject the secu-larization thesis. He recognized that both old and new forms of religion were still vital and vibrant, particularly in the United States, though he notes that Western Europe and Western academia are exceptions. In *The Deseculari-zation of the World*, he writes, ". . . the world today, with some exceptions . . . is as furiously religious as it ever was, and in some places more so than ever. This means that a whole body of literature by historians and social scientists loosely labeled 'secularization' theory is essentially mistaken."[47] More recent seculariza-tion theorists have taken a more global perspective in their analysis of the place of religion. Norris and Inglehart maintain that

> . . . the importance of religiosity persists most strongly among vulner-able populations, especially those living in poorer nations, facing personal survival-threatening risks . . . people who experience ego-tropic risks dur-ing their formative years (posing direct threats to themselves and their families) or socio-tropic risks (threatening their community) tend to be far more religious than those who grow up under safer, comfortable, and more predictable conditions. In relatively secure societies, the remnants of religion have not died away; in surveys most Europeans still express formal belief in God, or identify themselves as Protestants or Catholics in offi-cial forms. But in those societies the importance and vitality of religion, its ever-present influence on how people live their daily lives, has gradually eroded.[48]

This rather lengthy discussion of secularization theory is not for naught. We do not seek, here, to resolve the debate. Instead, secularization theory is presented in order to pose a question: To what extent has nursing been influenced by secularization thought in its own aspirations to become a recognized profession, rooted in science? In other words, have nursing's own social aspirations led it, implicitly, to embrace secularization thought to the neglect of religion?

NURSING ASPIRATIONS AND THE NEGLECT OF RELIGION

From its earliest days, modern nursing in the United States sought the social standing of a profession and the movement from an "art" to a "science," which it viewed as essential to accomplishing that end. In the late 1800s and early 1900s, when modern nursing moved into an educationally prepared occupation, nursing fought against its social image of a manual occupation requiring little more than apprenticeship-type training without education and against both medical and public opposition to advance nursing education. Writing in defense of rigorous nursing education, Isabel Adams Hampton Robb, an early U.S. nursing leader, writes,

> To distinguish between this popular idea of the care of the sick and to justify us in our pretensions to the rank of a profession we must consider the demands made by scientific medicine of today. . . . Not so long ago neither medicine nor nursing were scientific in character. But the evolution of the one created a necessity for the other. Modern medicine requires a thorough scientific training and modern methods of treatment require that the work of the physician be supplemented by the constant and intelligent service supplied by the trained nurse. . . . Nursing has thus become a matter of scientific discipline. . . . It is this education of the intelligence that constitutes the main difference between the trained nurse of today and the so-called nurse of former days, and that has rendered nursing worthy to rank as a department in scientific medicine.[49]

Here we can see how Robb, as did other nursing leaders, bound increased nursing education and the scientization of nursing to its hopes for social recognition as a profession. From its earliest days, nursing struggled with its own self-esteem and self-, social, and medical perception of nursing as a profession. Over the past 100-plus years, the American nursing literature is at times strident about nursing as a true profession, at times reflective, and almost always defensive. The discussion, or argument, of nursing's status as a profession continues in the literature today.

A few examples of the persistence of this concern will suffice. In 1940, the American Nurses Association (ANA) published *A Tentative Code for Nurses* in the *American Journal of Nursing (AJN)*, which was a proposed code of ethics for the profession. The publication called for submission of responses, which the ANA received. The first lines of the *Tentative Code* declare: "Nursing is a profession. The distinguishing characteristics of a profession have been described in many ways. The more fundamental attributes are included in the following compilation. . . ." The code then goes on to list six attributes of a profession, the fourth of which is "the ability of its workers to give a scientific and skilled service. . . ."[50] This is, of course, material that does not properly belong in a code of ethics. The *AJN* cites Abraham Flexner's criteria for a profession from his article *Is Social Work a Profession?*[51,52] In 1945, at the end of World War II, Genevieve and Roy Bixler published an *AJN* article *The Professional Status of Nursing* that assessed nursing's progress toward status as a profession using seven criteria.[53] Fourteen years later, they published a reassessment article of the same title in the *AJN* using those same criteria. Their two articles are typical of the virtual multitude of such articles in the nursing literature. Most such articles hang on issues of professional autonomy and a distinctive knowledge base rooted in science.

There are differing ways of defining a profession. Some construct "trait definitions" of professions that list attributes of professions then measure a specific occupational group over against those traits. Most of the articles in the nursing literature, in the past as well as in the present, approach professions in this way. Whether or not an occupational group is understood as a profession is based on the degree to which it displays the traits. Trait definitions assume that there are "true" professions that demonstrate all of the essential core traits.

> However, the attributes themselves are an untidy aggregation of overlapping, arbitrarily chosen, or undifferentiated elements, lacking in a unifying theoretical framework that explains their interrelationship. Trait theories tend empirically to generate a definition of a profession then ascribe to it a normative rather than a descriptive status.[54]

Functionalist definitions of a profession focus on the "functional value of professional activity for all groups and classes in society."[55] In functionalist models

> . . . there is no attempt to present an exhaustive list of 'traits': rather the components of the model are limited to those elements that are said to have functional relevance for society as a whole or the professional-client relationship.[56]

Johnson critiques functionalist models of professions as ahistorical and rationalistic, and causally linking professional function to social position and the upward social mobility of the profession's members. This presents a flawed model of the power of expertise and rationality to affect society. It fails to take into account the nonrational nature of social power relations that mitigate against social mobility and social power.[57] He maintains that neither approach provides an adequate explanation of professions. He asserts that "a profession is not . . . an occupation, but a means of controlling an occupation,"[58] emphasizing, instead, the consequences of the social division of labor for the client-professional relationship and their influence on the power differential between the producer and consumer and on occupational control. He posits three forms of occupational control: *collegiate* (*collegial* in American English), *patronage*, and *mediative*. In *collegiate* occupational control, members set the terms of their occupational work and "community-generated role-definitions and standards are maintained by a code of ethics and autonomous disciplinary procedures." In patronage occupational control, the profession is responsible to an individual or corporation who defines the parameters of their work. In *mediative* control, toward which Johnson sees collegiate occupations moving, a third, outside party (such as the state) exercises authority over both the producer and consumer of the occupation.[59] In this schema, considerably more social power resides in the hands of those in collegiate forms of occupational control. Despite some shifts away from trait and functionalist definitions of professions in the sociology of professions literature, for the most part, nursing persists in measuring itself over against trait definitions of professions.

Why seek to be identified as a profession? Occupational groups regarded as professions have social standing, power, respect, privilege, and authority. Indeed, a cynical view of professions is that they are "specialized, monopolistic, power elites that serve their own ends of social dominance, further power, privilege, exclusive authority, suppression of competition, and a secured position, through the exploitation of a social need."[60] The evidence would indicate that nursing's aspiration for status as a profession is tied to its concerns to gain autonomy of practice against medicine specifically, social regard, and to secure the economic and social welfare of the nurse. So nursing seeks to be regarded as a profession and sees science as the chief vehicle for realizing that aim. While society modernizes, rationalizes, scientizes, and secularizes, nursing, reflecting the society in which it is embedded, contemporaneously modernizes, rationalizes, scientizes, and secularizes as well. Nursing science gains ascendency and the journal *Nursing Research* begins in 1952. However much it may have affected patients and their decisions, religion is not among the topics that make it into nursing's research agenda. Yet nursing does not, historically, fall completely outside the purview of religion.

NURSING'S INTERACTION WITH RELIGION

Premodern nursing has some interaction with religion in the form of medieval religious nursing orders. Their *charism*, or spiritual gift, often formally included care of the sick, poor, widow, orphan, stranger, and the pilgrim. Although some orders were specifically devoted to nursing, one cannot assume that those who entered the order were committed to nursing. Their commitment may have been religious and devotional in nature, expressing a commitment to God and not specifically to those under their care. Some young girls were known to have been given to religious orders as a *tithe* (a tenth-part of what one has), particularly if they were the tenth child in a family. Some widows entered religious orders for reasons of survival, whether economic or political. For some, convents may have served as places of comfort for the "lovelorn." This is to say that we must be cautious in attributing a nursing motivation where perhaps none exists.

It is clear, however, that Florence Nightingale was possessed of a religious sensibility. Over the course of her life, she experienced a "call" from God on four occasions. Her journal has the following cryptic entry dated February 7, 1892:

> Calls to work, to holiness?
> Lea Hurst: shore's door. Behold the handmaid of the Lord.
> Embly, 7 February 1837 "the way to do good."
> Bridge Hill, 1844, call to hospital work, which have I followed?
> Lea Hurst, 1848, on my knees on Middle Hurst, not going to Hamburg nuns.
> Alexandria, 1850, to throw my body in the breach.[61]

Her first call occurred at the age of 16 at the family home at Embley, as a call to serve God, the nature of which was not further defined. She would refer to this date throughout her life. Her diary records six occasions on which "the Voice" spoke to her; some of which seem to have occurred when she was engaged in *lectio divina.* Lectio divina is a medieval tradition in which one prays with sacred scriptures in order to combine scriptural study with reflection, meditation, and prayer with listening for God. She felt herself called by God, and more specifically called to nursing as service. However, she also came to regard nursing itself as a calling and wrote to probationers (early nursing students) and nurses that "Nursing is said, most truly said, to be a high calling, an honorable calling."[62]

Nightingale was a devout Christian in the Anglican (Church of England) tradition with a Unitarian heritage. A large body of her writings has been preserved. It displays a deep and abiding interest in theology and in the Bible, a personal devotion to God, prayer, scripture, and service to God in the world and a rocky relationship with her Church. Just as some of her social beliefs were contrary to the social norms of the day, particularly for and as concerning women, likewise some of her theological beliefs could be regarded as heterodox. In a number of important ways (but not all) her decidedly feminist perspective, not to mention her own education and upbringing, placed her out of the mainstream or, more correctly, in advance of the eventual mainstream.[63] Showalter describes Nightingale's *Cassandra* as "a major text of English feminism, a link between [Mary] Wollstonecraft and [Virginia] Woolf."[64] Nightingale protested against the prevailing Victorian norm of feminine helplessness and socially useless life for women and was an ardent supporter of women's education. Nightingale's sometime departure from orthodox Christian theology can be seen in her work *Suggestions for Thought* as well as in others of her writings.[65,66] Although her theology may at points be found problematic in its heterodoxy, what is beyond question is that her Christian faith was devout and was lived out in service to God through her call to nursing and her embrace of nursing as a high calling in itself. As she moved into nursing education, she demanded a rigorous education for women who would become nurses. Surprisingly, however, she sought for a thoroughly secularized nursing education.

There seems to be three predominating reasons for this. The first is a disillusionment with nursing orders as well as the fact that, pragmatically, English Anglican religious orders for women never caught on. McDonald notes that "The young Nightingale's high opinion for religious communities of women did not survive later experience. As a nurse, Nightingale came to have a poor opinion of them."[67] Second, she loathed "saving souls" in the practice of nursing, though with greater nuance, it appears that making nursing subservient to *proselytizing* (attempting to convert others to one's own religion) was the particular irritant as opposed to proselytizing per se. Again, McDonald writes,

> The exacting workload, character, and devotion long required of the nurse go back to Nightingale's conceptualization of nursing as a religious *calling*, a calling to patient care and health promotion. She abhorred nurses acting as missionaries to save the souls of the sick or dying, which prompted her to insist that her training school for nurses be non-sectarian. Crimea had given her too much experience of people neglecting their nursing duties to gain another convert to their denomination. . . .[68]

Third, Nightingale wanted to accept students into her school independent of their religious commitment. Even so, while the school was to be nonsectarian, it was nevertheless Christian.

Nightingale wanted nurses to be ordinary women, not nuns, and the profession to be open to all without any religious test. But her letters to nurses and nursing students are full of religious material, advice and prayers, for she believed that nurses needed ongoing spiritual nourishment. . . . While nightingale insisted that her training school be non-sectarian, accepting students on the basis of merit regardless of religion, there was a significant Christian (indeed Church of England) element in the daily routine.[69]

Nursing schools were also to be based in science. Interestingly, however, Nightingale tied religion and science together. For her, observation of nature led to a recognition of the fixed laws that God had ordained as well as to a knowledge of God. However, she railed against positivism. In a "Note of Interrogation," *Fraser's Magazine*, in 1873, she wrote "By positivists, it is thought that, to learn laws of nature as far as we can, without troubling our heads about Him who made them, if indeed there be One (about whom, they say, we *can* know nothing), is the only course for man. Is not this leaving out of the most inspiring part of life?" For her, the study of the social sciences was coterminous with the study of God. She writes,

Is, then, moral science, the science of the social and political improvement of man, the science of education or administering the world by discovering the laws which govern man's motives, his moral nature, is synonymous with the study of the character of God, because the laws of the moral world are the expressions and solely the expressions of the character of God. . . .[70]

Science, in terms of nursing science, was a matter of observing God's laws of nature, of cooperating with them, and of both using them to prevent disease and promote health and to teach nursing students and nurses. Nightingale ". . . believed that nurses, with their responsibility for maintaining hygiene, had a unique opportunity for spiritual advancement, discovering the nature of God by learning his 'laws of health.'"[71] For Nightingale education, specifically nonsectarian education, and science were the soil of nursing, but faith was its bedrock.

A number of factors, *thus*, conspire toward modern nursing silence on the topic of religion: the legacy of Nightingale's nonsectarian and scientific educational structure, even if covertly religious; the modernizing and scientizing social context that surrounded the emergence of modern nursing in the 20th century, and nursing's own aspirations toward social recognition as a full profession based on scientific knowledge. Although Nightingale's viewpoints are not determinative of nursing's future, they are initiative. It remains a fertile point for historical research to ferret out more causative and less correlational factors, some of which receive attention in succeeding chapters. However, in view of the fact that nursing lays claim to whole person care, the absence of nursing discourse on religion that might inform practice is perplexing. The *American Nurses Association Code of Ethics for Nurses* states that

> An individual's lifestyle, value system and religious beliefs should be considered in planning health care with and for each patient. Such consideration does not suggest that the nurse necessarily agrees with or condones certain individual choices, but that the nurse respects the patient as a person.[72]

We would maintain that a consideration of or respect for the patient's religious beliefs necessitates at least a basic understanding of religions, religious beliefs, and religious ethics as they interact with health and nursing theory, practice, and health policy.

NURSING AND HOLISTIC, WHOLE PERSON CARE

The nursing scholarship examining religion is cachexic, a sharp contrast to the burgeoning nursing literature on the more generic concept of spirituality. A survey of nursing databases[73] for articles in English scholarly journals for the past 30 years (1982 to present) yields only 783 articles with religion and nursing coexisting as subject terms. When filtered to exclude articles principally on spirituality, not religion, that number drops precipitously. The most recent and prevailing themes for this body of literature include religion as an aspect of culture, as part of nursing history; and as a topic for ethical, philosophic, or conceptual discourse (usually about spirituality, but recognizing religion). Literature about faith community (parish) nursing, nurses' and nursing students' religious attitudes also exist to a lesser extent. An occasional article about religious restrictions pertaining to medical care can be found (e.g., how to care for the Jehovah's Witness whose tradition proscribes the acceptance of most blood products). Furthermore, only 330 of these articles were classified as research. This nursing research characteristically includes religion as one among many variables for study, often studies about factors related to coping and quality of life. Likewise, many introduction-to-nursing textbooks present a cursory discussion of religion, but only in terms of patients' religious behaviors or artifacts at the bedside that should be noted.[74] Often, nursing assessment tools do little more than to prompt the nurse to take note of dietary restrictions, artifacts, religious affiliation, or faith community. Actual attention—beyond stereotyping—to such things as the influence of religion on clinical moral decision-making, concepts of illness, understanding of suffering, motivations for caring, or nurse prescriptions for social justice in health care are remarkably absent. Nursing has made claims to whole person and holistic care. How can such a claim be made when religion does not substantively figure into the equation?

In tracing the holism discourse in nursing, Owen and Holmes take note of the fact that Nightingale promoted holistic principles. She "challenged nurses to identify the influences of the patients' social setting, and focused attention on prevention and 'natural' responses to disease. The concern was for the whole patient—mind, body, sprit—and the higher total environment . . ."[75] The nursing literature does not question that nursing is concerned about *the whole person* or that it approaches the patient *holistically*, giving *whole person care*. Nursing scholars neither challenge nor speak unapprovingly of either. Where the disagreement and debate resides is in how *holism* is defined and the varying definitions of holism that are employed. Kolcaba notes that "Holistic thinking is so diverse that practically every theorist can claim holistic credentials. The challenge for nursing, then, is not whether holism but which holism? As a practice-centered discipline, nursing gives a central role to whole person holism."[76] In a world where a nurse cannot escape caring for persons who are religious adherents, and in a world where religion plays a significant role in social, political, and economic life worldwide, as well as in the lives of individuals, families, and their communities, there is a critical need for nursing to engage in comprehensive study and research in order to understand religious traditions, values, questions, issues, and social perspectives. And, after 150 years of a whole-person holism in nursing, it is time for nursing to add religion into that equation by formally attending to the nature of religion and how it influences nursing theorists, educators, researchers, practitioners, and those whom nursing serves.

RELIGION AS OBJECT OF STUDY

Outside of nursing, the concept of *religion* has come under criticism among contemporary scholars in the social sciences and humanities, particularly in the past 20 years. The names of Daniel Dubuisson,[77] Russell McCutcheon,[78] Timothy Fitzgerald,[79] Tomoko Masuzawa,[80] and Talal Asad[81] are prominent in the debate about the legitimacy, coherence, and validity of the concept *religion*. Mercea Eliade writes of humans as *homo religiosus*, that is, of human religious behavior as a universal phenomenon by which the sacred could be apprehended through *hierophanies*, meaning through revelatory events and objects.[82] This would then make religion *sui generis* (of its own kind) a category of mind. It would seem that nursing's embrace of spirituality, shorn of religion, is in some way an embrace of a variant form of *homo religiosus*. Rejecting Eliade's perspective, in 2003, Daniel Dubuisson writes "Just like the notion itself, the most general questions concerning religion, its nature and definition, its origins or expressions, were born in the West. From there, they were transferred to all other cultures, however remotely prehistoric or exotic."[83] He asks three questions: (a) Is Christianity a Western form of a universal phenomenon? (b) Is religion a unique and original creation of Western civilization? and (c) Is religion the West's most characteristic and self-defining concept? Masuzawa, tracing the lineage of the field of world religions, maintains that "the modern discourse on religion and religions was from the very beginning—that is to say, inherently, if also ironically—a discourse of secularization; at the same time, it was clearly a discourse of othering." (p. 20).[84] She continues with the assertion that

> . . . world religions as a category and as a conceptual framework initially developed in the European academy, which quickly became an effective means of differentiating, consolidating, and totalizing a large portion of the social, cultural, and political practices observable among the inhabitants of regions elsewhere in the world.[85]

McCutcheon raises an additional critique that the study of religion is lacking in scientific rigor and method.[86]

Although the aforementioned scholars each address different questions, collectively they provide answers: yes, *religion* is a Western construct that is neither universalizable nor transcultural; yes, *religion* is distinctive of the West, and the concept by which the West defines itself; and yes, religious studies lack the rigor that science possesses. These lines of argument maintain that religion is an intellectual creation of the 19th century West that embeds a Christian vision of the world that functions to maintain a Western Christian intellectual hegemony, which further serves the function of "othering" non-Western cultures and peoples.[87] Dubuisson writes,

> In asserting the West invented religion and has continuously lived under its influence, we must, of course, understand that the West was not the only civilization to ask metaphysical questions, to try to understand the world in which it lived, to conceive of imaginary beings (gods, spirits, demons, ghosts), to develop theologies, organize worship, invent cosmologies and mythologies, support beliefs, defend morals and ideals, and imagine other worlds—but that it made this collection of attitudes and ideals an autonomous, singular complex, profoundly different from everything surrounding it. And it conferred on this distinct complex a kind of destiny or essential anthropological vocation: humans are held to be religious in the same way as they are omnivorous, that is, by nature, through the effects of a specific

inborn disposition. . . . While religion remains largely the incarnation of an atemporal notion or indestructible essence, it is . . . only the result of a discriminatory act performed in the West and there alone.[88]

For Dubuisson, other cultures asked similar metaphysical questions but did not then divide the world in secular and sacred categories.

In this view, religion is not a phenomenon *sui generis*, not a distinctive thing of its own, composed of a set of ahistorical, transcultural, even a priori features that form a distinctive and differentiated analytic category. The consequence of this perspective is that religion then becomes, not a field unto itself, but properly the object of study of any of the fields that study "nonreligious" social phenomena.[89] Dubuisson further sees religion as a tautological Western invention.

> Facts, of whatever kind, are not in themselves religious in the sense that they are endowed with some kind of specific, sui generis quality, come from who knows where. They only become religious at the point where individuals isolate them by invoking a certain number of criteria and then apply this distinct designation.[90]

In this view, *religion* is Eurocentric and Eurohegemonic in nature. The discourse of religion, then, becomes a discourse of othering that retains the center for the West and maintains all "others" at the margins. This perspective is less concerned with the nature of religion than with what religion means as a process.

Those who focus on the nature of religion present a contrasting approach. Riesebrodt asserts the universal applicability of religion cross-culturally.[91] He claims that religion has a referential legitimation, that is, the features of religion can be seen cross-culturally and that

> . . . religious actors and institutions recognize each other as similar. They mutually constitute, define, and transform each other; they compete with each other, polemicize against each other, and borrow from each other. In short: the systems of reference, in which religions emerge and interact with each other, resemble each other, a fact that we witness throughout history and across cultures.[92]

He gives as examples the three Abrahamic traditions of Judaism, Christianity, and Islam. The Biblical story of the ancient Hebrews is one of being constituted as a monotheistic people whose God is not that of the surrounding Ancient Near Eastern and Canaanite religions. Furthermore, early Christianity was seen to differentiate itself, first as a sect of Judaism, and thereafter over against Hellenistic mystery religions and Gnosticism. Islam too carved out a distinctive and contrasting identity over against both Judaism and Christianity. Riesebrodt also points to the emergence of Buddhism, distinguishing itself from both Brahmanism and other ascetic movements of the day. He concludes that religion, as an analytic category,

> . . . is not necessarily an imposition of a modern Western category on phenomena that are perceived and categorized totally differently in non-Western or premodern cultures. . . . These examples contradict the postmodern assumption that non-Western religions have been constituted as such only after they encountered the West and then began modeling themselves after the Western notion or religion.[93]

Neither Western hegemony nor Christian imperialism across history can be denied. However, the question is whether that history can bear the weight of rendering the concept of religion invalid as an analytic category.

DEFINING RELIGION

Despite these types of concerns regarding religion as a legitimate object of study, many have and continue to maintain that religion is a distinctive phenomenon capable of analysis.[94] However, religious scholars widely accept that there is no one essence of religion that is shared by all religions. Attempts to define religion in terms of a superhuman being have been rejected in the face of Buddhism and Jainism. Stark and Bainbridge, however, do distinguish between religion and other "ideological systems" by embracing Durkheim's notion that "religions involve some conception of a supernatural being, world, or force, and the notion that the supernatural is active, that events and conditions here on earth are influenced by the supernatural."[95] In *Dimensions of the Sacred: An Anatomy of the World's Beliefs*, Ninian Smart identifies seven *dimensions* (not an essence) of religion.[96] They include: ritual, narrative, experiential, institutional, ethical, doctrinal, and material dimensions. Religions tend to demonstrate these dimensions, though some religions may emphasize one dimension over another. Even within a given religion there will be diverse subtraditions, family members, so that one can only say that a particular religion "tends to" emphasize certain dimensions. No definitive set of characteristics or properties can be given that is broad enough to encompass all religions without at the same time folding in philosophies that are not religions. Attempts to precisely define *religion* have largely been abandoned. Even attempts to describe or define a specific religion (as opposed to religion per se) are often essentializing. Yet, there are good reasons not to abandon altogether an attempt to define religion if only to delimit the phenomenon of concern to avoid inconsistency, vagueness, narrowness, confusion, and bias.

There are, broadly, two types of definitional approaches: substantive and functional. These approaches are not unique to religion, but characterize attempts to define any basic term e.g., *person, profession, nursing,* or *religion.* Substantive definitions attempt to identify what religion *is*, its content, substance, or essence. Functional definitions attempt to identify what religion *does* relative to something such as culture, society, or the psyche. Both approaches have problems. Substantive definitions tend to incorporate terms such as the *sacred, numinous, transhuman,* or *transcendent* and consequently to be less verifiable by empirical research. Functional definitions tend to be reductionistic, reducing religion to its social or psychological or cultural function, making it an aspect of these. The often unspoken part of the debate arises from the prior understanding of whether the study of religion belongs to the humanities, or to the sciences. In the United States, this debate is reflected in the differences between the Society for the Scientific Study of Religion, over against the American Academy of Religion, both of which are devoted to the study of religion but do so from largely different perspectives. Although it ought not to go unexamined, Nursing's predisposition will be toward science and toward definitions with empirically verifiable terms, thus toward functionalist definitions.

Geertz offers a functionalist definition of religion that is perhaps more satisfactory than many:

> Religion is (1) a system of symbols that acts to (2) establish powerful, pervasive, and long-lasting mods and motivations in [people] by (3) formulating conceptions of a general order of existence and (4) clothing these conceptions with such an aura of factuality that the moods and motivations seem uniquely realistic.[97]

The virtues of this definition are several. It is holistic and a system; it encompasses moral feeling, disposition, and action; it allows for the construction of a larger worldview; and its "aura of factuality" permits the human symbol system to have a realism beyond the subjective experience of the religion's community of adherents. It seemingly maintains an "empathetic objectivity" (over against hostile disbelief) toward those human symbol systems that point toward the sacred, transcendent or transhuman.[98]

An additional point remains to be addressed: the popular tendency to reduce all religions, collectively, as paths to the same destination. However much religions might converge on certain ethical perspectives, neither their central theological questions and concerns, nor the theological ends that they seek redound to the same thing. Prothero writes that "what the world's religions share is not so much a finish line as a starting point: something is wrong with the world."[99] In discussing their differences, Prothero characterizes several religions, their central questions and aims, and summarizes their distinctiveness in a phrase. Although this runs the risk of essentializing traditions, it does point to content in each that is not of mutual religious concern. For example, he refers to Islam as "The Way of Submission;" to Christianity as "The Way of Salvation;" to Daoism as "The Way of Flourishing;" to Buddhism as "The Way of Awakening," and so on.[100] This is to say that some central concepts in one religion do not find resonance in another. *Sin*, so central to Christian theological understanding, is not a central concern in Buddhism. Even more, central theological concerns in one religion may not be shared by its own subtraditions. For example, theological questions that burned hot in Western Christianity found no ready connection in the theology of the Eastern Christianity. Religions only collapse into oneness when their understanding is based on stereotypes, stereotypes that can ultimately have negative consequences for patient care. In the face of this flawed understanding, religious literacy needs to be strengthened.

We return now, for a moment, to the acknowledged founder of modern Western Nursing, Florence Nightingale. She was born into a wealthy, upper-class, English family almost 200 years ago. Her social station in English society encumbered her with a set of expectations for her role as an adult woman in society. However, her family was a mix of convention and unconvention that served Nightingale well as she kicked against the social goad, seeking to achieve an active and educated life over against the ideal of "uselessness" of Victorian womanhood. She developed her statistical abilities and engaged in theological reflection. She was not satisfied with simple devotion to her Christian faith but became a lifelong student of theology. Her family wealth allowed her to travel, and in her travels she learned experientially as well as through readings of other religions and sects, both ancient and modern. Nightingale's writings speak analytically of Zorastrianism, Manichaeism, Socinianism, Jansenism, Muhammadanism (Islam), Judaism, Sufism, and more. Born into the British Empire, a vast 19th century empire "upon which the sun never set," her writings also reflect that she both transcended and was captive of her social station, gender, culture, religion, time, and empire.[101] Nightingale's religion was of surpassing importance to her. She saw fit, however, to move nursing both into formal education and into formally secular education. This would not have precluded the study of religion for the improvement of patient care. Even so, nursing has neglected religion for the past 150 years. There are many reasons for nursing to engage in religious study. Such study lends itself to a greater understanding of the geopolitical world and the larger societies in which nursing is situated. Engaging with religion would also afford nursing a glimpse into millennia of religious discourse—and wisdom—on the human condition, and alternative perspectives on *person, health, society*, and *environment*, care of the stranger, global health, and ethics. Even greater self-understanding of our profession might result. And, not least of all, for the sake of patients, it is time that today's nursing education, research, and practice take from Nightingale a measure of her intellectual commitment to the exploration of religion.

NOTES

1. Twain, Mark [Samuel Clemens]. Letter of May 1897. Web. http://www.twainquotes. com/Death.html
2. Twain, Mark [Samuel Clemens]. *New York Journal.* 4 May 1907.
3. Twain, Mark [Samuel Clemens]. *New York Journal.* 5 May 1907.
4. Time Magazine. 87.14 (8 Apr. 1966): cover.
5. Nietzsche, Friedrich. *The Gay Science [Die fröhliche Wissenschaft]: With a Prelude in Rhymes and an Appendix of Songs.* Trans. with commentary Walter Kaufmann NY: Vintage Books, March 1974, Section 125 (The Madman). See also: section 108 (New Struggles) and section 343 (The Meaning of our Cheerfulness). See also: Nietzsche, Friedrich. *Thus Spoke Zarathustra: A Book for All and None. [Also sprach Zarathustra: Ein Buch für Alle und Keinen].* Trans. Walter Kauffman. 3rd ed. 1882. New York: Random House, 1955.
6. Nietzsche. Section 108. Trans. Thomas Common, 1882. Sydney, Australia: George Allen & Unwin, 1967.
7. Nietzsche. *Zarathustra,* Part I, Section XXII. 3.
8. Oxford University Press. *Oxford German Dictionary.* New York: Oxford University Press, 2008.
9. Vahanian, Gabriel. *The Death of God: The Culture of Our Post-Christian Era.* New York: George Braziller, 1961.
10. Van Buren, Paul M. *The Secular Meaning of the Gospel: Based on an Analysis of Its Language.* 3rd ed. New York: Macmillan, 1966.
11. Hamilton, William. *A Quest for the Post-Historical Jesus.* London, New York: Continuum International Publishing Group, 1994.
12. Cox, Harvey. *The Secular City: Secularization and Urbanization in Theological Perspective.* New York: Collier Books, 1965.
13. Vahanian, Gabriel. *The Death of God: The Culture of Our Post-Christian Era.* New York: George Braziller, 1961.
14. Altizer, Thomas J. J. *The Gospel of Christian Atheism.* Philadelphia: Westminster, 1966.
15. Altizer, Thomas J. J., and William Hamilton. *Radical Theology and the Death of God.* Indianapolis: Bobbs-Merrill, 1966.
16. Rubenstein, Richard. *After Auschwitz: Radical Theology and Contemporary Judaism.* Indianapolis: Bobbs-Merrill, 1966.
17. Shiner, Larry. "Toward a Theology of Secularization." *The Journal of Religion* 45.4 (1965): 283.
18. Straumann, Benjamin. "The Peace of Westphalia as a Secular Constitution." *Constellations* 15.2 (2008): 173–188.

19. Simpson, John, and Edmund Weiner, eds. *Oxford English Dictionary*. New York: Oxford University Press, 1989.
20. Stallmann, Martin. *Was ist Säkularisierung?* Tübingen: JCB Mohr, 1960. 5–17.
21. Kaplan, Oscar. "Prediction in the Social Sciences." *Philosophy of Science* 7.4 (1940): 492–498.
22. Comte, Auguste. *Introduction to Positive Philosophy*. Trans. Frederick Ferré, 1844. Indianapolis: Hackett, 1988.
23. Spencer, Herbert. *The Principles of Ethics* (1897). Ann Arbor: University of Michigan Press, 2009.
24. Durkheim, Émile. *The Elementary Forms of Religious Life: A Study in Religious Sociology*. Trans. Carol Clausman and Mark Cladis, 1912. New York: Oxford University Press, 2001.
25. Weber, Max. *The Protestant Ethic and the Spirit of Capitalism*. New York: Oxford University Press, 2010.
26. Troeltsch, Ernst. *Protestantism and Progress* (1906). Boston: Beacon Press, 1958.
27. Marx, Karl, and Frederick Engels. *The Communist Manifesto* (1848). Ed. David McLellan. Oxford: Oxford University Press, 2008.
28. Freud, Sigmund. *The Future of an Illusion*. Trans. James Strachey, 1927. New York: WW Norton, 1989.
29. Hadden, Jeffrey K. "Toward Desacralizing Secularization Theory." *Social Forces* 65.3 (1987): 590.
30. Weber.
31. Mills, C. Wright. *The Sociological Imagination*. 1959. New York: Oxford University Press, 2000.
32. Shiner. 279.
33. Bruce, Steve. *God is Dead: Secularization in the West*. Malden, MA: Blackwell Publishing, 2002. 1–43.
34. Weber.
35. Bruce. 30.
36. Weber.
37. Norris, Pippa, and Ronald Inglehart. *Sacred and Secular: Religion and Politics Worldwide*. Cambridge: Cambridge University Press, 2004. 3–79.
38. Bruce. 1–44.
39. Stark, Rodney. "Secularization, R.I.P." *Sociology of Religion* 60.4 (1999): 249–273. See also: Dobbelaere, Karel. "Towards and Integrated Perspective of the Processes Related to the Descriptive Concept of Secularization." *Sociology of Religion* 60.4 (1999): 229–247.
40. Stark, Rodney, and William Bainbridge. *The Future of Religion: Secularization, Revival, and Cult Formation*. Berkeley: University of California Press, 1985. 2.
41. Ibid.
42. Ibid.
43. Cox, Harvey. *The Secular City: Secularization and Urbanization in Theological Perspective*. Collier Books, 25th anniversary edition. New York: Collier Books, 1990.
44. Berger, Peter. *The Sacred Canopy: Elements of a Sociological Theory of Religion* (1967). New York: Knopf Doubleday, 1990.
45. Berger, Peter, and Thomas Luckman. *The Social Construction of Reality: A Treatise in the Sociology of Knowledge*. New York: Knopf Doubleday, 1967.
46. Berger, Peter. *The Heretical Imperative: Contemporary Possibilities of Religious Affirmation*. New York: Doubleday, 1979. See also: Berger, Peter, ed. *The Other Side*

of God: A Polarity in World Religions. New York: Anchor, 1981. See also: Berger, Peter, ed. *The Capitalist Spirit: Toward a Religious Ethic of Wealth Creation.* San Francisco: ICS Press, 1990. And: Berger, Peter, Brigitte Berger, and Hansfried Kellner. *The Homeless Mind: Modernization and Consciousness.* New York: Random House, 1973.

47. Berger, Peter, ed. *The Desecularization of the World: Resurgent Religion and World Politics.* Grand Rapids: Wm. B. Eerdmans Publishing, 1999. 2.

48. Norris, Pippa, and Ronald Inglehart. *Sacred and Secular: Religion and Politics Worldwide.* Cambridge: Cambridge University Press, 2004. 4.

49. Robb, Isabel Adams Hampton. *Nursing Ethics: For Hospital and Private Use.* New York: Koeckert, 1900.

50. American Nurses Association. "A Tentative Code." *American Journal of Nursing* 40.9 (1940): 977.

51. Flexner, Abraham. "Is Social Work a Profession?" *The New York School of Philanthropy Studies in Social Work* 4 (1915): 10.

52. American Journal of Nursing. "The Flexner Criteria." New York: American Journal of Nursing 48.9 (1948): 589.

53. Bixler, Genevieve, and Roy Bixler. "The Professional Status of Nursing." *American Journal of Nursing* 45.9 (1945): 730–735.

54. Fowler, Marsha. "Social Ethics and Nursing." *The Profession of Nursing: Turning Points.* Ed. Norma Chaska. St. Louis: CV Mosby, 1990. 24.

55. Johnson, Terrance. *Professions and Power.* London: Macmillan, 1972. 37.

56. Ibid., 23.

57. Ibid.

58. Ibid., 45.

59. Ibid.

60. Fowler. 25.

61. McDonald, Lynn, ed. *Florence Nightingale's Spiritual Journey: Biblical Annotations, Sermons and Journal Notes. Collected Works of Florence Nightingale.* Vol. 2. Waterloo, Ontario: Wilfrid Laurier University Press, 2001. 516. See also: Bostridge, Mark. *Florence Nightingale.* London: Penguin Books, 2008.

62. Nightingale, Florence. *Florence Nightingale to her Nurses: A Selection from Miss Nightingale's Addresses to Probationers and Nurses of the Nightingale School at St. Thomas's Hospital.* London: Macmillan, 1914. 116.

63. Florence Nightingale. *Cassandra.* Ed. Myrna Stark. New York: The Feminist Press, 1979.

64. Showalter, Elaine. *Norton Anthology of Literature by Women: The Traditions in English.* Vol. 1. New York: WW Norton, 2007. 1016.

65. Calabria, Michael, and Janet Macrae, eds. *Suggestions for Thought by Florence Nightingale.* Philadelphia: University of Pennsylvania Press, 1994.

66. McDonald, Lynn, ed. *Florence Nightingale's Theology: Essays, Letters and Journal Notes. Collected Works of Florence Nightingale.* Vol 3. Waterloo, Ontario: Wilfred Laurier University Press, 2002. See also: Vallée, Gérard, ed. *Florence Nightingale on Mysticism and Eastern Religions. Collected Works of Florence Nightingale.* Vol. 3. Waterloo, Ontario: Wilfred Laurier University Press, 2003.

67. Ibid., 69.

68. Ibid., 74.

69. Ibid., 74–75.

70. Ibid., 28.
71. Attewell, Alex. "Florence Nightingale." *Prospects*. Paris: UNESCO 28.1 (March 1998): 156.
72. American Nurses Association. *Code of Ethics for Nurses with Interpretive Statements*. Washington, DC: American Nurses Association, 2001. 7. Section 1.2.
73. Medline, ISI web of science (including the science citation index, the social science citation index, and the arts and humanities index), Embase, PsycINFO, CINAHL, NAHL, PubMed.
74. Pesut, Barbara, Marsha Fowler, Elizabeth J. Taylor, et al. "Conceptualizing Spirituality and Religion for Healthcare." *Journal of Clinical Nursing* 17.21 (2008): 2803–10. See also: Pesut, Barbara, Marsha Fowler, Sheryl Reimer-Kirkham, et al. "Particularizing Spirituality in Points of Tension: Enriching the Discourse." *Nursing Inquiry* 16.4 (2009): 337–46.
75. Owen, Martin, and Colin Holmes. "'Holism' in the Discourse of Nursing." *Journal of Advanced Nursing* 18.11 (1993): 1689.
76. Kolcaba, Raymond. "The Primary Holisms in Nursing." *Journal of Advanced Nursing* 25.2 (1997): 290.
77. Dubuisson, Daniel. *The Western Construction of Religion: Myths, Knowledge, and Ideology*. Trans. William Sayers. Baltimore: Johns Hopkins University Press, 2003.
78. McCutcheon, Russell T. *Manufacturing Religion: The Discourse on Sui Generis Religion and the Politics of Nostalgia*. New York: Oxford University Press, 1997. See also: McCutcheon, Russell. *Insider/Outsider Problem in the Study of Religion: A Reader (Controversies in the Study of Religion)*. New York: Continuum, 1999.
79. Fitzgerald, Timothy. *The Ideology of Religious Studies*. New York: Oxford University Press, 2000. See also: Fitzgerald, Timothy. *Religion and Politics in International Relations: The Modern Myth*. New York: Continuum, 2011.
80. Masuzawa, Tomoko. *The Invention of World Religions: Or, How European Universalism Was Preserved in the Language of Pluralism*. Chicago: University of Chicago Press, 2005.
81. Asad, Talal. *Genealogies of Religion: Discipline and Reasons of Power in Christianity and Islam*. Baltimore: Johns Hopkins University Press, 1993.
82. Eliade, Mircea. *The Sacred and The Profane: The Nature of Religion*. Trans. Willard Trask. San Diego, CA: Harvest/Harcourt, 1957.
83. Dubuisson. 9.
84. Masuzawa. 20.
85. Masuzawa.
86. McCutcheon, Russell. *The Discipline of Religion: Structure, Meaning, Rhetoric*. London: Routledge, 2003. See also: McCutcheon, Russell. *Critics Not Caretakers: Redescribing the Public Study of Religion*. Albany: State University of New York Press, 2001.
87. Dubuisson. 10.
88. Ibid., 14.
89. Wiebe, Donald. "Theory in the Study of Religion." *Religion* 13.3 (1983): 303.
90. Ibid., 15.
91. Riesebrodt, Martin. "Religion": Just another Modern Western Construction? http://divinity.uchicago.edu/martycenter/publications/webforum/122003/riesebrodtessay.pdf.
92. Ibid., 2.

93. Ibid., 9.

94. Pals, Daniel. "Is Religion a Sui Generis Phenomenon?" *Journal of the American Academy of Religion* 55.2 (1987): 259–282.

95. Stark and Bainbridge. 5.

96. Smart, Ninian. *Dimensions of the Sacred: An Anatomy of the World's Beliefs.* Berkeley: University of California Press, 1996.

97. Geertz, Clifford. "Religion as a Cultural System." *Reader in Comparative Religion: An Anthropological Approach.* Eds. Lessa, William, and Evon Vogt. New York: Harper Collins Publishers, 1979, 79–80.

98. Smart, Ninian. *The Phenomenon of Religion.* London: Macmillan, 1973.

99. Prothero, Stephen. *God Is Not One.* New York: Harper One, 2010. 11.

100. Prothero.

101. Vallée.

2

Religious Ethics, Religious Social Ethics, and Nursing

Marsha D. Fowler and Sheryl Reimer-Kirkham

For the last few decades, nursing literature has tended to represent religion as a subset of spirituality, often as a narrow (and usually negative) construct of institutional and ideological beliefs and rituals. Such a perspective misses the complexity of religion and the millennia of richness of ethical discourse and moral guidance to be found in religion. This is to nursing's detriment, particularly in a globalized world where nursing could make common cause with many religious traditions to address social ills, such as poverty, which are chief determinants of morbidity and mortality worldwide. Not only do many religious traditions address bioethical issues, they also embrace a social ethics that reaches out to "repair the world."

In this chapter, we provide an overview of the potential contributions of religious ethics to nursing. Notably, nurses who attempt to fit religious ethics into the standard Western nursing construct of principle-based versus virtue-based versus caring-based ethics may find themselves perplexed. Although it is possible to fit some aspects of religious ethics into these categories, it is a square peg being mashed into a round hole: it just does not work. Religious ethics tends to be far more fulsome, often worked out over centuries, and focused on the lived experience of humankind. Thus elements of duties, expectations for virtue, ideals of human flourishing and community, ends of justice, compassion, caring, hospitality, recompense, gratitude and much more will all be found in the ethics of most religious traditions. Of course, because they may have been developed over centuries by "many hands," religious ethics may not present the most tidy package and may not have the neatly mitered corners of a pristine armchair ethics. Beyond general moral guidance, religious ethics also provides specific guidance for day-to-day life of the faithful individually and collectively. This wealth of moral guidance is in part a consequence of the wide range of moral authority and ethical sources from which believers might draw direction or construct responses to novel moral quandaries.

Before embarking on a discussion of religious ethics and religious social ethics, a few broad comments about religion are in order. Religions are not univocal. Their geography, historicity, and cultural situatedness make for a diversity of belief, expression, and practice, even within a single religion. In a number of instances, these diverse forms have come to bear different names such as Orthodox, Conservative, Reform, Reconstructionist, Hassidic, and Haredi, all of which are Judaism. Buddhism includes Theravada, Mahayana, Tibetan, Zen, PureLand, Son and other. We must, then, approach an understanding of religion with a few caveats in mind.[1]

First, we acknowledge that both good and evil have been and continue to be done in the name of religion. Religion has been used to mask personal ambition; to legitimate slavery, colonialism, patriarchy, and imperialism; and to subjugate peoples on the basis of race, ethnicity, or gender. Religion can be toxic at the personal level as well, as seen in the mass suicides/murders of the Solar Temple (Canada, 1997), People's Temple (Guyana, 1978), and Heaven's Gate (USA, 1997), and the Movement for the Restoration of the Ten Commandments of God (Uganda, 2000). Isolation, projection, and pathological anger, the "lethal triad," have been identified as the attributes shared by separatist extremist religious groups that predispose to death by suicide/murder.[2] Religion has had a hand in the suppression of cultures, the oppression of peoples, and the death of innocent persons. We do not dismiss this aspect of religion. However, we set it aside in part in order to explore the other side of religion, the side that works to heal and repair the world, to meet the needs of the poor, to heal the ill, to care for the orphan, to respond to natural disaster, to comfort the grieving, and to guide and nurture the living.

Second, although religion may arise within a very particular social context, it often migrates and, in diaspora, takes on its own distinctive character. That character is shaped by the new cultural context, the social location of the immigrant community, the desire to retain identity and tradition, and many other factors, some so simple as the nature of the foods that are available in the new land. Religion and culture are reciprocating and interpenetrating so that Reform Judaism in England may not be an identical twin of Reform Judaism in Israel and Sikhism in Vancouver, British Columbia, and Canada will not look like Sikhism in the Indian Punjab.[3]

Third, some cultures retain a religious metaphysics that may historically have shaped the nation, its laws, its culture, and its people, even if that religion no longer prevails or is no longer widely embraced. For example, the communitarian emphasis of communism in Russia did not originate in communism, but rather reinforced a preexistent communal emphasis found in Russian Orthodox Christianity that predated communism by almost a millennium. Despite the official atheism of the Soviet State, Russia was nevertheless Orthodox in its worldview. In those instances where a religious metaphysics is operative subliminally in the culture, it may work to the disadvantage of those groups possessed of a different philosophical ground.

Fourth, religions fall along a continuum of religious belief, adherence, and expression that may also be reflected in social expression. For example, some Jews may observe the dietary laws of *kashrut* fully, partially, or not at all. Some Christians may attend worship services weekly, or perhaps only on the major religious holidays of Christmas or Easter. Some Hindus may eat meat, or perhaps only fish and poultry, or be vegetarian. This continuum may be characterized in various ways, including: ultraconservative to liberal; traditional to progressive; fundamentalist to mainstream, and so on. These continua may also incorporate and be expressed in social and political views.

Fifth, individuals may pick and choose their beliefs over against the formal beliefs, standards, and practices of the religious tradition to which they belong. Some who affiliate with a religious tradition may even reject the religion itself and identify themselves as "cultural Christians," "cultural Hindus," and so on. In addition, the nuanced understanding and arguments of clergy and scholarly circles within a tradition may become a less subtle set of proscriptions and prescriptions by the time they are received by the ordinary follower.

Sixth, religion may commingle with "civil religion," that is, the "folk religion" of a nation and its political culture. Civil religion makes use of religious language and symbols to evoke shared national values, to promote national unity, and perhaps to call the people to act together. It is devoid of actual religious content; it is cultural content cloaked in religious language. Political civil religion may include rituals and expressions specifically linked to patriotism: in the United States, presidential exclamations such as "God bless America," "a national day of prayer," and the phrase "one nation under God" evoke not so much religious faith as nationalistic fervor. However, some religious traditions may so commingle with culture that the actual religious content may, in an accommodationist syncretism, become a variant form of nationalism.[4,5]

Seventh, many religions, or more specifically their organized forms, have had an enduring interest in matters of health. They may offer formal guidance to individuals in matters of life, death, illness, and health. They may prompt governments to act in specific ways regarding health care, and they may work on the world stage to seek health for all either directly or indirectly through addressing poverty, oppression, war, and injustice.

Eighth, religion can hold hands with power and it can provide an independent and powerful critique of power. It can call for action by its followers, by governments, nations, and world secular organizations such as the United Nations. It can stand apart from prevailing norms that work for harm and say "this must not continue." And, it can partner with other faith traditions to effect change. Religious organizations can also play a role in addressing national and international issues, events, and crises. For example, the Jewish Coalition for Disaster Relief, Islamic Aid Worldwide, Buddhist Global Relief, Church World Service, and many other religious organizations are actively involved in disaster relief in Japan, Christchurch, New Zealand, and elsewhere around the globe where humanitarian assistance is needed. However, before we can engage in a fuller discussion of religious social ethics, it is necessary first to explore the topic of religio-moral authority in religious traditions.

RELIGION AND RELIGIOUS MORAL AUTHORITY

An understanding of religious authority and ethics serves not only to inform our understanding of ethical decisions by nurses or their patients, but also informs our understanding of the world of which we are a part. The world is smoldering and aflame with religious strife that includes terrorism and suicide bombing, religious-ethnic cleansing, religious oppression, torture and war, and the imposition of stringently restrictive interpretations of particular faiths, and more. Although these conflicts are more than purely religious (combining as they do power, politics, greed, ambition, oppression, patriarchy, and culture), they do overshadow the more irenic and nurturant aspects of religion that foster human flourishing, sustain human community, guide the perplexed, and comfort the grieving. Much treatment of religion neglects the fact that many religious traditions are moral traditions as well. The question of sources of religious authority and their uses in moral reflection has enormous import in the world today, particularly for our understanding of that world. The discussion that follows is specifically focused on sources of authority in religious ethics that provides guidance for the faithful, individually and collectively. We will then turn to examine the collective ethics, the social ethics of religious traditions. But first we look at sources of moral authority upon which religious traditions might draw for moral reflection, analysis, action, and evaluation. We will examine four such sources: (a) sacred writings and sacred stories, (b) religious tradition, (c) reason, and (d) religious experience.[6] For nurses, understanding religious sources of moral authority for various faith traditions can give greater insight into how ethics function within a particular tradition, or the sources a particular patient might turn to for guidance, or a greater understanding of the moral position a patient might take. It can also assist the nurse in understanding what a patient might find more or less persuasive in moral deliberation. However, nursing too draws upon a corollary of these same four sources so that understanding plural sources of religious moral authority indirectly assists nurses to understand their own moral decision making. It helps to understand how purely deductive ethics do not work, as they do not take into account nursing's codes of ethics, nursing's moral tradition, and other sources of moral authority in nursing.

Sacred Writings and Sacred Stories as a Source of Religious–Ethical Authority

Religious stories, or narrative, predate religious writings. In some instances, these stories are retained as oral tradition in oral cultures, and resistant to codification in writing, even today. That is, they remain a living tradition held in common and passed orally from generation to generation in stories, songs, poems, and chants. These stories are sometimes a recitation performance for the community, passing cultural knowledge, values, and identity within the community. In such cultures, there may be a specific person, family, or class of persons charged with the responsibility of preserving and passing the oral tradition.[7–9] Where religious writings arise, they typically do so in the shift from a hunter-gatherer culture to an agrarian society, or with the rise of a monarchy. With monarchy, there is an attendant rise of a scribal class—and accountants. After all, even in ancient times the monarch kept records of his (sometimes her) great feats, and an accounting of his great wealth.

Religious writings often embed the early oral stories of a tradition. They have varying levels of authority and varying purposes, ranging from *scriptures*, that is *sacred* or *canonical* writings, to writings of a largely devotional nature. *Sacred writings* are those that the faith community in which they arise or to which they "belong" regard as having prior, or perhaps absolute, authority. These collected works are referred to as the *canon* of a community (Old English, Latin, and Greek for "rule"). A canon is considered *closed* if "books" cannot be added or removed and *open* if its contents may still be altered by the community. *Canonical writings* are seen as having their ultimate origin in God, or the divine, or the transcendent, and are customarily deemed as bearing a surpassing authority based upon their transcendent origin. They are given or revealed by the divine to humankind. In some cases, these writings are viewed as having been dictated by the divine; in other cases, such writings are seen as divinely inspired through the vehicle of human expression; in yet other cases, they are not understood to be from a divine source, but rather reflect divinity in having been set down by a singular individual who has reached a transcendent state of spiritual progress. The fact that some of these sacred writings began as oral tradition, passed through many generations and were redacted (edited with a theological purpose) across hundreds of years by many persons (or schools of persons) before being written down (displaying many compositional layers) is not seen as altering their sacredness. For example, the Hindu Mahabharata is thought to have originated in oral tradition around the eighth to ninth centuries BCE, passing into writing no earlier than about 400 BCE, reaching its final redacted form in the early Gupta period of the fourth century CE.[10,11] Examples of sacred writings, or scriptures, that are canonical are presented in Table 2.1.

Some religions, such as Shintoism, have no written scriptures. Many of the scriptures listed here began as an oral tradition, passed down verbatim for generations (or centuries) before being recorded so that the life of the sacred scriptures is often considerably longer than its life in written form. In cultures, whether ancient or more recent, where the primary mode of transmission remains through oral tradition, that transmission should not be regarded as less accurate than contemporary written transmission. These sacred writings are primary texts for the followers of their respective religious traditions. As such, they are read and followed as the basis for the tradition's worldview, as authoritative and trustworthy guides to the religious life and its practices, and as a source of moral authority, teachings, and guidance.

The development of the field of *textual studies*, as well as the rise in the 1800s of modern *critical methods* of study of ancient texts have served to advance the modern understanding of sacred scriptures by their respective scholars. These include literary, form, redaction, source, canonical, and other specialized forms of critical method. Textual studies attempt to recover the "original text," the actual words, of a work. "Higher" critical methods serve to assist the modern reader to read the text as it was intended to be understood within the literary form that the writers used. For example, these methods uncover passages that are poetry, hyperbole, puns, and other literary forms so that they may be read rightly; e.g., neither poetry nor the excess of hyperbole are to be understood literally. Critical methods also uncover the layers of a text where multiple writers or schools of writers may have converged in a single document, each writing with a different purpose. For example, in a book with many writers, such as this one, or in a chapter with more than one author, redaction and source criticism would be able to unravel which author wrote what segments and to what purpose through an examination of themes, motifs, vocabulary, and style. The ultimate task of critical methods is to assure that the reader is reading the text rightly and to assist the modern reader to remove the 21st century lens through which the text is read in

TABLE 2.1   Examples of Sacred Texts

Religion	Sacred Text (Canonical)	Description
Hindu	Mahabharata	The Hindu sacred scriptures fall into two categories, the Śruti (or Shruti; Sanskrit for "hearing" or "listening," that is, "that which is heard") that includes the Vedas and Upanishads, and Smriti (Sanskrit for "that which is remembered"), which includes the post-Vedic Hindu Mahabharata and the Ramayana. The authority of the Śruti is given greater weight. The Bhagavad Gita, widely known in the non-Hindu world and considered to be sacred text by almost all Hindus, combines elements of both Śruti and Smriti.
Buddhism	Tipitaka Mahayana Sutras	Theravada Buddhists regard the Tipitaka as the complete teachings of the Buddha, whereas the Mahayana Buddhists regard the Tipitaka and the Mahayana sutras, together, as sacred scripture.
Daoism/ Taoism	Tao De Ching	The Tao De Ching (or Daodejing) are writings attributed to Laozi (Lao Tzu; dates disputed possibly circa sixth or fourth century BCE), considered the founder of Taoism and regarded as a deity in much of Taoism. Taoism began as a nonreligious philosophy and psychology but was eventually accepted as a state religion in China.
Judaism	Torah Tanakh	The Jewish Torah refers to the Five Books of Moses, also called the Pentateuch (from *penta*, meaning five). However, the term Torah may be more widely applied to the whole of the Jewish Bible, known as the Tanakh, or even more broadly to the entire historical tradition of the Law and its exposition. Tanakh is an acrostic for Torah (Law), Niviim (Prophets) and Ketuvim (Writings), the three categories of works that are combined into the Jewish Bible.
Christianity	Bible	The Tanakh, with very few minor variations, forms the basis for the first section of the Christian Bible, commonly referred to by Christians as the "Old Testament" or the "Old Covenant." The second section of the Christian Bible is the "New Testament" or "New Covenant." Both the Tanakh and the Christian Bible are understood to be descended from oral tradition, the work of multiple writers and redactors with layers of composition, yet inspired by God in their recording of the sacred writings.
Islam	Qur'an	The Qur'an precisely records the words of God revealed by the angel Jibril (Gabriel) to the prophet Muhammad and are the sacred writings of Islam. The Qur'an is, thus, recorded as the word of God communicated through a single individual to the followers of Allah who memorized the text. It was set in writing shortly following Muhammed's death, when differing dialects of Arabic began to lead to variations.
Sikhism	Guru Granth Sahib	The Guru Granth Sahib is a collection of sacred hymns and sayings (*baanis*), compiled and composed during the period of Sikh gurus, from 1469 to 1708. It is the final and eternal guru of the Sikhs.

order to understand the ancient lenses through which the writers looked upon their situation. Today, sacred scriptures are understood by scholars to be works of faith, not works of science, history, or geography, and as being shaped by the language, culture, literary genera, setting-in-life (sitz-im-leben), and redactional purposes of the writers and redactors of the work. Scholars within the related tradition conduct much of this critical work on sacred writings. These studies make it clear that there is no such thing as a "plain and simple" reading of ancient texts. That is to say that a *precritical reading* of sacred writings runs the risk of doing violence to the text.

There are three fundamental phases of interpretation of sacred writings. They are *exegesis, interpretation* (together, a process that is referred to as "hermeneutics"), and *application. Exegesis* is the process of examining a text in order to uncover how the text's first readers would have understood its meaning. *Interpretation* involves discerning how we are to understand the text today in the light of what it meant to the first readers. Exegesis is, thus, prior to interpretation. In the same way, interpretation precedes application. Application addresses the question of how we should live in the light of this interpretation. Understanding of the texts customarily requires that some study accompany reading if one is to see how, for instance, the *sitz-im-leben* (setting in life) or the literary genera/ subgenera serve to limit potential exegetical interpretations of the text, and *eisegesis*, that is, reading into the text what is not there. Exegesis and interpretation tend to be the domain of a tradition's scholars. Customarily, the interpretation and some general application are then passed to the followers of a tradition to apply within their own life setting. For those who wish to dig deeper into a tradition's exegesis and interpretation, it is fortunate that for those not adept at ancient languages, works such as "commentaries" can be used to shed considerable hermeneutic light on passages of sacred writings, from which the members of the faith community may draw guidance.

Many religious traditions also have written works that are revered though not regarded as canonical, that is, as authoritative, reliable, and worthy, yet subordinate to sacred scriptures. In most instances, these works serve as general guides, or further explication, for the life of faith, but are not necessarily considered to be "binding" in the same sense as scriptures. These include the writings of faithful persons, leaders, and heroes of their respective traditions, or devotional or spiritual works. Persons within a given faith community will draw upon the sacred writings as well as these other religious works for guidance in the moral life. But the question remains, "How do those who live an intentionally religious life actually draw upon sacred writings for moral guidance?"

There are several approaches to the derivation of ethical precepts from scriptures. One way is to view sacred writings as moral cookbooks, that is, as books of rules that provide concrete moral specifications that are universally applicable. This is an unsatisfactory and methodologically unsound means of deriving moral norms, on at least four grounds. First, it is a precritical approach to sacred writings that interprets scriptures literally without contextual understanding. It wrests portions of scripture from their broader and immediate context, a context that specifies the nature of the communal context in which these norms are operative. Second, it neglects the interpretive boundaries that are set by such things as literary genera and original setting-in-life, applying them to contexts that do not bear the same hallmarks. Third, it grants normative stature to particular portions of sacred writings without "testing" those portions over against the whole of the corpus. Fourth, this approach is often a means of *proof texting* a preexisting disposition in the reader. Rather than seeking an accurate interpretation of the text, it is a disposition in search of a justification, utilizing scripture to make an argument or assert a conclusion that the passage does not actually support. This is to use sacred writings in such a way as to make them mean what the "user" wishes them to mean rather than what they actually mean, a form of *eisegesis*. Precritical readings of sacred writings tend to characterize less interpretive traditions or fundamentalist movements. On the other hand, some persons simply reject the use of sacred scriptures as sources of moral authority, on the grounds that their antiquity makes them dated and inapplicable to contemporary life. This dismissive approach is flawed in the same way in that it, too, treats sacred writings as a cookbook but now with ingredients past their expiration date.

Religious scriptures do contain concrete, material prescriptions and proscriptions for moral behavior, but such specifications customarily give way to the authority of more formal norms. For instance, concrete norms against misrepresentation in the marketplace would give way to formal norms enjoining us to treat one another as we ourselves would wish to be treated. At the level of formal norms, there is considerable concurrence among world religions. For instance, many religions have a similar norm about the way in which we are to treat others, often called "the golden rule." A story is told of Rabbi Hillel:

> A certain heathen came to Shammai and said to him, "Make me a proselyte, on condition that you teach me the whole Torah while I stand on one foot." Thereupon he repulsed him with the rod which was in his hand. When he went to Hillel, [he also asked Hillel to teach him the entire Torah while standing on one foot] he said to him, "What is hateful to you, do not do to

your neighbor: that is the whole Torah; all the rest of it is commentary; go and learn." (Talmud, Shabbat 31a)

A similar formal norm is found in many other religions[12]:

Buddhism: ". . . a state that is not pleasing or delightful to me, how could I inflict that upon another?" Samyutta NIkaya v. 353; also: "Hurt not others in ways that you yourself would find hurtful." Udana-Varga 5:18

Baha'i: "And if thine eyes be turned towards justice, choose thou for thy neighbour that which thou choosest for thyself." Epistle to the Son of the Wolf.

Christianity: "Teacher, which is the great commandment in the law?" Jesus said to him, "You shall love the Lord your God with all your heart, and with all your soul, and with all your mind. This is the great and first commandment. And a second is like it, You shall love your neighbor as yourself. On these two commandments depend all the law and the prophets." Bible, Matthew 22.36–40

Confucianism: Tsekung asked, "Is there one word that can serve as a principle of conduct for life?" Confucius replied, "It is the word shu—reciprocity: Do not do to others what you do not want them to do to you." Analects 15.23; See also: "Try your best to treat others as you would wish to be treated yourself, and you will find that this is the shortest way to benevolence." Mencius VII.A.4

Hinduism: "One should not behave towards others in a way which is disagreeable to oneself. This is the essence of morality. All other activities are due to selfish desire." Mahabharata, Anusasana Parva 113.8

Islam: "Not one of you is a believer until he loves for his brother what he loves for himself." Forty Hadith of an-Nawawi 13

Jainism: "A man should wander about treating all creatures as he himself would be treated." Sutrakritanga 1.11.33; See also: "In happiness and suffering, in joy and grief, we should regard all creatures as we regard our own self." Lord Mahavira, 24th Tirthankara

Pima Native American tradition: "Do not wrong or hate your neighbor. For it is not he who you wrong, but yourself." Pima proverb

Sikhism: "Do not create enmity with anyone as God is within everyone." Guru Arjan Devji 259

Taoism: "The sage has no interest of his own, but takes the interests of the people as his own. He is kind to the kind; he is also kind to the unkind: for Virtue is kind. He is faithful to the faithful; he is also faithful to the unfaithful: for Virtue is faithful." Tao Teh Ching, chapter 49

Yoruba: "One going to take a pointed stick to pinch a baby bird should first try it on himself to feel how it hurts." Yoruba proverb

A caution is in order at this point. Although similar core material may be found in a number of religions, religions cannot be reduced or collapsed into one another as simply differing cultural expressions of the same religious impulse. It only indicates that there may be some agreement in the moral norms that religious persons will use. These norms may bring about similar applications and similar conclusions such that the religious worldview resident behind them is imperceptible in moral discourse. Similar norms may also produce divergent interpretations—even within one tradition. In some instances, the divergence relates to a difference in interpretation of a fact, rather than the value itself. Formal principles such as these require reflection in order to be applied. In a very accessible book on religion, Prothero has recently argued that "God is not one." More specifically, he writes that

> . . . as Hindu teacher Swami Sivananda writes, "The fundamentals or essentials of all religions are the same. There is difference only in the nonessentials." This is a lovely sentiment but it is dangerous, disrespectful, and untrue . . . the idea of religious unity is wishful thinking nonetheless, and it has not made the world a safer place. In fact, this naïve theological groupthink . . . had made the world more dangerous by blinding us to the clashes of religions that threaten us worldwide. . . . The world's religious rivals do converge when it comes to ethics, but they diverge sharply on doctrine, ritual, mythology, experience, and law. . . . One of the most common misconceptions about the world's religions is that they plumb the same depths, ask the same questions. They do not. Only religions that see God as all good ask how a good God can allow millions to die in tsunamis. Only religions that believe in soul ask whether your soul exists before you are born and what happens to it after you die. And only religions that think we have one soul ask after "the soul" in the singular. Every religion, however, asks after the human condition. Here we are in these human bodies. What now? What next? What are we to become?[13]

Despite the differences between and among religions, they do, as Prothero notes, often converge at the point of ethics. Setting aside the less adequate means of deriving moral norms from scripture outlined above, at least three different general approaches emerge. Sacred scriptures may be seen as divinely reveled moral law that should govern the actions of the faithful; as a glimpse of the nature of the divine or transcendent from which one derives moral norms in accord with the attributes, character, or nature of the transcendent; or as providing a moral context and vision for the life of faith from which themes (such as destiny, hope, oneness, and salvation) inform and guide moral deliberation and choice.[14] Within these three basic approaches, formal and moral norms are given concrete specification for particular settings by means of reflection that employs reason, tradition, and experience and the sacred writings themselves to give further specification in a particular context or situation.

Religious Tradition as a Source of Religious–Ethical Authority

Religions are, by nature, lived within a community of faith. Customarily these communities have one or more religious leaders and not infrequently a hierarchy of religious leadership, whether formal or informal. The authority that accrues to these leaders, or the leadership collectively, is that of the interpretation of all aspects of the faith including whatever sacred writings there may be. The extent to which "ordinary followers" are at liberty to interpret the tradition and its sacred writings varies widely within as well as among religions.

Although religions are situated within a particular culture, they themselves have their own "religious culture." Civil culture and religious culture can become so commingled as to be one-and-the-same in the minds of the followers. Under these conditions, it may become difficult for followers of a religion to sort out what is "religion" and what is "culture" and how culture may actually shape and even supplant aspects of the religion. Aspects of the culture may even become *de fide*, or essential tenets of the faith, even while they have no actual foundation in the faith. H.R. Niebuhr (1951) wrote of five paradigmatic relationships between "Christ and culture."[15] Although he applies his typology to Christianity and American culture, it is useful to employ the typology to think about other relationships between a religious tradition and its surrounding culture. One relationship, "Christ against culture," is a rejectionist, separationist isolative stance where the group opts out of society and forms its own community in isolation. The Essene community in ancient Israel or the Amish community in the Unites States are examples of this. Perhaps more troubling is the "Christ of culture" position whereby a faith community so commingles American culture with Christian faith that they are seen as one and the same—American culture *is* Christian faith. The consequences of this for international relations are both profound and potentially devastating.

The culture of a religion, rather than its actual tenets, may govern many aspects of nonmoral behavior, including how one reacts with joy or sorrow, success or disappointment, forgiveness or anger. The culture may even govern the specific foods to be eaten at community gatherings, apart from festivals or feasts. In many instances, religion and culture can be difficult to disentangle.

Our concern here is with the more formal aspects of a religious tradition, per se, wherein the official statements, beliefs, rules, customs, or policies of a tradition are "handed down" to the faithful. This would include formal authoritative teachings regarding religious ethics, moral issues, and moral expectations of followers individually or collectively. Such proclamations may be issued orally or in writing, or both. Today, a considerable amount of information detailing various religious perspectives on bioethical issues can be found on the Internet. A search of the terms "Sikh" and "end-of-life" produces a number of pages across the Internet that set forth Sikh theology and then discusses it in relation to end-of-life issues such as euthanasia, physician-assisted-suicide, and suicide. There are a number of clearly articulated, formal statements by widely respected Sikh scholars, clerics, and ethicists and organizations representing the Sikh tradition. The Internet can also provide access to official religious sites. For instance, there are Web sites for the Office of His Holiness the 14th Dalai Lama of Tibet; the Office of the Chief Rabbi (Chief Rabbi Professor Lord Jonathan Sacks) of the United Hebrew Congregations of the Commonwealth (British); as well as Web sites for The Vatican (in six languages), the Church of Scotland; the Jain Global Resource Center; the Sikh Network and the Golden Temple Kar Seva; the Baha'i International Community; His Holiness Patriarch Kirill of Moscow and all Russia; the Pagan Federation; The British Druid Order; The Tay Ninh Holy See of the Cao Dai faith, and so on. It is now possible to obtain official statements and teachings on a wide range faith-based questions and concerns on the Internet, including bioethical issues of interest to nurses, for virtually all major and not so major world religions. It is characteristic of religious traditions to detail the religious foundation first before tackling explicating a position on a particular issue. Thus one will typically find the religious rationale, not simply the position per se, on an issue. In addition to these statements on bioethical issues, a number of religious traditions have scholarly journals available online as well. For example, the *Journal of Buddhist Ethics* is available online, free, in the current as well as back issues. Volume 2 contains articles on human rights, virtue, justice, medical ethics, unwholesomeness of action, peace, social engagement, statecraft, and environmentalism, all obtainable in full-text format without fee.[16]

Because religions always deal with "the stuff of life," they often develop tradition-specific (or subtradition-specific) perspectives and statements on major life issues, including childbirth, death, bodily practices, sexual behavior, permitted or prohibited foods and beverages or larger social issues such as hunger, poverty, homelessness, or child labor. Some of these positions began in ancient times and were renewed and refined across centuries. In the realm of nursing and bioethics, religious traditions usually have an understanding of what constitutes "health," beliefs about disease, mental illness, suffering, death and dying, caregiving, health care, and medical treatment. They often formally address issues related to the end-of-life and end-of-life care, withdrawal of treatment, reproduction, congenital disabilities, care of the elderly, euthanasia, suicide, access to health care, health care delivery systems, recombinant DNA, cloning, and all the major bioethical "quandaries." The statements that are produced are fundamentally position statements for the tradition itself, and a means of guidance for individual believers. When a tradition issues such statements, there is an implicit or explicit expectation that adherents of the tradition will embrace and follow this guidance. Depending upon the gravity of the issue being treated, and its implications for the faith, some traditions allow a degree of variation among believers based on circumstances and the conscience of the individual adherent.

Within any single tradition, geography, history, and culture will serve to create a diversity of perspectives, some perspectives more extreme than others. That is to say that official statements of a tradition may not be embraced by all segments of that tradition, not because they are actually rejected, but because of the nonreligious influences that may shape a community. For example, nonliterate and rural or schismatic members of a tradition may have an earlier received or less changed form of a tradition that differs from that of urban members, and these subgroups may deal with a different range of personally pressing issues. These rural representatives may retain a "purer," or perhaps more historically rooted, or more "antique," form of the tradition and may also retain rituals and symbols lost to the general or larger body of believers. The "Old Believers" Bielaia Krinitsia Church of Russia (Ukraine), which broke away from the larger Orthodox Church in the mid-1600s, would be an example of such a group.

A number of religious traditions view personal health maintenance as a part of one's religious obligation, sometimes referred to as *stewardship* or *stewardship of the body*.[17] How a life is to be lived is not solely a matter of obedience to guidance or directives or rules. The particular ends of the religion also inform how one is to live life in relation to our bodily existence. Whether the *telos* (end) of the faithful life is salvation, or mukti, or nirvana, or paradise, or the beatific vision, or union with God, or oneness with the universe, the *teloi* (ends) of traditions will influence the tradition's, and hence the believer's, understanding of how life is to be lived. Moreover, there may be specific religious practices, such as fasting or vegetarianism, that the tradition encourages and might affect health. The degree to which an individual nurse or patient is influenced by the official teachings and statements of a tradition, its cultural aspects, its vision of human life and its ends; its views of health, illness, mental health, death, dying and suffering; its moral perspectives and guidance is dependent upon several factors. These include the degree of devotion or adherence of the believer, the level of religious integration, the tradition's limitations on the exercise of disagreement or conscience, the individual's level of self-reflection, and the personal religious support systems of the individual.

Reason as a Source of Religious–Ethical Authority

Discussions of reason in relation to religion often center on specific questions, such as proofs of the existence of God, or the possibility of a divine–human (i.e., personal) encounter, on the use of reason to discover or defend religious truth, on the relationship of reason to faith, on the reliability of reason, or on other questions of customary concern in that branch of study called "the philosophy of religion." These are not questions that we will address. Rather, the concern here is for the use of reason as a source of moral authority within the sphere of religious ethics.

Reason serves several general purposes within any religion. Religions in general give a systematic account of reality, a metaphysics, usually referred to as a "worldview." Within that worldview, there are epistemological claims about knowledge and its acquisition, ontological claims about the nature of humanity and its ends, and ethical and aesthetic claims about the way in which the life of faith should be lived. It is by way of reason that the individual believer can evaluate the claims of the religion for coherence, consistency, comprehensiveness, congruity, or compatibility with facts about the material world, their explanatory power, and sense-making potential. This is a critical rationalism applied to one's own faith for the purposes, not only of evaluation, but of deepening an understanding of the faith.[18] However, another use of reason is to reflect critically upon religious values, precepts, and guides for the purposes of moral decision making. For instance, a religion may contain a basic rule, "do not kill," in its sacred writings. Searching the context of the rule in sacred scripture leads one to believe that it refers to killing humans and not animals or plants or not, more broadly, something like "the environment." Yet, even with this clarification, the norm against killing cannot be applied as it stands, for we still do not know what is meant by "killing." A search of commentaries on this particular scriptural passage is of some assistance in that it clarifies that "do not kill" means "do not murder." That too is helpful, but it still does not take us far enough. Is withdrawal of treatment murder? Or abortion, euthanasia, suicide? What about killing another human being in war, or for self-defense, or in an accident? What about capital punishment, or if someone dies during surgery? Are any or all of these types of killing "murder"? Does this rule indicate moral blameworthiness for any of these types of killing? The difficulty with a formal rule is that it is contentless and, even after clarification, it still requires that reason be used in order to discern how and when it should be applied. However, many modern moral questions are not addressed in ancient writings or stories. New variations of old questions or altogether new questions may arise. Here, the follower or a religion must use reason to "construct" a response rooted in the faith. Such a process has been called *constructive theology* in some traditions. For example, the use of nuclear or biological weapons in war will obviously not have been discussed in ancient sacred writings. Yet discussions of peace and war can be brought forward and applied in a discussion of modern weapons. However, a question such as the acceptability of surrogate mothering, brain transplant, recombinant DNA, or genetically modified crops can take religious moral reasoning into new realms.

How then might reason be used within religious ethics in both exploring and employing moral norms? This is not a simple question both because particular traditions have affinities for particular methods or systems of reasoning, and because every conceivable method of reasoning is represented across and within religions. However, not unlike nursing research, two fundamental methods of moral reasoning may be broadly sketched. This is the point at which nurses might find themselves on more familiar moral ground.

The first method is essentially deductive and principle-based. It begins with abstract, formal principles drawn from sacred writings or stories, reason, or the tradition. These principles are seen within a tradition as timeless. As such, they can be applied, by reason, with rigor, clarity, coherence, consistency, and precision, independent of the context—at least in formal theological argument. Although not entirely formulaic, this approach shares with formulas a certain "tidiness" for its assumed degree of objectivity or impartiality. Reasoned evaluation and application thus show a degree of orderliness and stability and provide for a transhistorical continuity by moving from formal to concrete material norms applicable by all, everywhere, across time. On the other hand, these norms are not entirely objective or impartial and free of cultural influence. Neither is life generally known for "tidiness"; theological argument must negotiate the messiness of life. The purely deductive approach, for all its rigor and precision, fails to take account of the complexity and impreciseness of the human situation, of the social construction of reality, of the fluidity of human freedom, nonrational motivations, or the uniqueness of particular moral contexts.[19]

A second general method of moral reasoning in religions is *casuistic. Casuistry* is reasoning used to resolve moral problems by applying formal rules to particular instances. It takes greater account of the messiness of life by beginning more inductively with experience and particularity, rather than logic and supposed universality. It is empirical in nature and may draw intentionally upon the social sciences and scientific research in its reflection. Norms are important but are conditioned by circumstances in this approach. Unlike the deductive approach, which has its own limitations, casuistry can risk relativity at its farther end and a lack of rigor in its use. Casuistry may be more familiar as a form of legal argument from a paradigm case or precedent to a similar case at hand. It is important to note that some religious traditions (e.g., Judaism, Islam) are based in religious law; thus make heavy use of casuistry. For example, Jewish discussion of euthanasia today draws upon ancient cases: chopping wood outside the window of a dying person, removing the pillow from the head of a dying person, removing salt on the person's tongue, and closing the eyes of a dying person. The discussion proceeds in this fashion:

> The Talmud and rabbinic code state that a *goses*, a dying patient whose demise is imminent, is regarded as a living person in all respects. Nothing may be done to hasten his death. It is forbidden to wash the patient, remove the pillow from underneath him, to place him on the ground. It is also forbidden to close his eyes "for whoever closes the eyes with the onset of death is a shedder of blood." Furthermore, the keys of the synagogue may not be put under is head so that he may depart. (Shulhan Arukh, Yoreh Deah, 339.1)
>
> Each of these acts is forbidden because the slightest movement of the patient may hasten death. As the Babylonian Talmud puts it, "this action may be compared to a flickering flame; as soon as one touches it, the light is extinguished." This is called *hariga bayadayim*, literally "killing with one's hands" or in modern parlance, active euthanasia.[20]
>
> If there is anything that causes a hindrance to the departure of the soul, such as the presence near the patient's house of a knocking noise, such as wood chopping, or if there is salt on the patient's tongue, and these hinder the soul's departure, it is permissible to remove them from there because there is no act involved with this at all but only the removal of the impediment.[21]

The *Talmud* dates from 200CE to 500CE. The *Shulhan Aruch* was published in 1565. As an ancient question, Jewish bioethics draws upon millennia of casuistry to formulate its position on euthanasia today.

As examples within the nursing ethical literature, the deductive approach is more closely associated with what has been called "ethical principalism" and casuistry, which starts with experience and circumstances, is more familiarly seen in various approaches to "feminist ethics" or "contextual ethics" in the nursing literature. Both approaches are a part of religious moral reasoning.

These two basic approaches to religious ethics ought not to be cast in an either/or standoff. The deductive approach does indeed allow for rigor and precision, for the exploration of nuance, dispassionate discussion, resistance to relativization, and consistency and evenhandedness in application. These are strong reasons to retain a deductive approach. The casuistic approach pays close attention to the experience of the moral community and its members as a valid source of moral knowledge and judgment, to the complexity of moral dilemmas, to the nonuniversal aspects of those dilemmas, and to the fact that our reason is suffused with elements drawn from culture, tradition, and the historical context. For these strong reasons, an inductive approach should be retained as well. Although the deductive method has gained a dominant position in Western secular circles, both the principle-based and casuistic methods should be used, bringing their respective strengths to moral reflection, discourse, and decision making.

Religious Experience as a Source of Religious–Ethical Authority

Religious experience is an encounter with a transcendent reality and is understood by the person as an experience of something larger than the natural, perhaps a supernatural presence or being, or a sense of an *ineffable* reality (i.e., a reality incapable of being described by words). Such experiences tend to be intensely real, intimate, awe-filled, perhaps overwhelming or frightening, and as having a depth of mystery. These experiences may be, but are not necessarily, productive of religious moral insight. That moral insight may be greater clarity, self-understanding, illumination of the mind, or a sense of fittingness of a moral perspective. To speak of religious experience is, in the end, to address the issue of what is customarily called the inner or interior life, or more commonly, "spirituality." Although nursing tends to speak of spirituality as an ontological category, divorced from all religious content, religious traditions see spirituality as a matter of the life of faith in the way that it is lived. That is, as integral to the religious life. Spirituality may be defined in a number of ways, including definitions that are more formal than contentful. For instance, Wakefield defines spirituality as . . . "those attitudes, beliefs, practices that animate people's lives and help them to reach out towards super-sensible realities."[22] Fitchett, a hospital chaplain, defines spirituality as ". . . the dimension in life that reflects the need to find meaning in existence and in which we respond to the sacred."[23] Spirituality may also be defined in a more contentful way that more broadly points toward its ramifications for the moral life, that is, one that includes a stronger indication of the relationship between spirituality and its contiguity with the moral life:

> Spirituality is the way in which a person understands and lives life in view of her or his ultimate meaning, beliefs, and values. It is the unifying and integrative aspect of the person's life and, when lived intentionally, is experienced as increasingly pervasive and integrative, that is, as a process of growth and maturity. It integrates, unifies, and vivifies the whole of a person's narrative or story, embeds her or his core identity, establishes the fundamental basis for the individual's relationship with others and with society, includes a sense

of the transcendent, and is the interpretive lens through which the person sees the world. It is the basis for community for it is in spirituality that we experience our consanguinity and co-participation in the shared human condition. It may or may not be experienced or expressed in religious terms but when understood religiously it includes life in a community of faith that serves as a referent community for growth, nurture and discipline.[24]

By discipline is meant the potential for corrective that prevents the person from "going off the deep end." It is this element of discipline that is missing from the communities demonstrating the "lethal triad," which will be discussed shortly. It is the fact that one's spirituality (here, in this discussion, informed by religion) can serve as an interpretive lens that is important for a discussion of experience as a source of religious-ethical authority. For some persons and some traditions, however, religious experience is less a part of moral evaluation or outlook. Much of what has been said here is true primarily of traditions that overtly value religious experience, and primarily of persons who have determined to live their faith intentionally, that is, they have chosen to live employing the filter of their religious worldview and to act in a manner congruent with it. Those who affiliate more loosely with a faith tradition, or embrace it only nominally or culturally, will probably not demonstrate as full an attempt to draw upon its resources in the exercise of daily or professional life. Even so, those who are culturally, but not by belief, bound to a faith tradition may find themselves employing various aspects of the tradition's sources of authority in the moral life, perhaps unknowingly. Again, insofar as a religion is also a culture, those who have been reared, even nominally, in a faith but do not embrace it may find that they have internalized a substantial degree of its metaphysics and may even strongly represent its worldview.

Within religious traditions, spirituality is often discussed in terms of a journey, as ascent, or as a path. Spirituality is generally seen as a life journey, a process of development and maturation. Some religions may see this path as more intense for a season, for those called to nonreligious vocations. A second issue relating to the use of sources of religious ethical authority has to do with what might be called the "spiritual maturity" of the follower of the tradition. There are several theories of spiritual development, one of which follows the cognitive structural and developmental work of Piaget and Kohlberg, respectively.[25,26] Without exploring these theories, a few brief observations common to these theories might be helpful. In general, greater spiritual maturity demonstrates intentionality, critical reflection and reasoning, coherence of basic beliefs, a higher level of integration; familiarity with the tradition's history, literature, and practices; involvement with the religious community, personal practices of piety, a commitment to spiritual growth; and activities that foster growth. Such persons see the world through the lens of their religious worldview. Persons with less-developed spiritual lives tend to compartmentalize their faith to a greater degree. They may, for example, apply it to their religious activities, but not to their business practices. There is commonly a twofold direction of spiritual growth, the journey inward and then the journey outward into a concern for the world.[27] This is ultimately the basis for the individual's development of a personal social ethics and participation in the community of faith's social ethics.

There are several areas in which religious experience may influence the way in which one operationalizes, or more accurately lives, ethics. Devotional or spiritual readings, as well as sacred writings, and faith community ideals, often motivate and foster the production and exercise of specific virtues. These could include such virtues as faith, hope, love, peaceableness, equanimity, kindness, generosity, hospitality, goodwill, awareness, carefulness, wisdom, and so forth. Moral agency, then, would be rooted in the spiritual character of the person as much as in specific religio-moral duties. In general, religious traditions and their communities would seem to retain an overt emphasis on virtues, including specific moral virtues, to a greater degree than does the larger secular society at this time in history.

Religious experience may also be felt as an encounter with the divine, or the numinous, or the absolute, or the transcendent that is in and of itself religiously and morally authoritative and a source of moral knowledge. Here, the importance of a community of faith as a community of reference cannot be stressed enough. Individualized or privatized religious experience (as also with a privatized interpretation of sacred writings) that has no referent in the broader community and has no source of course correction. The People's Temple/Jim Jones, the Order of the Solar Temple/Luc Jouret and Joseph Di Mambro, the Branch Davidians/Vernon Wayne Howell (a.k.a. David Koresh), and Heaven's Gate/Marshall Applewhite are examples of groups with privatized religious experience and interpretation, and without a larger community of reference and thereby a source of correction. These religious groups demonstrate the "lethal triad" mentioned above. A larger community of faith that serves as a community-of-reference also serves as the guardrail at the edge of the cliff.

That community of reference should not, however, be a steel trap that holds timeless truths in a time warp. Where this is the case, the community is poorer for it: spiritual exemplars, sages, heroes, hell-raisers, and saints are less likely to emerge. Such persons, however much an irritant, can be forces for social change, forces for good, and forces for the benefit of the community. Their religious experience may give rise to a valid (it unwelcome) critique of the community itself. They may step out and boldly take risks that the world might be changed, or that those in need might receive help, or that good might be done for individuals, communities, the world, or even the environment. There are many examples of this, but Walter Rauschenbusch, Rheinhold Niebuhr, the Pastor's Emergency League in Nazi Germany, Mohandas Gandhi, the Dali Lama, Desmond Tutu, Dag Hammerskjold, and Mother Theresa come to mind.

Experience, especially experience within community, helps to nurture that faculty called conscience and helps to imbue a sense of duty and with that sense an understanding of specific duties that accrue to an individual within the faith tradition. It can foster virtues such as humility in the face of moral complexity, and grace or forgiveness for error that springs from human limitation. Experience, personally and within community, can also help to navigate those few instances in which religious and secular ethics come into conflict.

Bringing the Four Sources of Religio-Moral Authority Together

Although most religious traditions will draw from all of these sources of authority, some will draw more heavily from one or two sources than the others. Even within one tradition, subtraditions will draw more heavily from sources that are less used by others within the tradition. For example, in the American Pentecostal traditions, experience particularly and scripture weigh more heavily, almost to the exclusion of reason and tradition. Fundamentalist Christians rely heavily upon scripture (though a precritical reading of scripture) and rely little on other sources of authority. However, Roman Catholic Christians draw very heavily from tradition, reason, and scripture, but less so from religious experience. Yet, all of these groups are Christian, evidencing the diversity found within and between groups. Thus, the nurse caring for a Pentecostal Christian patient will not draw from the same resources that she or he might use for a Roman Catholic Christian patient. In addition, a nurse must never assume that all Muslims, or all Buddhists, or all Sikhs are the same.

Religious Ethics and Nursing Ethics

Those sources of religious–ethical authority that have been discussed— sacred writings, tradition, reason, and experience—are also the same categories of moral authority upon which nurses depend. Although not precisely "sacred writings," the codes of ethics and policy statements that have been formulated by provincial and national nursing associations (and the ICN) serve as authoritative moral standards for practice. The issue-based position statements produced by those nursing associations are documents that extend the codes of ethics, and comprise the subordinate standards of moral practice. The larger body of moral literature in nursing over the past 125 years of modern nursing comprises the "devotional readings" for the profession.

Nurses may also draw from the tradition of nursing for moral knowledge. Nursing has a long history of caring, and a much longer tradition of service. Within this tradition, nursing students are socialized into the norms of the profession such as keeping confidences, evenhanded treatment of patients, truth-telling, and so forth. These norms of tradition render "abandoning the patient" or "prejudicial treatment" abhorrent. The tradition inculcates its students with the ends that the profession seeks: of human dignity, well-being, human welfare, health care, and so on.

Reason is also a source of moral knowledge in nursing. One need only turn to the debate in the nursing literature over an "ethics of caring" to see the exercise of moral reason. Nursing, too, uses both deductive and casuistic moral reasoning. Increasingly, however, nursing has found itself more at home with both casuistry and virtue. The question of how much of this turn is methodological and how much of it relates to the identity, aspirations, and social location of nursing as a female-dominant profession warrants additional attention.

Experience, too, is a source of moral knowledge for nurses. Many of the dilemmas that nurses encounter, in practice, do not wait for graduation. Students begin their encounter with those human tragedies that we call moral dilemmas well before graduation. All too often, however, ethics education, at least within nursing education in the United States, is remanded to that "issues and ethics" course in the final year of nursing education. Students in nursing and nurses in practice are better served if their experience is undergirded by an ethics education that creates a community of moral discourse in both education and practice settings.

The question remains, "what about those instances in which religious ethics may come into conflict with professional ethics?" (Competing values are not new to nursing, particularly in an economically constrained environment where "cost" competes with "care," "quantity" competes with "quality," and economics trumps nursing values, beckoning nurses to collective action that demands change in the health care environment.) There are occasions where religious values or duties might conflict with professional values or duties. Basic values such as human dignity and well-being tend not to find conflict with religious values. More often, where they occur, the conflicts are specifically conflicts of duty, not value. For example, the nursing ethical literature deals extensively with "distributive justice," whereas many religious traditions emphasize a "preferential option for the poor" that is a justice that embeds a particular duty to care for underserved, marginalized, disadvantaged, and vulnerable persons, to rectify health disparities. In some religious traditions refusal, or withdrawal, of end-of-life treatment may be prohibited, potentially placing nurses who are assigned as caregivers in a morally difficult position. In conflicts such as these, the nurse must weigh the religious values and duties over against those of the profession or the setting, and must make difficult choices.

However, not to take the issue of conflict between religious and secular ethics lightly, it is nonetheless the case that such conflicts are infrequent. Several specific kinds of conflict (e.g., participation in a procedure the nature of which raises moral objections) have long been addressed in the moral literature of the profession, and nursing has made accommodation for these situations by specifying procedures for nurses to opt-out where they have moral objections, or for *conscientious objection* (refusal to participate in something legally required on the basis of moral grounds). More often, religious ethics affirms and sometimes expands professional ethics and presents more nuanced arguments. Where conflict occurs, the degree to which nurses or patients embrace a religious tradition, as well as their point of spiritual development will, in part, determine the scope and depth of their reliance upon that religion's moral norms in facing moral dilemmas in health care. If their level of commitment is less than moderate, then it is the case that other values may overwhelm their religious ethical values and claim priority. It is more frequently the case, however, that the religiously based ethics of the nurse or patient will produce moral responses, decisions, and actions that are similar to those of other practitioners. A mature and reflective religious worldview that undergirds and grounds a nurses' or patients' moral position may in fact remain transparent (transparent, not hidden) and unconflicted.

Nursing ethics is not simply an ethics "at the bedside." From the earliest days of modern nursing, nursing's ethics has involved a wide range of social action, advocating both for nursing practice and for patient welfare. Florence Nightingale, Mary Seacole, and Dasha Sevastopolskaya (Darja Lavrentjevna Mikhailova) changed nursing—and society—forever by taking nursing care to wounded soldiers in the Crimea. Nightingale subsequently became heavily involved in social legislation for health within the British Empire. Thus from the start of modern nursing, nurses have become involved in legislative processes, as consultants to governmental agencies, and (after women's suffrage) as informed voters. Nursing shares with religion a profound concern for social ethics.

SOCIAL APPLICATIONS OF RELIGIOUS ETHICS: SOCIAL JUSTICE AND SOCIAL ENGAGEMENT

When considering the intersections of religious traditions and nursing ethics, we do well to draw on centuries of thought in regard to ethics as socially embedded and socially enacted. Social ethics has been defined as the domain of ethics that deals with "issues of social order—the good, right, and ought in the organization of human communities and the shaping of social policies."[28] For nursing, there are three broad functions of social ethics: reform of the profession, value-based public discourse (referred to as epidictic discourse), and social reform.[29] These functions have traditionally been most often exercised through the profession and its professional organizations, rather than through individual nurses. Social ethics, as a field of study, lifts the gaze from the more narrow focus of bioethics (i.e., on clinical, typically biomedical concerns) to applications of concepts that concern social institutions and structures, discourses, and constructions. Within this framing, social ethics tackles social and global concerns such as poverty, hunger, violence, racialization, and oppression, access to health and health care, and social and health inequities. The historical, economic, political, religious, and institutional forces that shape these concerns are squarely within the purview of a social ethic.

The last decade has seen nurse scholars increasingly use the ethical lens of social justice to examine the social pathways and historical structures that contribute to health inequities (in access to services and disparities in health outcomes) and to advocate for social change at the level of populations (particularly groups of people made vulnerable by their social location). Social justice is advocated for collectively by the profession of nursing (e.g., professional nursing organizations) and is also enacted by individual nurses to challenge hegemonic structures and discourses, and to advocate and intervene to end health inequities. Current social justice discourse in nursing is referenced to the social mandate of nursing, and yet is often constrained by an individualistic focus.[30] Entrenched notions of society (fed by neoliberal ideologies) reinforce the view that individuals are freely choosing, autonomous, and exist in an essentially egalitarian environment.[31] Health is then seen as primarily an individual responsibility, dependent on healthy lifestyle choices, the genetics one has been dealt, and the resources one has at one's disposal (to access health care services). Operationalizing the social mandate of nursing to address the social conditions that constrain opportunities for health has become increasingly urgent, and yet difficult to do in sociopolitical contexts of neoliberal ideologies and cuts to health and social services.[32] To achieve the social mandate of nursing, critical perspectives and commitments beyond the classic interpretations of distributive justice are required. Simply put, distributive justice appeals for the fair distribution of resources, with little attention to the social conditions and relations of power that create opportunity and disadvantage. As a corrective, Iris Young's work, for example, has been pivotal in calling for broader and more critical interpretations of social justice that situate individuals in social groups, for people are oppressed not as individuals but as members of social groups.[33] Other feminist scholars, such as Fraser, have expanded social justice discourses to encompass not only redistribution but also participation and recognition, thus bringing together economic, political, and cultural dimensions of justice.[34] Benefitting from such perspectives, nursing scholars too are increasingly viewing the call of social justice as that of (a) addressing the social gradients imbued with oppression and disadvantage that result in health disparities, in order to (b) create the social conditions for human flourishing. Social justice thus becomes "inclusive participation in the common good," indicating the interdependence of all the just relations and institutions that make up the common good.[35]

The theoretical scaffolding for social justice discourses in nursing is increasingly found in critical social theories such as feminism or postcolonialism.[36] Rarely is the contemporary social justice discourse in nursing rooted in religious or theological traditions. The term and modern conceptualization of social justice was developed first in the 1840s by a Jesuit priest, based on the teachings of Thomas Aquinas (1225–1274), a Christian theologian and philosopher, and is found in many religions.[37] It was taken up as a secular concept more recently, led by philosophers John Stuart Mills and John Rawls. Given the origins of the concept, theological and/or religious ethics may well complement or enhance how social justice is taken up in the profession, and it is toward this point that this last section of this chapter is oriented.

Several themes that are shared across religious traditions support our case that nursing's social ethics can benefit from articulation with religious ethics. First, justice is a foremost value taught by many religions. As pointed out by Cahill, "a distinctive contribution of theology, especially but not exclusively Christian biblical theology, can be to challenge exclusionary systems of access to social and material goods under the aegis of 'love of neighbor', 'self-sacrifice', or 'the preferential option for the poor.'"[38] Illustrated earlier in this chapter, theological doctrines such as love of neighbor and community are shared by many traditions and provide a foundation for social justice. Liberation theology, for example, described as a convergence of Christianity and socialism, has taken fullest expression in Latin America with its analysis of poverty by an application of scriptural theology and critique of the social relations and global and government policies that have led to impoverishment of the southern hemisphere. Liberation theologians explain that the Christian message teaches a form of consciousness-raising that makes people aware of their oppression and results in a biblically mandated rising up against that oppression. While also criticizing oppression and violence, the peace theology of Mennonite, Amish, and other Anabaptist Christian traditions has them furthering social justice from quite a different interpretation of the Scripture. Christian theologian and ethicist Lebacqz notes that theological traditions extend views of justice from questions of allocation and distribution to social requirements for living in community and systematic issues, with attention to histories and systems of oppression and the ways in which social changes affect groups of people.[39] Here, the language of liberation takes its full expression. For example, the World Alliance of Reformed Churches (2004; representing 75 million members in 107 countries) met in Accra, Kenya. The resulting *Accra Confession* states,

> The root causes of massive threats to life are above all the product of an unjust economic system defended and protected by political and military might. Economic systems are a matter of life or death. We live in a scandalous world that denies God's call to life for all. The annual income of the richest 1 per cent is equal to that of the poorest 57 per cent, and 24,000 people die each day from poverty and malnutrition. The debt of poor countries continues to increase despite paying back their original borrowing many times over. Resource-driven wars claim the lives of millions, while millions more die of preventable diseases. The HIV and AIDS global pandemic afflicts life in all parts of the world, affecting the poorest where generic drugs are not available. The majority of those in poverty are women and children and the number of people living in absolute poverty on less than one US dollar per day continues to increase.[40]

The Accra confession concludes with a series of theological affirmations and rejections such as this one,

> We believe that God calls us to stand with those who are victims of injustice. We know what the Lord requires of us: to do justice, love kindness, and walk in God's way (Micah 6.8). We are called to stand against any form of injustice in the economy and the destruction of the environment, "so that justice may roll down like waters, and righteousness like an everflowing stream" (Amos 5.24). Therefore we reject any theology that claims that God is only with the rich and that poverty is the fault of the poor. We reject any form of injustice which destroys right relations—gender, race, class, disability, or caste. We reject any theology which affirms that human interests dominate nature.[41]

Similar instructions for social justice are abundantly articulated by other religions.

Second, justice in religious traditions is deemed a necessary virtue, a matter of character. Citing Lebacqz, in a biblical perspective justice is "first and foremost relational; the requirements of justice emerge out of a history of God's interaction with God's people. Justice is therefore fidelity to the demands of a relationship."[42] With this emphasis, religious ethics is often the grounding of virtue ethics (whether by implicit historical influence, or more explicit reference), a field of ethics that is receiving renewed attention in nursing. Engaged Buddhism provides an excellent example of the inter-dependence of personal virtue and social justice. This branch of Buddhism has emerged to distinguish itself from the traditional Buddhist emphasis of personal faith and enlightened disengagement to promote critique of social maladies and political injustices, and is articulated by the Dalai Lama as all having a "universal responsibility."[43] The core values of Engaged Buddhism speak of cultivated positive virtues: benevolence (compassion, loving kindness, and giving); putting Buddhist values into practice through active service; self-development toward enlightenment; and increasing altruism. King quoted Mett̄a Sutt̄a to illustrate the virtuous engaged benevolence that characterizes Buddhist social ethics,

> Just as a mother would protect her only child, even at the risk of her own life, so let one cultivate a boundless heart toward all things. Let one's thoughts of love pervade the whole world—above, beyond, across, without any obstruction, without any hatred, without any enmity.[44]

By way of further example, Judaism with social justice as a central tenet of its theology, brings together the concepts of *simcha* ("gladness" or "joy"), *tzedakah* ("the religious obligation to perform charity and philanthropic acts; acts of loving kindness"), and *tikkun olam* (repairing the world). More broadly, the seven core values of the Rabbinic tradition include: *chesed* (lovingkindness), *kavod habriot* (dignity of all creatures), *bakesh shalom* (seek peace), *lota'amod* (you shall not stand idly by), *darchei shalom* (the ways of peace), *ahavat ger* (loving the stranger), and *emet* (truth).[45] Schwarz writes:

The Jewish tradition teaches that even if you have not caused a certain injustice, nevertheless 'you are forbidden to hide your eyes from the situation.' (Deuteronomy 22.7). When a fellow human being is suffering persecution or is threatened with annihilation, 'you shall not stand idly by while the blood of your neighbor is being shed' (Leviticus 19.160). Judaism teaches that even if you are convinced that your efforts may fall far short of solving a given problem, you are forbidden to withdraw in despair over the futility of the mission. 'It is not incumbent upon you to complete the task, but neither are you free to desist from trying.'[46] (ethics of the ancestors)

Third, the mechanisms of social ethics that is theologically rooted and enacted through religious groups often take on a participatory, more democratic form. Religious ideals, especially when ecumenical, are participatory in essence and tend to be optimistic, resulting in greater investment for real social change. With a source of moral authority other than the state (although typically also respecting the state), religious groups tend to act to reclaim democratic authority over actions and policies that reflect special interests, consolidate elite privileges and biases, or base their assumptions on pragmatic cost-benefit calculations rather than moral principle. They usually reflect communalistic rather than individualistic sensibilities. Hence they can be seen as important catalysts for participatory democracy, embodying a force for practical equality, inclusiveness, reciprocity, and empowerment of socially marginal groups, even though their substantive agendas vary.[47]

The potential contributions of religions to social justice are strengthened by the global networks that characterize many of them and that offer a "politics of solidarity and alliance formation," a point noted by Muslim scholar Abdullahi An-na'im.[48] Reflecting this global participatory motivation, religious organizations play a role in addressing national and international issues, events, and crises. For example, the Presbyterian Church (USA) has an Advisory Committee on Social Witness Policy that, at the behest of its General Assembly (similar to a House of Delegates) formulate social policies that are then formally adopted by the denomination and become policy for its three million members. In the past several years, the Committee has prepared policies on gun violence in the United States, torture, serious mental illness, homelessness, globalization, national health, U.S. energy policy and global warming, domestic violence, care giving and older adults, human rights, and much more.[49] These policies and study papers are used for the church's members and to inform governmental agencies, decision makers, and legislators. Going farther, this denomination holds official "special consultative status" with the United Nations Economic and Social Council (ECOSOC). This permits representatives of the Church to have "voice," to consult on and be signatory to U.N. statements arising from the work of ECOSOC. This includes the work of the nine commissions under the purview of ECOSOC including, for example, the Commission on the Status of Women. In the case of international natural disasters, this same church devotes millions of dollars to the Presbyterian Disaster Assistance Agency, which partners with other religious traditions to bring immediate disaster relief intervention anywhere in the world. Such involvement, at all these levels, is by no means unique to the Presbyterian Church (USA), but rather points to extensive engagement in social ethics by many institutions representing different religions.

In sum, these three themes—social justice as foremost concern, social justice as virtue, and social justice as participatory and democratic—evident in religious traditions, provide a depth and diversity of theological, philosophic, and pragmatic foundations that can be accessed by nurses committed to social justice. Religious organizations offer a vast array of examples of social engagement. Our last point in this chapter is to provide an incomplete sampling to underline the scope of religious social justice commitment with the suggestion that the nursing profession could benefit from aligning its efforts for social justice with the many existing social initiatives.

Examples of Social Engagement: Opportunities for Nursing

Religious organizations—whether linked to specific faith traditions such as Catholicism or Islam or Judaism, or whether more ecumenical—are engaged in social ethics, moving beliefs and sacred teachings into action across the spectrum of disaster relief, community development, social advocacy, and community service. We offer a few examples with the observation that many nurses are engaged with these types of religiously based efforts, and with the proposition that nurses might find more ways to take advantage of the initiatives already in place as sites to make the type of contributions to social justice for which nurses are well equipped.

Disaster Relief

When Haiti was devastated by an earthquake in 2010, many faith-based organizations responded with aid and relief efforts. Bergman in his survey of religious disaster relief notes that the techniques utilized demonstrate both the practicality and potency of faith-based initiatives.

> Through a preexisting network of churches in the United States, the United Methodist Committee on Relief (UMCOR) provides volunteer services for reconstruction and ministry development, effectively leveraging local knowledge and personnel supported by a modern infrastructure. The Church World Service, whose presence in Haiti began in the aftermath of Hurricane Hazel in 1954, coordinates development aid, food security programs, training, and technical assistance. They also provide cutting edge agricultural programs and sustainability measures thus enabling Haiti to provide for the needs of its own citizens. Islamic Relief USA and the International Red Crescent constitute a major part of the response campaign. Volunteers from these groups shored up damaged structures with parent organizations providing seed money for local rehabilitation strategies. The Jewish Distribution Committee has a long history in Haiti going back to World War II when the island nation provided a safe harbor to Jews fleeing the Holocaust. It currently offers medical and counseling services for the injured and amputees in a brand new rehabilitation center.[50]

Community Development

Mennonite Central Committee (MCC, http://mcc.org) is a worldwide ministry of Anabaptist Christian churches responding to basic human needs and working for peace and justice. MCC approaches its mission by addressing poverty, oppression, and injustice and their systemic causes; accompanying partners and the church in a process of mutual transformation, account-ability, and capacity building; building bridges to connect people and ideas across cultural, political, and economic divides; and caring for creation. MCC has community development initiatives in 17 African countries (in-cluding Burundi and Sudan), 12 countries in Asia (including Myanmar, Afghanistan, Bangladesh, and North Korea), eight countries in Europe (such as Croatia and Ukraine), 10 Latin American and Caribbean coun-tries (including Haiti and Guatemala), and eight countries in the Middle East (including Palestine and Israel, Syria and Iraq) and Canada and the United States.

Social Advocacy

Drawing on their own history of slavery in Egypt about 3,500 years ago, and more recently the Holocaust genocide (Holocaust), a strong response has arisen in the Jewish community against the ongoing genocide in Darfur. Working with Jewish congregations and community councils, Jewish federa-tions, campus Hillels, the American Jewish World Service, and the Jewish Council for Public Affairs rallied tens of thousands to protest the violence in Sudan. It is estimated that more than half of the 75,000 protestors at the Save Darfur: Rally to End Genocide in Washington, DC in April 2006 were Jewish.[51]

Community Service

There are a many Islamic women's groups around the world that serve to illustrate community engagement for advocacy and service, such as the Muslim Women's National Network Australia and the International League of Muslim Women (with nearly 30 chapters in the United States and be-yond). For example, the Buffalo Chapter has initiated the Bonding Series Programs for women and youth in an interfaith community forum and acted as a liaison for refugees in schools, clinics, and social service agencies to expedite their acclimation to the new American culture. The Birmingham, Atlanta, Chicago, Los Angeles, Norfolk, and Memphis Chapters have worked with battered, incarcerated, mentally ill, and homeless women and have established social outreach programs that have been highly effective and of great benefit to their respective communities.[52]

In India, the Hindu organization, the Sevabharati, was founded in 1980 and now administers thousands of service projects in education, health care, rural development, and rehabilitation of differently abled and special needs children. Their primary focus is on urban slums and impoverished rural villages, where they have established medical aid centers, mobile clinics, tuberculosis eradication programs, urban counseling services, and numer-ous other service initiatives.[53] This small sampling of religiously based orga-nizations committed to social justice through disaster relief, social advocacy, community development, and service give witness to global movements of great interest to nurses.

Many religious social ethics concerns—concerns for the poor, socially disadvantaged, those who suffer, those in need—are also central concerns of nursing. Although religious sources of moral authority provide guidance for their own people, they also serve as rich sources of moral reflection and wisdom from which nursing might benefit. As nursing scholars contemplate the intersections of religion, ethics, and nursing, we do well to consider how to draw on the religious themes of an expanded view of social justice, the character of each moral agent, and the liberatory, participatory potential of religious discourses to create community, facilitate shared action against injustice, and to offer hope.

NOTES

1.   Fowler, Marsha D. "Religion, Bioethics, and Nursing Practice." *Nursing Ethics* 16.4 (July 2009): 393–405. Caveats are adapted from this journal article.
2.   Gilmartin, Kevin M. "The Lethal Triad: Understanding the Nature of Isolated Extremist Religious Groups." *FBI Law Enforcement Bulletin* 65.9 (Sept. 1996): 1–5.
3.   Reimer-Kirkham, Sheryl. "Lived Religion: Implications for Nursing Ethics." *Nursing Ethics* 16.4 (July, 2009): 406–417.
4.   Bellah, Robert. *Varieties of Civil Religion*. San Francisco: Harper, 1982.
5.   Niebuhr, H. Richard. *Christ and Culture*. San Francisco: Harper, 1951.
6.   Fowler, Marsha. "Religion in Clinical Ethics." *Essentials of Teaching and Learning in Nursing Ethics: Perspectives and Methods*. Ed. Davis, Anne, Louise de Raeve, and Verena Tschudin. London: Elsevier. 2006. 37–48.
7.   Vansina, Jan. *Oral Tradition as History*. London: James Currey Publishers, 1985.
8.   Ki-Zerbo, Jacqueline ed. *General History of Africa: Methodology and African Prehistory*. Paris: UNESCO, 1990. See also: Ki-Zerbo, Joseph ed. *General History of Africa: Methodology and African Prehistory*. Berkeley: University of California Press, 1981.
9.   Tonkin, Elizabeth. "Investigating Oral Tradition." *Journal of African History* 27.2 (1986): 203–213.
10. Fitzgerald, James. "The Great Epic of India as Religious Rhetoric: A Fresh Look at the Mahabharata." *Journal of the American Academy of Religion* 51.4 (Dec 1983): 611–630.
11. For an example from the Islamic tradition: The Hadith records the process: Narrated Anas bin Malik: Hudhaifa bin Al-Yaman [early convert to Islam] came to 'Uthman [companion of Mohammed] ... Hudhaifa was afraid of their differences in the recitation of the Qur'an, so he said to 'Uthman, "O chief of the Believers! Save this nation before they differ about the Book [Qur'an] as Jews and the Christians did before." So 'Uthman sent a message to Hafsa [widow of Muhammed] saying, "Send us the manuscripts of the Qur'an so that we may compile the Qur'anic materials in perfect copies and return the manuscripts to you." Hafsa sent it to 'Uthman. 'Uthman then ordered Zaid bin Thabit, 'Abdullah bin AzZubair, Said bin Al-As and

'AbdurRahman bin Harith bin Hisham to rewrite the manuscripts in perfect copies. 'Uthman said to the three Quraishi men, "In case you disagree with Zaid bin Thabit on any point in the Qur'an, then write it in the dialect of Quraish, the Qur'an was revealed in their tongue." They did so, and when they had written many copies, 'Uthman returned the original manuscripts to Hafsa. 'Uthman sent to every Muslim province one copy of what they had copied, and ordered that all the other Qur'anic materials, whether written in fragmentary manuscripts or whole copies, be burnt. From: The Hadith Translation of Sahih Bukhari. Virtues of the Qur'an. Trans. M. Muhsin Khan Volume 6, Book 61, Number 510 University of Southern California Center for Muslim-Jewish Engagement, Web. 23 April 2011.

12. Ontario Consultants on Religious Tolerance, Religious Tolerance.org. The Golden Rule. Web. 23 April 2011.
13. Porthero, Stephen. *God Is Not One: The Eight Rival Religions that Run the World—and Why Their Differences Matter.* New York: Harper One, 2010. 2–3, 24.
14. Gula, Richard. *What Are They Saying About Moral Norms?* Mahwah, NJ: Paulist Press, 1982.
15. Niebuhr, H. Richard. *Christ and Culture.*
16. Journal of Buddhist Ethics. Web. 23 Accessed 28 April 2011. http://blogs.dickinson.edu/buddhistethics/
17. Schaefer, Valentin. "Science, Stewardship, and Spirituality: the Human Body as a Model for Ecological Restoration." *Restoration Ecology* 14.1 (March 2006): 1–3.
18. Peterson, Michael, William Hasker, Bruce Reichengach, and David Bassinger. *Reason and Religious Belief.* Oxford: Oxford University Press, 2003. 51.
19. Jonsen, Albert, and Stephen Toulmin. *The Abuse of Casuistry: A History of Moral Reasoning.* Berkeley: University of California Press, 1988.
20. Jacob, Walter, and Moshe Zemer, eds. *Death and Euthanasia in Jewish law: Essays and Responsa.* New York: Rodef Shalom Press, 1994. 192.
21. Ibid., 18.
22. Wakefield, Gordon S. "Spirituality." *Westminster Dictionary of Christian Spirituality.* Philadelphia: Westminster John Knox Press, 1983. 361.
23. Fitchett, George. *Assessing Spiritual Need: A Guide for Caregivers.* Minneapolis: Augsburg Fortress Press, 1983. 11.
24. Fowler. Definition of Spirituality.
25. Piaget, Jean. *The Child's Conception of the World.* Lanham, MD: Rowman & Littlefield, 1929. See also: Piaget, Jean. *The Psychology of Intelligence.* Trans by Malcom Piercy and D.E. Berlyne. New York: Routledge & Kegan, 1950.
26. Kohlberg, Lawrence. "Moral Stages and Moralization: The Cognitive-Developmental Approach." *Moral Development and Behavior: Theory, Research and Social Issues.* Ed. Tom Lickona. Holt, NY: Rinehart and Winston, 1976.
27. Fowler, James. *Stages of Faith.* New York: Harper & Row Fowler, 1981. See also: Deloria, Vine. *God is Red,* 2nd ed. Golden, Co: North American Press, 1992; Azeemi, Khwaja Shamsuddin. *Muraqaba: The Art and Science of Sufi Meditation.* Houston: Plato, 2005; Bolman, Lee G., and Terrence E. Deal. *Leading With Soul.* San Francisco: Jossey-Bass, 1995.
28. Fowler, Marsha. *Guide to the Code of Ethics for Nurses. Interpretation and Application.* Silver Spring, MD: American Nurses Association, 2008. 123.
29. Fowler, Marsha. "Social Ethics and Nursing." *The Nursing Profession: Turning Points.* Ed. Norma Chaska. St. Louis: CV Mosby, 1990. See also: Fowler, Marsha. *Guide to the Code of Ethics for Nurses. Interpretation and Application.*

30. Bekemeier, Betty, and Patricia Butterfield. "Unreconciled Inconsistencies: A Critical Review of the Concept of Social Justice in 3 National Nursing Documents." *Advances in Nursing Science* 28.2 (2005): 152–162. See also: Reimer Kirkham, Sheryl and Annette Browne. "Toward a Critical Theoretical Interpretation of Social Justice Discourses in Nursing." *Advances in Nursing Science* 29.4 (2006): 324–339.

31. Neo-liberalism is a term used by many critics to describe the liberalization and globalization of market forces. This prevailing ideological paradigm leads to social, economic, and political approaches that emphasize individualism, individual freedom and responsibility; efficiency; egalitarianism; and free market economies that, in effect, shift risk from governments and corporations onto individuals. See: Ong, Aihwa. *Neoliberalism as Exception: Mutations in Citizenship and Sovereignty.* Duke University Press, 2006. See also: Browne, Annette. "The Influence of Liberal Political Ideology on Nursing Science." *Nursing Inquiry* 8.2 (2001): 118–129.

32. Bekemeier, Betty, and Patricia Butterfield. "Unreconciled Inconsistencies: A Critical Review of the Concept of Social Justice in 3 National Nursing Documents."

33. Young, Iris Marion. *Justice and the Politics of Difference.* Princeton, NJ: Princeton University Press, 1990.

34. Fraser, Nancy. "Redistribution or Recognition? A Critique of Justice Truncated." *Redistribution or Recognition? A Political Philosophical Exchange.* Eds.Nancy Fraser and Axel Honneth. London: Vorso, 2003. 9–25.

35. Cahill, Lisa Sowle. *Theological Bioethics. Participation, Justice, Change.* Washington, D.C.: Georgetown University Press. 2005. p. 7.

36. Reimer Kirkham, Sheryl and Annette Browne. "Toward a Critical Theoretical Interpretation of Social Justice Discourses in Nursing." See also: Anderson, Joan, Koushambhi Basu Khan, Heather McDonald, Adrienne Peltonen, Annette Browne, Sheryl Reimer-Kirkham, Judith M. Lynam, Paddy Rodney, Elsie Tan, Colleen Varcoe, Sabrina Wong, Jennifer Baumbusch, Joanne Reimer, Pat Semeniuk, Victoria Smye, and Anureet Brar. "The Uptake of Critical Knowledge in Nursing Interventions: Insights from a Knowledge Translation Study." *Canadian Journal of Nursing Research* 42.3 (2010): 106–122.

37. Zajda, Joseph. *Education and Social Justice.* New York: Springer, 2006.

38. Cahill, Lisa Sowle. "Theology's Role in Public Bioethics." *Handbook of Bioethics and Religion.* Ed. Robert Guinn. Oxford, UK: Oxford University Press. 2006. p. 51.

39. Lebacqz, Karen. "Philosophy, Theology, and the Claims of Justice." *Handbook of Bioethics and Religion.* Ed. Robert Guinn. Oxford, UK: Oxford University Press. 2006. 253–264.

40. World Alliance of Reformed Churches. The Accra Confession: Covenanting for Justice in the Economy and the Earth. 2004. Web. http://www.warc.ch/documents/ACCRA_Pamphlet.pdf.

41. Accra Confession, 2004.

42. Lebacquz, Karen. "Philosophy, Theology, and the Claims of Justice." 255.

43. Edelglass, William, and Jay L. Garfield. *Buddhist Philosophy: Essential Readings.* Oxford: Oxford University Press. 2009.

44. King, Sallie. *Being Benevolence: The Social Ethics of Engaged Buddhism.* Honolulu: University of Hawaii Press, 2005. 239.

45. Schwarz, Sidney. *Judaism and Justice: The Jewish Passion to Repair the World.* Woodstock, VT: Jewish Lights, 2002. 63–82.

46. Ibid., 249.

47. Cahill, Lisa Sowle. "Theology's Role in Public Bioethics." 53.

48. Cahill, Lisa Sowle. *Theological Bioethics. Participation, Justice, Change.* 62.

49. These policies have been posted and can be downloaded from the Web. Accessed 28 April 2011. http://gamc.pcusa.org/browse/resources-resource/ministries/acswp/?page=2

50. Bergman, Jonathan. 2011. Sightings 2/3/2011 The Haiti Earthquake One Year Later: A Survey of Religious Disaster Relief. Belief and Beyond Home. Accessed April 25th from: http://www.yorkblog.com/faith/2011/02/sightings-the-haiti-earthquake.html

51. Schwarz, Sidney. *Judaism and Justice: The Jewish Passion to Repair the World.*

52. http://www.ilmwintl.org/aboutus.html

53. http://www.sevabharathi.org/index.htm

3

Religion and Theoretical Thinking in Nursing

Barbara Pesut

To mention nursing theory elicits responses from nurses that can range from incomprehension to boredom. Nursing theory is not well understood, in part, because the nature of nursing theory has changed much over the evolution of the discipline. More significantly, nurses may have difficulty in seeing the relevance of theory to practice. Theory is viewed as peripheral to the *real* world of nursing. However, in its broadest sense, nursing theory is about ideas, and ultimately ideas have the power to change the world. When those ideas are religious, that is they are seen to have a sacred origin, the effect becomes even more powerful. Religious individuals hold the tenets of their religion in highest value and so religious ideals pervade all aspects of their lives and thinking. My goal in this chapter is to discuss how religion has influenced nursing's theoretical thinking and to address some of the ethical implications of the use of religious ideas in a diverse society. I will begin with a brief discussion of the influences of religion on early nursing theory, including nursing models, metaparadigm development, and nursing diagnosis. I will then discuss some of the current trends in religion and spirituality in the broader society and their influence on nursing theory. The ethical issues of proposing theoretical views in nursing that do not adequately encompass the religious views of patients will be outlined. I will conclude with an approach to incorporating religion into nursing theoretical thinking that allows for both the diverse experience of religious individuals and the scientific basis of the nursing discipline. In this chapter, the terms religion and spirituality will be used interchangeably to describe what individuals would identify as special experiences or things, as opposed to the ordinary,[1] and that have their origin in the divine or sacred. Nursing theory is understood as a logical structuring of ideas that provide an undergirding philosophy and science for the discipline.[2]

THE POWER OF IDEAS

To appreciate the power of ideas fully, it is interesting to reflect on how our lives have changed as a result of certain ideas. CNN (Cable News Network) once did an article on 10 ideas that changed the world.[3] Farming, relativity, human rights, and the unconscious have become such an ingrained part of our experience that it is difficult to appreciate their impact. Yet, what about those more recent developments, like the Internet first conceptualized by Tim Berner-Lee, in 1989? Who can forget the days of being a student without electronic online sources and having to spend hours in the library searching for references? Families would spend significant amounts of money for an Encyclopedia set so that their children could have access to knowledge. Now with the Internet, it is possible to have quality information, including academic resources at our fingertips, from anywhere in the world. Indeed, now our challenge is having too much information and evaluating its quality. Beyond the acquisition of knowledge, the Internet has restructured the way we relate to one another. Anyone who has entered the worlds of Facebook, Twitter, or online dating can appreciate just how much our social interaction has changed. Individuals have the capacity to construct electronic identities that bear little resemblance to the embodied individual. Truly, the idea of one scientist and his successors has revolutionized how we access information and enact social relationships.

The influence of the Internet is only one example of the importance of ideas for humanity. For some philosophers, the power of the human spirit is evidenced by the ability to originate and create. Willard in his book *Renovation of the Heart* suggests that the human spirit is the "capacity of the person to originate things or events that would not otherwise be or occur. By *originate* here we mean to include two of the things most prized in human life: freedom and creativity."[4] When we understand the generative and creative capacity of our spirits, we understand that each of us holds great potential to contribute to the betterment of society. Yet, it all begins with an idea. This same ability to create through the world of ideas is what has shaped the development of the discipline of nursing. Nursing theory, in its broadest sense, is simply the generation of ideas significant to nursing. It is nursing's best attempt to grapple with the nature of nursing practice and how one goes about engaging with that practice. Some of these earliest ideas originated from religion.

THE INFLUENCE OF RELIGION ON EARLY NURSING THEORY

Florence Nightingale is credited with being one of the first formal theoretical thinkers in nursing.[5] Prior to her work in nursing, she was deeply concerned about the religious issues of her day. In particular, she was concerned that scientific knowledge was turning some individuals toward atheism. Her response was a voluminous 829 page work entitled, *Suggestions for Thought*, which she referred to as "her stuff."[6] Written while she was in her 30s, it was a sweeping commentary on the religious issues of her day. It was this theology that informed some of her later understandings of nursing. Of particular relevance are her ideas about universal law and the role of women in society. Her belief that God had ordered the world in such a way that natural laws determined the cause and effect drove her search for the natural laws that would regulate healing. Her famous *Notes on Nursing: What it is, and what it is not* outlines the natural conditions under which she felt that healing could occur.[7] Her frustration with the limited role afforded to women in Victorian society, coupled with her theological beliefs that God gave individuals gifts to be used for God's purposes (in her case a profound intellect), caused her to work to establish nursing as a means for women to use their gifts to serve the broader society.[8] Above all, her deepest motivations for nursing were religious a desire to serve humanity in response to her calling from God.

Little formal theorizing occurred in the years between Florence Nightingale and the nursing theorists of the 1960s. However, Hamilton suggests that despite the absence of formal theorizing, influential nurses such as Lillian Wald, Lavinia Dock, and Annie Goodrich were still in the process of "constructing the mind of nursing."[9] These nurses, unlike the religious nursing sisters of the time, rejected formal religion as a basis for nursing and instead focused on the spirit of nursing itself. Their desire to distance nursing from the influence of religion was a reflection of the broader society where unbelief was becoming an option for the first time, which was a trend that Florence Nightingale had so astutely observed. In their minds, the spirit of nursing was not religious, but rather a natural response to the human condition. Hamilton suggested that even though these nurses envisioned their work differently in relation to religion, ultimately, the path led to the same place, that is, a deep sense of meaning for the nurse as she (in that day) worked to mount a compassionate response to the needs of humanity.

Formal nursing theorizing developed in the late 1950s and early 1960s. By this time, science had replaced religion as the authoritative source for much of modern society. Nurses sought a scientific basis for the profession and so began to ask themselves what nursing's unique contribution was to scientific knowledge. Since that time, a rich body of nursing theoretical thinking has emerged. Two theoretical developments intersect most significantly with religion. First, there is a broad range theory that has been referred to more recently as nursing philosophy. Within nursing philosophy, nurses grapple with defining for nursing's purposes the metaparadigm concepts of nursing: person, health, nursing, and the environment. Nurses have engaged in model building, using these metaparadigm concepts to describe nursing and nursing work. Second, there has been theory development that explicitly seeks to incorporate religion and spirituality as a focus of nursing practice. The nursing process and the related diagnostic categories often form the cognitive vehicle whereby nurses describe how this should be done.

RELIGION AND NURSING PHILOSOPHY

It was in the late 1950s and early 1960s that nursing began to formalize theory about the nature, scope, and object of the discipline. Over the next two decades, nurses produced over 20 new theoretical models.[10] Those models made claims about the nature of nursing with the goal of providing direction for nursing practice, education, and research. During the early 1980s, this work focused more specifically on defining what have been considered the metaparadigm concepts of nursing: nursing, person, health, and the environment.[11] An important belief undergirding this model and concept building work was that nursing required a common philosophic foundation upon which to build the theoretical structure of the discipline.[12]

The development of these nursing models occurred in the wake of the countercultural movement of the 1960s, a movement that included reactions to dominant biomedical approaches. A loss of trust in progress, and in the progress of science in particular, was reflected in a greater emphasis on holism and personal responsibility for health.[13] In the United States, the 1960s also brought a loss of trust in and respect for authority, specifically physicians as authority figures. An emergent distaste of medical paternalism, greater awareness of medical abuses, and revelations of profound sexism in medical research and practice resulted in informedness and respect for autonomy becoming ensconced as guiding principles. Subsequently, economic concerns pressed toward *self-care* under the guise of *respect for autonomy* that masked economic motivation. As such, nursing models reflected a biopsychosocial approach to the person and emphasized ways in which nurses could work with individuals to facilitate the meeting of their own needs. For example, Dorothea Orem's self-care deficit theory focuses on nurses filling gaps in care that individuals could not fill themselves. However, explicit attention to spirituality and religion were remarkably absent from many of these models.[14] In a review of the concept of spirituality in 12 nursing models, Martsolf and Mickley[15] find that little or nothing was said in four models and that it was implied or embedded in four other models. Only Betty Neuman, Margaret Newman, Rosemary Parse, and Jean Watson included it as a central concept in their models. The holistic approach did not necessarily extend to the spiritual aspect of the person, a development that may have reflected the discomfort between religion and science evident at the time.

Nursing has deep roots within Christianity, and a number of models have been developed from a Christian perspective.[16] These models draw upon theology to describe the nature of persons, health, and the environment within which nursing work occurs. The work of the nurse is often described in theological terms, such as Bradshaw's covenantal caring, O'Brien's standing on holy ground, or Shelly and Miller's restoration of relationship between God and humankind. More recently, a strand of nursing theoretical thinking, sometimes referred to as the *simultaneity strand*, has become more prominent. Models developed within the simultaneity perspective have largely been influenced by Eastern, or more specifically, Chinese and Indian worldviews.[17] Theorists who have written from this perspective include Martha Rogers, Margaret Newman, and Rosemary Parse.[18] Although these are often characterized as philosophic rather than religious positions, this is basically a semantic difference. Theorists writing within this strand locate themselves within specific understandings about the cosmos and humanity's place within that cosmos, and share common understandings of holism, the evolution of consciousness, self-transcendence, open systems, harmony, relativity of space–time, and patterns in the universe.[19] As such, one could argue that they are proposing religious or quasi-religious answers to metaphysical questions.

It is within theorizing about the metaparadigm concepts of nursing that the religious influence has been present but perhaps less explicit. Indeed, it is unlikely that any form of theorizing that attempts to make claims about the nature of persons, health, and the environment can escape religious influence. Whether those influences are explicitly acknowledged or not, claims about the nature of reality are often religious claims, simply because religion has traditionally sought to provide answers to what cannot be fully known empirically.

Claims about the nature of persons and health are a good example. The concern for the nature of persons is a relevant one for nurses because of the effect of illness on personhood and the relational nature of practice. Green provides an interesting overview of how nurses have theorized the concept of persons over time. Nursing has shifted from an understanding of persons as an abiding, natural substance, such as viewed by Nightingale, to "beings who can have knowledge."[20] This shift toward epistemology, or the knowing between the nurse and the patient, positions nursing away from physical actions and more toward ways of being in relationship. Religious thinking is evident in nursing's view of persons as being inter-related parts, which reflects religious and, specifically, Christian, Jewish, and Buddhist theological thinking about persons being an integration of body, mind, and spirit. Persons are also perceived as having a common nature and a normative state of health or well-being. As such, persons can make good and bad choices about their overall health. This idea is consonant with and perhaps reflects Christian religious thinking of persons having a nature that consists of both good and evil. This was evident within Nightingale's thinking of natural law theology. In this view of persons, the nurse could look at the various parts, identify areas of need, and implement nursing interventions for health. More recently within the simultaneity strand of nursing theoretical thinking, there has been a shift away from characterizing health choices as being inherently good or bad toward simply being ways that individuals choose to co-construct their reality.[21] Health is not normative, but rather self-defined in terms of quality of life. Nurses are encouraged to withhold judgment over those choices. The emphasis becomes one of being in relationship. One could argue that this reflects a broader societal discourse that has rejected religion in favor of a type of spirituality whereby all of life (including individuals) is sacred and inherently good.[22] This is only one example of how nurses use the generative capacity of ideas, and in particular their own ideas about the nature of reality, to construct theory for the nursing discipline. Many of these ideas about the nature of reality have been derived from religion. The largely Christian ethos of Western nursing, particularly in the late 19th and early 20th centuries, lent itself to infusing nursing theory, either intentionally or inadvertently, with Christian theological formulations.

RELIGION AND NURSING DIAGNOSES

Over the past two decades, there has been an attempt to theorize, more purposefully, about religion and spirituality in practice. This theorizing has often been evident in the language of nursing process and diagnosis.[23] Historically, the nursing process came into being as a nursing response to the diagnostic language of other professions. Medicine focused on diagnostic categories of physical illness, psychiatry focused on the diagnostic categories of mental illness, and nursing sought to categorize its own unique responses to illness. However, with its commitment to holism, nursing's problem focused categories sought to include both bio/psycho/social/

spiritual concerns as well as the potential for enhanced wellness. Therefore, spiritual diagnoses include "spiritual distress" and the "potential for enhanced spiritual well-being." Religious diagnoses include "religiosity, impaired," and "religiosity, ready for enhanced."[24] More specifically, O'Brien's research reveals seven nursing diagnoses that could be manifestations of the broader category of "alterations in spiritual integrity": spiritual pain, spiritual alienation, spiritual anxiety, spiritual guilt, spiritual anger, spiritual loss, and spiritual despair.[25]

These diagnoses rest largely upon religious thinking. For nursing diagnoses to be useful, there must be some agreement about what problematic responses are, how a nurse might intervene to solve those problems, and what an effective outcome will look like.[26] This normative frame of reference for constructing these diagnostic categories is often derived implicitly or explicitly from Christian theology. For example, the following is O'Brien's explanation of the diagnosis of spiritual pain: "The loss of or separation from God and/or institutionalized religion; the experience of evil or disillusionment; a sense of failing God; the recognition of one's own sinfulness; lack of reconciliation with God; and/or perceived loneliness of spirit."[27] One can see that this diagnosis contains theological ideas about a personal God, sin, evil, fallen humanity, and redemption. It might be entirely appropriate for a Christian patient but inappropriate for a patient who holds a different worldview. The following is an excerpt from Walsch's *Tomorrow's God*, a best-selling book on spirituality, which reflects quite a different theological understanding: "Tomorrow's God does not require anyone to believe in God . . . Tomorrow's God will be unconditionally loving, nonjudgmental, noncondemning, and nonpunishing."[28] Here, God is not an essential part of the worldview, and there is no sense of sinfulness or the need for redemption. I point this out not to assert one view over the other, but rather to show how nursing diagnoses related to the spiritual matters can be inherently religious and, even more, reflective of a particular religion. Indeed, if we do not recognize that they are inherently religious, we may find ourselves operating out of certain assumptions in relation to spiritual well-being and spiritual distress that have little relevance for our patients.

CURRENT RELIGIOUS INFLUENCES ON NURSING THEORY

The above discussion of how nursing ideas about persons and health have intersected with religious ideas illustrates how nursing derives much of its theoretical thinking from the broader social context. The extent to which religion plays a role in the broader society influences the extent to which those ideas are taken up in nursing. It is therefore useful to understand some of the current trends and understandings of religion in society.

In the first half of the 20th century, when religions were fairly "easily categorized" into Western and Eastern, religious studies' departments in universities offered courses entitled Eastern or Western world religions. However, global migration has challenged the validity of these categories—presenting a much more complex picture of religion.[29] For example, many cities in Western Canada now have diasporic populations in which the major religious influence from their country of origin remains a strong unifying force.[30] Second and third generation individuals from these families often develop a religious perspective that is informed by the religious and cultural traditions of both their homeland and their adopted country.[31] Therefore, Eastern and Western categories are no longer sufficient to describe the melding of religions and the expressions that may range from conservative to liberal within the same religion, all of which attend worldwide immigration movements.

Another trend has been the rise of new spiritualities. As the influence of institutional religion has declined in some modern societies, there has been a more individualized pursuit of spirituality. Individuals draw from different traditions and practices to craft a spirituality that represents their search of the divine. Although it is difficult to categorize this form of religious thinking, Lynch provides an overview, albeit cautiously, of what characterizes progressive spirituality in Western culture.[32] He positions his work within two important understandings. First, he acknowledges that whenever one writes about spirituality or religion there is a tendency to infuse those writings with one's own beliefs. He likens it to a Rorschach test whereby we tend to layer our own cultural and religious understandings on what might be quite ill-defined. Second, he describes the new spirituality as an ideology rather than a worldview. It provides a framework for how to make sense of experiences and dictates more of a pragmatic response to how one should live within the world rather than propose a set of doctrinal beliefs.

According to Lynch the new spiritualities have arisen out of a need to learn how to live within the ideas of a liberal society that incorporates feminist issues, new scientific developments in relation to cosmology, and the relationship of humanity to the natural order.[33] Despite its pragmatic emphasis, there are key tenets that inform this new spirituality. The divine is seen as an ineffable unity that is unknowable and encompassing all of life. This is in contrast to some theological understandings of a patriarchal God who exists separately from life. Feminist theological understandings are an important part of this ideology. Nature and the self are seen as sacred. This sacredness has important implications for our obligations to care for self and nature. Emphasis is placed on developing mystical union with a sacred source. Lynch notes that these ideas are crossing religious traditions and tend to be shaped by each unique cultural, religious, and political context.

Although not necessarily antireligious, individuals who espouse the ideas of the new spirituality tolerate religion only insofar as that religion would honor these particular understandings of the world.

An example of a new spirituality that has been influenced by the cultural, religious, and political context is put forward in Todd's book, *Cascadia*.[34] This edited volume portrays a spirituality informed by the unique context of Oregon, Washington, and British Columbia, which has often been referred to as "Cascadia." Shaped largely by the spectacular beauty of this region and the unique history that includes a large First Nations influence, many individuals residing in this geographic area resist organized religion. Instead, they embrace a spirituality that is characterized by a sacred sense of place and a desire to create a utopian existence characterized by health, healing, and wellness. A connection to the arts, an eclectic variety of spiritual practices, and an emphasis on environmentalism help to foster this utopian ideal.

These cultural flows of religion and spirituality suggest that nursing theoretical thinking shaped by binaries that seem to reflect Eastern and Western religious perspectives may no longer be relevant. Instead, there is a need to reflect the type of diversity that would characterize modern, globalized societies. This leads us to a difficult question. If nursing operates from the assumption that a single theoretical perspective should inform the discipline, and if nurses draw upon religion to inform that perspective, how do we ensure that the discipline remains ethically responsible to the religious diversity operating in society?[35]

ETHICAL IMPLICATIONS OF RELIGIOUS INFLUENCES ON NURSING THEORY

Until now, nursing has been somewhat uncritical of the ethical implications of putting forward various views derived from religion for the discipline.[36] For example, the body of literature on spirituality in nursing is largely based, implicitly, upon Christian theological assumptions. Only recently have Eastern worldviews been included in the discourse. However, again, these views are often being put forward as normative for the discipline rather than as one possible view. For example, Chan, Ng, Ho, and Chow argue for interventions in practice based on religious ideas derived from Confucianism, Taoism, and Buddhism.[37] They propose these interventions on the basis that they are religiously neutral, which is an important factor given that many individuals are no longer religious. However, the authors fail to recognize that the claims they make are essentially religious claims, only the nomenclature has changed. For example, they begin with the assumptions that humans are innately altruistic that suffering should be accepted and seen as a means to release control, and that letting go of attachments to possessions and relationships is essential to overcoming loss.[38] These are not religiously neutral claims. Rather, to position them as such only increases the risk that they will be used to impose a view on others who may see the world differently.

A solution that has been proposed in the literature is that naturalism should be the common basis for nursing practice, although the nature of this naturalism differs depending upon who is writing.[39] Paley argues for naturalism whereby all religion is regarded as "positive illusion." Nurses begin from the assumption that religion is an illusion but are free to support those aspects of it that contribute to positive outcomes, such as hope in their patients. However, Paley's ideas have generated significant debate.[40]

A different approach to naturalism has been put forward by Willis et al.[41] They recently proposed a unifying model for the discipline. Implicit in their model is the understanding that although diverse religious views will necessarily be a part of the practice context, nurses should ground their practice within the human–natural paradigm. They argue that all religious experiences will be embodied and therefore it is at the embodied level that issues relevant to nursing arise. For example, a patient who holds a religious view that suffering is redemptive and should be endured may make a decision to refuse opioids. This is where the nurse responds at the level of embodied decisions. This naturalistic approach is different than that put forward by Paley in that it makes no judgment about the truth value of religion, but rather anchors practice within the natural realm.

However, one could argue that even the naturalistic approach is not religiously neutral, but is based upon an underlying assumption that what is most fundamentally true about the world is what can be accessed empirically. Nurses are still left with the thorny challenge of privileging either religious or scientific claims, should there be a conflict between the two. What position do nurses take if the scientific evidence for a practice decision contravenes their or patients' religious beliefs? How do we negotiate personal beliefs at a disciplinary level?

RELIGION INFORMING THE NURSING DISCIPLINE

Nurses' religious views are important factors in how they construct meaning in their lives and work. However, upon entering the discipline, nurses must also take on a professional identity. At this point, they must (but often do not) ask the difficult questions of how those religious views affect their understanding of nursing and its basic concepts, how it should be integrated into practice, whether they can uphold disciplinary values, and how those values may be informed, critiqued, interrogated, or enriched by religious values.[42] This issue is most difficult for those nurses whose beliefs may diverge from popular disciplinary theory. For example, a nurse who holds Christian beliefs may struggle with the integration of what is perceived to be Eastern religious influence into nursing theory or to enact *Christian* nursing in a discipline that upholds the values of a multifaith society.[43,44] In some cases, this challenge may be exacerbated by a religious perspective that defines faith as living out principles and beliefs without question.

From a theoretical perspective, we are faced with several decisions in relation to religion and disciplinary theory. Do we incorporate religion into theoretical perspectives or rather choose to adopt a naturalistic approach as recommended by some? It is unlikely given the meaning that religion provides for many nurses that neglecting it completely or severely compartmentalizing it within the theoretical development in nursing is realistic. The popularity of the nursing models that incorporate the sacred and transcendent aspects of practice suggests that there is little appetite for a purely naturalistic approach.[45] However, if we do choose to integrate religion, how do we do it in a way that remains respectful of the diverse ideas held by both patients and providers?

Taves provides an approach for the disciplinary study of religion that may be useful for the theoretical development of religion in nursing.[46] Acknowledging that religion can be difficult to define; she begins instead by focusing on the experience of religion. In nursing, religion has often been defined in terms of institutional practices. In contrast, Taves describes religion in terms of special experiences to which individuals ascribe value, existence, or intentionality. These special experiences can be categorized into experiences of agency (e.g., spiritual beings or deities), ideal things (e.g., absolutes), and anomalous places, objects, experiences, or events (e.g., something having mystical or spiritual qualities). Individuals will attribute special outcomes to the intervention of spiritual beings (e.g., healing), some objects will be considered beyond price (e.g., sacred scriptures or a crucifix), and some ideals or qualities will be held to be sacred (e.g., not receiving blood). From Taves' perspective, what is more important than the religious label is seeking to understand the special goal that individuals seek and the practices that they employ to reach that goal. For example, a Christian patient might seek the goal of eternal salvation and will enact spiritual disciplines such as prayer, scripture reading, and charitable action to reach that goal. From a nursing theoretical perspective, this would allow for the development of knowledge across diverse religious and spiritual perspectives. Rather than only dealing with religious categories, nurses would seek to develop theory around religious goals and practices that go across the boundaries of religions. This theory would be inclusive of individuals who, though distant from institutional religion, may still embrace a spiritual path that would recognize sacred goals and seeking practices independent of religion. It is important to note that this does not nullify the legitimacy of institutional religious traditions, but rather focuses nursing's theoretical development at the more fundamental building blocks of *special* experiences that cross and exist outside of religious traditions.

Yet, nursing is still left with the challenging task of negotiating scientific and religious claims should they conflict in the context of practice. To illustrate this, I will draw upon a recent qualitative study that explores quality of life in individuals with bipolar disorder.[47] One young woman for whom spirituality was integral to her life described her experiences with psychosis and religious delusions. Throughout her battle with bipolar disorder, she was aware that although delusions were always a potential during her experiences, she was conscious of an enduring *healthy* spirituality that provided an important resource for her life. She struggled with health care providers who dismissed the importance of this spirituality and instead pathologized it as part of her bipolar disorder. In frustration, she turned away from traditional medicine to seek spiritual healers. Having found someone who could help to make sense of her *spiritual emergency*, she drew upon both traditional biomedical approaches and alternative spiritual approaches as part of her *personal* medicine to cope with her illness.

This is an excellent example of the types of difficulties that arise as nurses try to navigate the difficult terrain between evidence-based practice and the phenomenological experiences of the patient—or that difficult dialectic between the general and the particular in a practice-based discipline. Nurses hold many professional values such as spirituality and cultural safety that are difficult to know how to enact in practice.[48] Scientific knowledge in this case would suggest that religious delusions are characteristic of bipolar disorder and so should be treated. On the other hand, this woman's phenomenological experience is that there is also a healthy aspect to what is occurring. Perhaps best practice entails holding both ideas in appropriate tension by continuing to rely upon the best available evidence for the treatment of the bipolar disorder while acknowledging fully the legitimacy of the patient's account.[49] Indeed, it makes for a unique partnership where each contributes a particular expertise. Above all, it is important in complex situations such as this to resist simple solutions.[50] In performing the complex task of integrating religion into nursing theoretical thinking, we must seek to construct generalizable theory that respects the diversity of religious views in society while holding to the idea that the phenomenological experience of religion may indeed be quite unique.

CONCLUSION

Ideas are powerful. Religious ideas are particularly powerful because of their origin in a divine or sacred source. With strong roots in religion, nursing has often drawn upon religion, whether Western or Eastern, in its disciplinary theoretical thinking. It is unlikely that nursing can ignore the contributions of religion as long as it continues to generate theory in the areas where religions have traditionally been the source of answers. Religions propose answers to metaphysical questions that remain otherwise largely unanswerable. The nature of persons, health, and the environment has been the fodder of philosophers and theologians for centuries. However, nursing theorists can become more thoughtful and explicit about from where their ideas originate. In the spirit of intellectual humility, theorists can propose their ideas as one possible answer to the questions of life. Scientific understandings partnered with a creditable patient phenomenological account of special experience is an important ethical approach to the potential complexity of religious ideas in nursing. In doing so, theoretical thinking in nursing can be sensitive to the religious diversity that characterizes modern globalized societies.

NOTES

1. Taves, Ann. *Religious Experience Reconsidered: A Building Block Approach to the Study of Religion and Other Special Things.* Princeton, NJ: Princeton University Press, 2009.
2. Thorne, Sally. "Theoretical Issues in Nursing." *Canadian Nursing: Issues and Perspectives.* Ed. Janet C. Ross-Kerr and Marilyn J. Wood. Toronto: Mosby, 2003. 116–34.
3. Mackay, Mairi. "10 Ideas that Changed the World." *CNN.com.* Cable News Network, 12 December 2008. Web. 20 Mar. 2011.
4. Willard, Dallas. *Renovation of the Heart: Putting on the Character of Christ.* Colorado Springs, CO: Navepress, 2002. 33.
5. Thorne, Sally. "Theoretical Issues in Nursing." *Canadian Nursing: Issues and Perspectives.* See also: Meleis, Afaf I. *Theoretical Thinking and Practical Wisdom: Challenges for the Future.* 3rd ed. Philadelphia: Lippincott, 1997.
6. Calabria, Michael D., and Janet A. Macrae, eds. *Suggestions for Thought by Florence Nightingale.* Philadelphia: University of Pennsylvania Press, 1994. Print.
7. Nightingale, Florence. *Notes on Nursing: What It Is, and What It Is Not.* New York: D. Appleton and Company, 1860.
8. Grypma, Sonya. "Florence Nightingale's Changing Image. Part 1: Nightingale the Feminist, Statistician and Nurse." *Journal of Christian Nursing* 22.3 (2005): 22–8. Print.
9. Hamilton, Diane. "Constructing the Mind of Nursing." *Nursing History Review* 2 1994:3–28.

10. Thorne, Sally. "Theoretical Issues in Nursing." *Canadian Nursing: Issues and Perspectives.*

11. Meleis, Afaf I. *Theoretical Thinking and Practical Wisdom: Challenges for the Future.*

12. Sarter, Barbara. "Philosophical Sources of Nursing Theory." *Nursing Science Quarterly* 1.2 (1988): 52–9. See also: Holmes, Dave and Denise Gastaldo. "Rhizomatic Thought in Nursing: An Alternative Path for the Development of the Discipline." *Nursing Philosophy* 5.3 (2004): 258–67. See also: Fawcett, Jacqueline. "From a Plethora of Paradigms to Parsimony in Worldviews." *Perspectives on Nursing Theory.* Ed. Pamela G. Reed and Nelma C. Shearer. Philadelphia: Lippincott Williams and Wilkins, 2004. 179–83.

13. Boschma, Geertje. "The Meaning of Holism in Nursing; Historical Shifts in Holistic Nursing Ideas." *Public Health Nursing* 11.5 (1994): 324–30.

14. Oldnall, Andrew S. "On the Absence of Spirituality in Nursing Theories and Models: Guest Editorial." *Journal of Advanced Nursing* 21.3 (1995): 417–8.

15. Martsolf, Donna S., and Jacqueline R. Mickley. "The Concept of Spirituality in Nursing Theories: Differing World-views and Extent of Focus." *Journal of Advanced Nursing* 27.2 (1998): 294–303.

16. Bradshaw, Ann. *Lighting the Lamp: The Spiritual Dimension of Nursing Care.* Middlesex, England: Scutari Press, 1994. See also: O'Brien, Mary Elizabeth. *Spirituality in Nursing: Standing on Holy Ground.* 3rd ed. Sudbury, Mass: Jones and Bartlett, 2008. See also: Shelly, Judith A. and Arlene B. Miller. *Called to Care: A Christian Theology of Nursing.* Downers Grove, IL: InterVarsity Press, 1999.

17. Sarter, Barbara. "Philosophic Sources of Nursing Theory." *Nursing Science Quarterly* 1.2 (1988): 52–9.

18. Ibid.

19. Ibid.

20. Green, Catherine. "A Comprehensive Theory of the Human Person from Philosophy and Nursing." *Nursing Philosophy* 10.4 (2009): 273.

21. Parse, Rosemarie R. *The Human Becoming School of Thought: A Perspective for Nurses and Other Health Professionals.* Thousand Oaks, CA: Sage, 1998.

22. Lynch, Gordon. *The New Spirituality: An Introduction to Progressive Belief in the Twenty-First Century.* London: I. B. Taurus, 2007. See also: Walsch, Neal Donald. *Tomorrow's God: Our Greatest Spiritual Challenge.* New York: Atria, 2004.

23. Pesut, Barbara. *A Philosophic Analysis of the Spiritual in Nursing Literature.* Unpublished doctoral dissertation, University of British Columbia; 2005. See also: Pesut, Barbara. "Spirituality and Spiritual Care in Nursing Fundamentals Textbooks." *Journal of Nursing Education* 47.4 (2008): 167–73.

24. North American Nursing Diagnosis Association. *Nursing Diagnoses: Definitions and Classifications.* 7 ed. Philadelphia: NANDA, 2007.

25. O'Brien, Mary Elizabeth. *Spirituality in Nursing: Standing on Holy Ground.* 68–9.

26. Pesut, Barbara and Rick Sawatzky. "To Describe or Prescribe: Assumptions Underlying a Prescriptive Nursing Process Approach to Spiritual Care." *Nursing Inquiry* 13.2 (2006): 127–34.

27. O'Brien, Mary Elizabeth. *Spirituality in Nursing: Standing on Holy Ground.* 71.

28. Walsch, Neal Donald. *Tomorrow's God: Our Greatest Spiritual Challenge.* 386.

29. Wuthnow, Robert. *America and the Challenges of Religious Diversity.* Princeton, NJ: Princeton University Press, 2005.

30. Canefe, Nergis. "Commentary: Religion and Politics in the Diaspora: The Case of Canadian Muslims." *Journal of Community and Applied Psychology* 18.4 (2008): 390–4.

31. Bramadat, Paul and David Seljak. "Charting the New Terrain: Christianity and Ethnicity in Canada." *Christianity and Ethnicity in Canada.* Ed. Paul Bramadat and David Seljak. Toronto: University of Toronto, 2008. 3–48.

32. Lynch, Gordon. *The New Spirituality: An Introduction to Progressive Belief in the Twenty-First Century.*

33. Ibid.

34. Todd, Douglas, ed. *Cascadia: The Elusive Utopia.* Vancouver, BC: Ronsdale Press, 2008.

35. Pesut, Barbara, Marsha Fowler, Sheryl Reimer-Kirkham, and Elizabeth Johnston Taylor. "Particularizing Spirituality in Points of Tension: Enriching the Discourse." *Nursing Inquiry* 16.4 (2009): 1–10.

36. Pesut, Barbara. "Ontologies of Nursing in an Age of Spiritual Pluralism: Closed or Open Worldview." *Nursing Philosophy* 11.1 (2009): 15–23.

37. Chan, Cecilia L. W., Ng, S. M., Ho, Rainbow T. H., and Chow, Amy Y. M. "East Meets West: Applying Eastern Spirituality in Clinical Practice." *Journal of Clinical Nursing* 15.7 (2006): 822–32.

38. Ibid.

39. Paley, John. "Spirituality in Nursing: A Reductionist Approach." *Nursing Philosophy* 9.1 (2008): 3–18.

40. Pesut, Barbara. "A Reply to 'Spirituality and Nursing: A Reductionist Approach' by John Paley." *Nursing Philosophy* 9.2 (2008): 131–7. See also: Nolan, Steve. "In Defence of the Indefensible: An Alternative to John Paley's Reductionist, Atheistic, Psychological Alternative to Spirituality." *Nursing Philosophy* 10.3 (2009): 203–13. See also: Betts, Clinton E., and Andrea F. J. Smith-Betts. "Scientism and the Medicalization of Extistential Distress: A Reply to John Paley." *Nursing Philosophy* 10.2 (2009): 137–41.

41. Willis, Danny G., Pamela J. Grace, and Callista Roy. "A Central Uunifying Focus for the Discipline: Facilitating Humanization, Meaning, Choice, Quality of Life, and Healing in Living and Dying." *Advances in Nursing Science* 31.1(2008): E28–E40. See also: Willis, Danny G., and Pamela J. Grace. "A Response to 'Ontologies of Nursing in an Age of Spiritual Pluralism: Closed or Open Worldview.'" *Nursing Philosophy* 11.1 (2010): 24.

42. Pesut, Barbara, and Sally Thorne. "From Private to Public: Negotiating Professional and Personal Identities in Spiritual Care." *Journal of Advanced Nursing* 58.4 (2007): 396–403.

43. Salladay, Susan A. "Healing is Believing: Postmodernism Impacts Nursing." *The Scientific Review of Alternative Medicine* 4.1 (2000): 39–47.

44. Fawcett, Tonks N., and Amy Noble. "The Challenge of Spiritual Care in a Multifaith Society Experienced as a Christian Nurse." *Journal of Clinical Nursing* 13.2 (2004): 136–42.

45. Parse, Rosemarie R. *The Human Becoming School of Thought: A Perspective for Nurses and other Health Professionals.* See also: Watson, Jean. *Caring Science as Sacred Science.* Philadelphia: FA Davis, 2005.

46. Taves, Ann. *Religious Experience Reconsidered: A Building Block Approach to the Study of Religion and Other Special Things.*

47. Michalak, Erin E., Lakshmi N. Yatham, Sharlene Kolesar, and Raymond W. Lam. "Bipolar Disorder and Quality of Life: a Patient-centered Perspective." *Quality of Life Research: An International Journal of Quality of Life Aspects of Treatment, Care and Rehabilitation* 15.1 (2006): 25–37.
48. Thorne, Sally. "Ideas and Action in a Terrain of Complexity: Editorial." *Nursing Philosophy* 10.3 (2009): 149–51.
49. Taves, Ann. *Religious Experience Reconsidered: A Building Block Approach to the Study of Religion and Other Special Things.*
50. Thorne, Sally. "Ideas and Action in a Terrain of Complexity: Editorial."

4

Feminist and Religious Ethics in Nursing

Barbara Pesut

Religion provides important moral guidance for many nurses' lives. It informs their deepest beliefs about what is good and right to do and what it means to live well. This understanding of the good is the essence of morality. Ethics, however, is the normative and theoretical approach to morality.[1] Ethical theories outline those areas in life that require intentional choices about rights and responsibilities, provide judgments about the values that should underpin those choices, and reason about what is right or wrong within particular choices.[2] Health care ethics is the systematic attempt to determine what is good and right to do in health care contexts. Likewise, nursing ethics seeks to determine what is good and right to do in the context of the delivery of nursing care.

Devettere[3] suggests that there are two main types of ethical theories: those that assume that individuals by nature *do not* seek the good and those that assume individuals *do* seek the good. Theories derived from the first assumption focus on ethical obligations and from the second assumption focus on the moral capability of the person performing the action. Nursing ethics to date has been shaped largely by the perspective of ethical obligations. The codes of ethics created by the Canadian Nurses Association and the American Nurses Association[4] focus on values, responsibilities, and commitments expected of nurses in the context of their practice. More recently, nursing ethics have been influenced by feminist ethics that focuses more on Devettere's second type of ethical theory, the moral capability of the nurse.

In this chapter, I shall illustrate some of the contributions that feminist ethics can make to religious ethics in nursing and reveal how each provides an important lens to understand what is good and right to do within the discipline. Religious ethics considers the ways in which religion informs our understandings of the most important values in life, the obligations we have in response to those values, and the way those values should shape our decisions. Indeed, this book is about religious ethics and how various traditions inform how nurses seek to live and nurse well. However, I need to begin with a caution about the concept of religious ethics. Fowler[5] outlines important considerations when we speak of religious ethics. We cannot assume that religions are homogenous, even within their own traditions. For example, individuals within a religious tradition will fall along a continuum from liberal to conservative in their beliefs; where one falls on that continuum will determine what is considered morally right. Also, individuals may not embrace all the tenets of their tradition. For example, a Roman Catholic nurse may decide that confession is not an important part of her or his living out of Catholicism. It is impossible to separate religion from culture. A religious ethic will be shaped by the culture within which it is lived. A Christian living in North America may embrace a different religious ethic than a Christian living in Africa. The important point is that the same limitations of any conceptual label (e.g., Protestant, Catholic, and Muslim) are relevant to conceptualizations of religion as well. There may be more diversity within a category than between categories. When it comes to deciding what is morally right, a conservative Christian may have more in common with a conservative Muslim than a liberal Christian. In the everyday ethical decision making informed by religion, the landscape of right and wrong, good and bad, obligations and rights are more complex than religious categories would suggest.

As the goal of this chapter is to illustrate the intersections and contributions of religious and feminist ethics to nursing, an important starting point is the relationship between religion, feminism, and nursing. Only when one understands some of the tensions that have surrounded religion, feminism, and nursing, can one understand the challenges to realizing the potential for feminist ethics to contribute to religious ethics in nursing. However, first it is important to define feminism. There are many diverse strands of feminism, including but not limited to, Liberal, Marxist, Radical, Psychoanalytic, Socialist, and Postmodern.[6] Those who write within a feminist tradition generally need to locate themselves because these strands are so diverse. Across that diversity, however, there is a common consciousness that women have been oppressed and a common goal to eliminate that oppression.[7] The diversity arises out of the differing ideas of the origins of and solutions to the oppression. Feminist ethics is a branch of feminist philosophy, which seeks to philosophize within a particular understanding of women's place in the world.[8] This way of philosophizing includes both the questions one asks and the tools one uses to answer those questions.

NURSING AND FEMINISM: A COMPLEX RELATIONSHIP

Although feminist ideas are now extensively integrated into nursing theory, research, and ethics, this has not always been the case. Nursing's reluctance to affiliate with feminism may be attributed, in part, to its roots in religion and the military,[9] patriarchal institutions that have afforded few opportunities for women. With such strong affiliations with what have been predominantly patriarchal organizations, it may have been difficult for nursing to embrace feminism; although a primarily female occupation, it was an oppressed group.

Another factor that has inhibited nursing's relationship to feminism was its quest for professionalism. Wuest[10] argues that the idea of professionalism has been shaped largely by masculine ideals of rationalism, science, and objectivity. Nursing assimilated these same ideals in its pursuit of professional status. The knowledge that was to characterize the developing profession was anchored in a scientific, reductionistic, and biomedical perspective. This was facilitated by academic preparation within university settings where scholarly achievement was understood within these masculine ideals. This led to a theory–practice gap and divided nurses between those who taught and those who practiced. In contrast to a masculine model of professionalism, feminist thinkers would focus on caring, social action, and reflexivity. Rather than viewing knowledge as gained within academic structures, it would be the nurse at the bedside who would have the "more legitimate perspective of nursing."[11] Knowledge in a feminist perspective is held to be much less certain than masculine perspectives would suggest, being shaped by gender, social, historical, and political contexts.[12]

Despite the contention that nursing has been reluctant to embrace feminism, others argue that nursing has contributed to advancing the feminist agenda. For example, many early and influential nurses such as Lavinia Dock, Isabel Stuart, Adelaide Nutting, Lillian Wald, and Wilma Scott Heidie supported women's suffrage.[13] Profiles of early nurses who worked in religious orders reveal how powerful these women were, even within male-dominated systems. The Grey Nuns, founded in Montreal in 1737 (long before first wave feminism), influenced the development of hospitals and health care services in Canada.[14] Nineteenth century Catholic Nuns and Mormon women created influential places for themselves in the public realm of health care during a time when most women were confined to the domestic sphere.[15]

They administered hospitals by providing oversight, handling budgets, and supervising the buying and selling of property. This was no simple task. They held the difficult task of providing leadership within male-dominated systems while continuing to give lip service to the feminine ideals of subservience. In this situation, "gender roles reflected a complex integration of obedience to authority and use of power that emerged uniquely from gender."[16] Although nursing may have held itself somewhat distant from feminism, nurses themselves were carving out significant positions of influence and leadership within society, and within powerful religious institutions. In doing so, these women were helping to realize the ideals of the feminist movement.

Whether or not Florence Nightingale was a feminist has been a matter of some debate. She has been criticized for not supporting women's suffrage[17] even though she clearly struggled with the role of women in Victorian society. She likened the family to a prison where women were forced into mindless roles that belied their gifting and role in the world.[18] This situation was particularly acute for her. Unlike the majority of women during the Victorian era, she had the benefit of an excellent education, but felt she had no legitimate outcome for that intellectual development. This went against her religious beliefs that God had important roles for women to play in society and that Christ had elevated women to their rightful status.[19] She had a strong sense of her own destiny and felt that the constraints on women contradicted her religious calling. However, this did not necessarily mean that she supported women's suffrage, as indicated from the following quote from a letter to John Stuart Mill:

> That women should have the suffrage, I think no one can be more deeply convinced than I. . . . But it will probably be years before you obtain the suffrage for women. And, in the meantime, are there not evils that press much more hardly on women that not having a vote?[20]

She cites the problem of married women not being able to own property. Indeed, this was an important issue for her as it was her financial dependence on her family that initially prevented her from realizing her dream of serving God. Nightingale's own feminist values stood against the Victorian values of the day. Her own values centered around the rights of women to achieve their maximal potential in the context of meaningful employment.[21] She resisted a dualistic masculine and feminine view of the world, acknowledging the importance of a meaningful existence for all individuals.[22] From this perspective, even though she chose not to give her energies to women's suffrage, she worked against women's oppression.

The relationship between feminism and nursing has been a complex one and perhaps one could argue that nursing has contributed both to the liberation and oppression of women.[23] However, it might be more useful to think of the various ways that nurses have chosen to advance the causes of women in society. Some nurses overtly embraced feminism, whereas others held positions of power within largely patriarchal institutions, advancing the role of women in a more hidden fashion. Either way, most feminists would agree that what was once a rather tenuous relationship has now developed into a highly intertwined one. Feminism has influenced all aspects of nursing's philosophy and theory. More recently, feminism has begun to profoundly influence nursing ethics.

FEMINIST ETHICS IN NURSING

Nursing's ontology and ethics are deeply intertwined. Ideas about what nursing is determine what is perceived to be good and right to do within the profession.[24] Historically, nursing first perceived itself as a calling, then a profession, and more recently as a practice.[25] Although this was a historical progression, it is important to note that all three ideas about what nursing is still exist today. Nurses who view their profession as a calling from God will often derive their ideas of good practice from religious ethics. They seek to do what is good and right as described by their religion. For example, Bradshaw[26] envisions nursing as covenantal caring. Nursing is a moral response to God's covenant to care for humankind. As nursing began to view itself more as a profession than a calling, ethical guidance came from codes of ethics that outlined values and principles of responsibility (e.g., Canadian Nurses Association Code of Ethics and American Nurses Association Code of Ethics). More recently, there has been a shift to viewing nursing as practice as a moral way of being that contributes a good to society. From this perspective, ethical guidance has been derived from the virtues of caring and relationship.

Two feminist ethicists, Carol Gilligan and Nel Noddings, have influenced nursing's ethical focus of caring and relationships. Carol Gilligan in her book, *A Different Voice*,[27] critiques Kohlberg's stages of moral development as too masculine in their focus on justice, rights, and rules. Instead, she proposes that when making decisions about good and right, women focused more on responsibilities in the contexts of their relationships. Similarly, Nel Noddings in her book *A Feminine Approach to Ethics and Moral Education*,[28] published just 2 years after Gilligan, argues that ethics is about the caring that occurs with relationships. She believes that there was a pattern of care whereby the one caring imparted real goods to the one being cared for in situations of concrete interactions. This was in contrast to the more disembodied rule-oriented focus of ethics popular at the time. These ideas of caring in the context of relationships have strongly influenced both nursing theory and philosophy from the 1990s onward.

There are multiple, and sometimes competing, approaches to ethics in nursing. These differences may be useful, given the diversity inherent in the world.[29] Each approach provides a different lens by which to view a situation. However, there have been some important difficulties with traditional principle-based approaches to ethics that feminist ethicists have sought to redress. Liaschenko nicely summarizes some of the feminist critiques of bioethical approaches, which are driven primarily by advances in science and technology, and therefore focus on rules and legal structures to address these advances. The resulting approach to decision making is impartial, disinterested, and universal, ignoring important character aspects of moral life.[30] In the same way, the biomedical approach is also disembodied and often fails to take into account the real experiences of individuals.[31] Because morality and ethics are developed within social relationships, it is often those who are most socially powerful who define what a moral issue is. Biomedical ethics, largely shaped by the medical profession, has tended to focus on the crisis points experienced by medicine rather than the process points experienced by nursing.[32] This renders the particular ethical issues experienced by nurses invisible. For example, end-of-life decision making is an ethical issue. From a biomedical perspective, the ethical questions often surround what is good and right to do in the light of the outcome of that decision. In contrast, what often concerns nurses is the process that individuals and families pursue as they seek answers about what is good and right. The physician might ask, "Is terminal sedation ethical?" and the nurse might ask, "What are the consequences for this family of having to make the decision to terminally sedate their loved one?" From a biomedical perspective, the ethical issues most relevant for nursing are often the hidden ones. This is where feminist ethics makes an important contribution to nursing ethics.

As in most theoretical understandings, ideas about feminist ethics are diverse. Those who work with feminist ethics have quite different ideas about the nature of the human self (an important consideration in ethics) and the nature of knowledge and how one obtains it. However, the unifying goal of feminist ethics is to raise consciousness about, and eliminate, gender oppression.[33] An important distinction is made between *feminine* and *feminist* ethics.[34] *Feminine* ethics draws on and values feminine traits such as caring, compassion, and nurture to inform what is good and right to do. The underlying assumption is that feminine characteristics have been devalued and need to be reclaimed as an important contribution to the moral development of society. *Feminist* ethics, on the other hand, seeks for equal rights and to redress the inequities inherent in patriarchal institutions and systems of thought. It seeks to transform society at the political level. More recently, feminine and feminist ethics have been termed "care-focused" versus "power-focused" ethics.[35] For the remainder of this chapter, I will be using the term *feminist* ethics to refer to both strands.

Feminist ethics can inform health care ethics in a number of ways.[36] First, traditional questions of ethical inquiry can be answered using a feminist lens. In particular, these questions are answered from the perspective of those who are less powerful in health care, such as the patients or those who occupy the less prestigious professions. Second, the types of ethical questions are expanded in the light of women's concerns. Commonly, these additional questions focus on women's childbearing experiences, such as abortion or reproductive technologies. Third, ethical analytic tools that reflect feminist perspectives are used to answer these questions. Typically, these tools resist dichotomies such as fact or value and theory or practice, because what is positioned as an objective fact may only reflect the values of a particular social context. Feminist ethics brings important new questions and perspectives to health care and nursing ethics.

The work of feminist ethicist, Margaret Urban Walker,[37] illustrates the potential of feminist ethics to inform nursing ethics.[38] Four main assumptions underlie her approach to ethics. First, morality needs to be understood as practices, not theories. Morality cannot be an objective endeavor that we simply think about, but rather something that is inextricably related to how we live our lives. Second, morality is always enacted within a social setting. What is good and right to do within a situation is informed by the social practices of that context; there is no such thing as an objectivity that stands apart from context. Third, morality is essentially about practices of responsibility. We seek to know what our responsibilities are in contributing to the good. Fourth, when we assume that there is some ideal or pure morality, we make some people's moral lives invisible by inhibiting their ability to see their own moral dilemmas and choices.

These underlying assumptions illustrate some of the challenges that nurses have with traditional biomedical approaches.[39] A principle-based approach tends to ignore the health care conditions within which nurses work. Nurses often practice within institutions where gender and class profoundly influence nurses' abilities to make moral choices. The dilemmas that arise because of nurse's location in these institutions are rendered invisible. Walker's work points to the importance of examining the social context of health care. For nurses, this means recognizing that moral worlds are inseparable from the social worlds in which morality is enacted. Nursing is largely about practices of responsibility to vulnerable patients, and therefore this ethical focus resonates with the work they do. For example, many ethicists would not identify excessive workloads as an ethical dilemma. Yet, for nurses, if excessive workloads constrain their responsibility to give good care and vulnerable patients suffer as a result, this becomes a pressing ethical issue. Feminist ethics provides a powerful lens for examining what is good and right to do for professionals, such as nurses who practice largely within hierarchal institutions.

However, the feminist assumptions that there are no absolute truths about human persons and knowledge, and in particular moral knowledge, are assumptions that may not sit well with religious nurses. Religion seeks to answer the moral questions of life, and often does so in codified, principled ways. Seeing those principles as situation-dependent might be experienced as a conflict with faith. I will now turn to this dilemma.

FEMINIST AND RELIGIOUS ETHICS IN NURSING: CONTRIBUTIONS AND TENSIONS

To understand the tensions between religious and feminist ethics, it is necessary to think about the nature of religious ethics. I will be drawing primarily on my own tradition of Christianity, as I know this best. Christian morality and ethics are grounded in sacred writings. Religious people study these writings to derive principles that enable them to grow in character and to live more responsibly in relation to others. However, because these writings are often considered to be both sacred and infallible, it is difficult for some religious people to subject them to critical analysis. Indeed, some might claim that it is the essence of faith; to take these ideas at face value and to obey them without discussion. Clearly there are challenges to this claim, but that is not my focus here. Devettere[40] suggests that the perspective of unquestioning faith is sometimes played as the "trump card" in health care decision making. He further argues that, ultimately, religious individuals must make a decision about whether their ethical basis for what it means to live a good life comes from religious faith or from human reason. Even those individuals who claim that faith and reason are complementary must ultimately resort to one or the other, should there be a contradiction between the two. From a virtues-based approach, religious individuals would ask themselves whether or not their religion supports their ability to live virtuously in the pursuit of a good life.

Religious perspectives are further complicated by gender issues. Feminists writing from a Christian outlook (and this would apply to many other religious perspectives as well) have pointed out the difficulties of a theological view that has been largely constructed by white, celibate males who had the privilege of position and status. This perspective does not adequately represent the experiences of non-white people, women, poor people, and those whose sexuality is different from the mainstream.[41] Theology is largely a language of male intellectuals. Male images of God and Christ tend to encode morality with a particular gender that disenfranchises women.[42] As a result, the voices representing morality and ethics are not informed by the full spectrum of human interest, which is ultimately dehumanizing.[43]

One can appreciate the difficulties that religious ethics presents for feminist ethics. Not only has religious ethics been shaped largely by male intellectuals, but when enshrined as sacred, these ideas are not open to critical analysis. Some people would argue that feminist ethics holds exciting possibilities for revitalizing and transforming religious ethics. Feminist ethics can provide a counterpoint that critiques traditional religious ethics and provides alternative ways of understanding that can inform and enrich religious thinking.[44] For example, Keller suggests that the Holy Spirit, rather than the Father or the Son (the three "persons" of the Christian God), is an image of the Divine that most resonates with women's interests.[45] The Holy Spirit represents an embodied knowing that seeks to relate, to create, and to connect across difference as ethical ideals that better represent women's lives and responsibilities.

It is interesting to reflect on the relationships between feminist ethics, caring, and spirituality in nursing over the past several decades. Caring and spirituality have been enormously popular concepts in nursing. The popularity of caring predated the popularity of spirituality and one could argue that the interest in spirituality arose in part because of deficiencies in caring as an ethics for nursing. As discussed previously, the ethics of care was an important contribution of feminism to nursing and represented a shift away from masculine ideals. However, individuals have argued that these ideas of caring have been ungrounded from any moral tradition, such as those found in religion, and hence there is no real guidance on how to care ethically.[46] Spirituality (as opposed to religion) may have arisen as an ideal to reground the moral basis of caring. For example, some nursing models[47] have partnered caring with the sacred, thus lending divine authority to the moral imperative of caring. Further, nursing ideas about spirituality suggest that the environment in which nursing practices is somewhat mysterious, in which connectedness plays a vital role in the healing relationship.[48] This nursing spirituality is largely free of institutional religion, although many of the basic ideas remain informed by Christian theology.[49] By embracing the ideas of caring and spirituality, nursing has seen itself as moral practice informed by a feminized form of spirituality that is clearly removed from institutional religion with its patriarchal origins. Nurses' care then becomes enacted, in a mysterious spiritual context that is independent of institutional religious ethics. This context-dependent, epistemologically flexible ethic, enacted through relational practices of responsibility, is characteristic of feminine or care-focused ethics. However, both the ethic of care and the ethic of spirituality have come under criticism for their inability to provide a normative and grounded perspective that has the political leverage to address issues of marginalization and social justice.[50] Yet, it is interesting to see how spirituality and caring have been used within nursing as the basis for an ethical approach that has been informed both by religion and feminism.

The potential tensions between religious ethics and feminist ethics might suggest that nursing needs to adopt one approach or the other. Perhaps a more useful way to integrate the two would be to see how each provides the other with important analytical mileage for considering ethical issues. Gadow's[51] framework is one that is particularly useful for considering multiple aspects to inform an ethical problem.[52]

A TRI-PARTITE FRAMEWORK FOR EXPLORING ETHICAL ISSUES

Gadow[53] suggests that the nursing profession requires an ethical cornerstone to guide its practice and proposes a three-level ethical framework to serve as such. It is important to note that ethical frameworks can serve either to provide a basis for normative decision making or to provide guidance for a fuller description of an ethical situation. Her framework seeks to fulfill the latter. She calls the three layers of her framework "subjective immersion," "objective detachment," and "relational narrative." She sees these layers as corresponding to historical turns in nursing ethics. *Subjective immersion* is characteristic of premodern ethics. From this perspective, individuals tend to have an uncritical certainty about the good derived from influences such as family, religion, tradition, or community. *Objective detachment* is characteristic of modern ethics. From this perspective, people use universal principles and theories to determine the good. *Relational narrative* characterizes the "postmodern turn" in nursing ethics and sees the good as co-constructed between individuals. It is this final layer that is most characteristic of feminist ethics.

Interestingly, the majority of nursing authors who draw on Gadow's work focus solely on the relational narrative level of the framework. However, Gadow suggests that the three levels were not meant to be subsequent stages of development whereby one level was transcended in favor of the next. Rather, these levels were meant to operate together in a dialectic fashion that allowed individuals to gain a broader depth and appreciation of the circumstances at hand. It is this understanding of her framework that provides such a useful integration of religious ethics, principle-based ethics, and feminist ethics. This framework is used here in the context of a clinical situation.

Justin is an RN who works in a rural community on an acute medical floor that has one palliative bed. It is the night shift and a young male patient with a palliative cancer diagnosis is admitted in severe pain. Justin knows this young man well, having lived in the same community for many years. They have had many conversations about how he would like the end of his life to go. Justin knows that his young patient has two wishes, to die without pain and without conscious suffering. In their conversations Justin had promised that he would do his best to fulfill those wishes. On admission, Justin tries everything within the palliative orders to ease the pain and suffering of this young man, but nothing works. The patient is in severe intractable pain and suffering, the very situation that Justin committed to alleviate. Justin calls the GP for further orders, reiterating his patient's request not to be conscious or in pain at end of life. The GP curtly replies "I don't believe in euthanasia" and provides an analgesic order that Justin knows is well within the safe limit but will not provide the needed relief. Justin knows the GP from his church and is aware that she is a passionate advocate of sanctity of life is-sues and so it is unlikely he will get any further with her. He hangs up the phone, feeling frustrated and desperate to help his patient and friend. He immediately thinks of the old adage from nursing school "physicians cure and nurses care" and is angered by the physician's uncaring response. He begins to "work the system" to find the needed pain relief for his patient. He contacts the emergency physician on call, the palliative hotline, and the community physician who specializes in palliative care. No one is willing to over-ride the GPs' orders, but the community physician agrees to contact the GP to advocate for the patient. The GP finally calls back and agrees to more aggressive opioid therapy as long as it is only given every 10 minutes and the patient is carefully monitored. However, by this time two of Justin's other acute medical patients have crises and his workload is overwhelming. Justin is unable to return to his friend to provide the 10 minute analgesia, although he does his best to give it as frequently as possible. His friend dies that night in unremitting pain. Justin completes his shift, devastated by his inability to fulfill the final wishes of his patient and friend.

An in-depth discussion of this scenario is beyond the scope of this chapter, but it is useful to see how Gadow's framework would illuminate the ethical issues at play. The first level of the framework is concerned with the certainties in life that tend to be unquestioned and derived from cultural sources. They are characterized by a certainty about what is good. In this scenario, the GP has a certainty about her beliefs in relation to any form of sedation that might end life prematurely. The nurse has an uncritical certainty about physician–nurse relationships that lead him to believe that the physician really does not care. The second level of the framework is based on the principles that can be derived from professional or religious sources. In this scenario, the nurse may be operating from a principle of patient choice and the physician may be operating from a principle of sanctity of life. The third layer of relational narrative is characterized by a co-construction of the good. "The ethical knowledge created through a relational narrative is particular, contextual and nongeneralizable."[54] In this situation, the good has been constructed between the patient and the nurse; they have envisioned a death without suffering or pain. However, this good has not been enacted because of other perceived goods. Ideally, discussions with the physician would have included her in the co-construction of the good, but that may not be possible, either because of her own reluctance to question her certainty about the good, or because the nurse dismissed her too quickly based on his professional stereotype of physicians as not caring. A feminist ethical lens would look at the contextual factors that place power in the hands of physicians who are located away from the actual patient suffering and the organizational factors that create workloads that prevent the nurse being presentable to provide adequate analgesia. Even this brief description of how Gadow's framework might be used illustrates the complexity of the factors that come into play in a scenario like this, and how individuals draw on multiple sources to determine what is good and right in a particular situation. The beauty of the framework is that it focuses attention on certainties, principles, and relational factors, thus providing a more nuanced and grounded picture of the context.

CONCLUSION

Religious ethics has been, and will continue to be a powerful shaper of what many nurses consider to be good and right in the context of nursing practice. Indeed, it was religious ethics, expressed in the commitment to care, that provided the motivation for many early nurse pioneers. Over the last decades, nursing ethics has been shaped largely by feminist ethics. A feminized form of caring and a political focus on social justice have characterized nursing's ideas of good practice. However, the feminist perspective of situated knowledge and context-dependent values is one that may conflict with religious ethics. Religious nurses in particular may experience dissonance between the ethical frameworks provided by their religion and those proposed by their profession. However, rather than seeing these as dichotomous frameworks, it is perhaps more useful to see them as complementary. Feminist ethics can provide a nuanced lens that illuminates the context of a situation. Religious ethics can help to anchor that nuanced picture within normative values. These perspectives together can provide powerful analytical mileage for the complex ethical situations that confront nurses daily in practice.

NOTES

1. Walker, Margaret U. *Moral Understandings: A Feminist Study in Ethics.* 2nd ed. Oxford: Oxford University Press, 2007.
2. Devettere, Raymond J. *Practical Decision Making in Health Care Ethics: Cases and Concepts.* Washington, DC: Georgetown University Press, 2010.
3. Ibid.
4. Canadian Nurses Association. *Code of Ethics for Registered Nurses.* Ottawa: Canadian Nurses Association, 2008. Web. And: Fowler, Marsha D., ed. *Guide to the Code of Ethics for Nurses.* Silver Spring, MD: American Nurses Association, 2008.
5. Fowler, Marsha D. "Religion, Bioethics and Nursing Practice." *Nursing Ethics* 16.4 (2009): 393–405.
6. Tong, Rosemarie. *Feminine and Feminist Ethics.* Belmont, CA: Wadsworth Publishing Company, 1993.
7. Tong, Rosemarie. *Feminist Approaches to Bioethics: Theoretical Reflections and Practical Applications.* Boulder, CO: Westview Press, 1997.
8. Jaggar, Alison M., and Iris M. Young, eds. "Introduction." *Blackwell Companion to Philosophy: A Companion to Feminist Philosophy.* Oxford: Blackwell Publishers Ltd, 2000. 1–6.
9. Bunting, Sheila, and Jacquelyn C. Campbell. "Feminism and Nursing: Historical Perspectives." *Advances in Nursing Science* 12.4 (1990): 11–24.
10. Wuest, Judith. "Professionalism and the Evolution of Nursing as a Discipline: A Feminist Perspective." *Journal of Professional Nursing* 10.6 (1994): 357–67.
11. Ibid., 365.
12. Doering, Lynn. "Power and Knowledge in Nursing: A Feminist Poststructuralist Approach." *Advances in Nursing Science* 14.4 (1992): 24–33.
13. Bunting, Sheila, and Jacquelyn C. Campbell. "Feminism and Nursing: Historical Perspectives." See also: Wuest (1994). See also: Doering, Lynn. "Power and Knowledge in Nursing: A Feminist Poststructuralist Approach." See also: Hampson, M.O. "A Review of the Relationship Between Feminism and Nursing: From an Evolutionary, Historical, Paradigmatic, Theoretical, and Intrapsychic Perspective." *Nursing Leadership Forum* 2.4 (1996): 120–25.
14. Paul, Pauline. "The Contribution of the Grey Nuns to the Development of Nursing in Canada: Historiographical Issues." *Canadian Bulletin of Medical History* 11 (1994): 207–17.
15. Marshall, E. Sorenson, and Wall B. Mann. "Religion, Gender, and Autonomy: A Comparison of Two Religious Women's Groups in Nursing and Hospital in the Late Nineteenth and Early Twentieth Centuries." *Advances in Nursing Science* 22.1 (1999): 1–22.
16. Ibid., 3.

17. Selanders, Louise C. "Florence Nightingale: The Evolution and Social Impact of Feminist Values in Nursing." *Journal of Holistic Nursing* 16.2 (1998): 227–43.
18. Calabria, Michael D., and Janet A. Macrae, eds. *Suggestions for Thought by Florence Nightingale*. Philadelphia: University of Pennsylvania Press, 1994.
19. Grypma, Sonya. "Florence Nightingale's Changing Image. Part 1: Nightingale The Feminist, Statistician & Nurse." *Journal of Christian Nursing* 22.3 (2005): 22–28.
20. Calabria and Macrae, (1994). 103.
21. Selanders, (1998).
22. Holliday, Mary E., and David L. Parker. "Florence Nightingale, Feminism and Nursing." *Journal of Advanced Nursing* 26.3 (1997) 483–88.
23. Wuest, Judith. "Professionalism and the Evolution of Nursing as a Discipline: A Feminist Perspective." 365.
24. Liaschenko, Joan, and Elizabeth Peter. "Nursing Ethics and Conceptualizations of Nursing: Profession, Practice and Work." *Journal of Advanced Nursing* 46.5 (2004): 488–93.
25. Ibid.
26. Bradshaw, Ann. *Lighting the Lamp: The Spiritual Dimension of Nursing Care*. Middlesex, England: Scutari Press, 1994.
27. Gilligan, Carol. *In a Different Voice*. Cambridge, MA: Harvard University Press, 1982. Print.
28. Noddings, Nell. *Caring: A Feminist Approach to Ethics and Moral Education*. Berkeley: University of California Press, 1984.
29. Tong, Rosemarie. (1993).
30. Liaschenko, Joan. "Feminist Ethics and Cultural Ethos: Revisiting a Nursing Debate." *Advances in Nursing Science* 15.4 (1993): 71–81.
31. Peter, Elizabeth, and Liaschenko, Joan. "Whose Morality is it Anyway: Thoughts on the Work of Margaret Urban." *Nursing Philosophy* 4.3 (2003): 259–62.
32. Liaschenko, Joan, and Elizabeth Peter. (2004).
33. Tong, Rosemarie. (1993).
34. Ibid.
35. Tong, Rosemarie. (1997). 96.
36. Sherwin, Susan."Health Care." *Blackwell Companion to Philosophy: A Companion to Feminist Philosophy*. Eds. Alison M. Jaggar and Iris M. Young. Oxford: Blackwell Publishers, 2000. 420–428.
37. Walker, Margaret Urban (2007).
38. Peter, Elizabeth, and Joan Liaschenko. (2003).
39. Ibid.
40. Devettere, Raymond J. (2010).
41. Keller, Catherine. "Christianity." *Blackwell Companion to Philosophy: A Companion to Feminist Philosophy.* Eds Alison M. Jaggar and Iris M. Young. Oxford: Blackwell Press, 2000. 225–35.
42. Ibid.
43. Haney, Eleanor H. "What is Feminist Ethics? A Proposal for Continuing Discussion." *Feminist Theological Ethics: A Reader.* Ed. Lois K. Daly. Louisville, KY: Westminster John Knox Press, 1994. 3–12.
44. Ibid.
45. Keller, Catherine. (2000).
46. Bradshaw, Ann. "Yes! There is an Ethics of Care: An Answer for Peter Allmark." *Journal of Medical Ethics* 22.1 (1996): 8–12.

47. Bradshaw, Ann. (1994). See also: Watson, Jean. *Caring Science as Sacred Science.* Philadelphia: FA Davis, 2005.
48. Watson, Jean. (2005). See also: Burkhardt Margaret A., and Mary Gail Nagai-Jacobson. *Spirituality: Living Our Connectedness.* New York: Delmar Thomson Learning, 2002.
49. Pesut, Barbara, Marsha Fowler, Elizabeth Johnston Taylor, Sheryl Reimer-Kirkham, Rick Sawatzky. "Conceptualizing Spirituality and Religion for Healthcare." *Journal of Clinical Nursing* 17.21 (2008): 2803–10.
50. Bradshaw, Ann. (1996). See also: Pesut, Barbara, Marsha Fowler, Elizabeth Johnston Taylor, Sheryl Reimer-Kirkham, Rick Sawatzky. (2008).
51. Gadow, Sally. "Relational Narrative: The Postmodern Turn in Nursing Ethics." *Scholarly Inquiry for Nursing Practice* 13.1 (1999): 57–70.
52. Pesut, Barbara. "Incorporating Patients' Spirituality into Care Using Gadow's Ethical Framework." *Nursing Ethics* 16.4 (2009): 418–28.
53. Gadow, Sally. (1999).
54. Ibid., 65.

5

A Critical Reading Across Religion and Spirituality: Contributions of Postcolonial Theory to Nursing Ethics

Sheryl Reimer-Kirkham

Global patterns of migration, against the backdrop of historical colonial relations, have resulted in unprecedented religious diversity in many nations. Secularism and the rise in alternative or emergent spiritualities (typically outside of organized religions) have added further complexity to the religious/spiritual landscape of contemporary societies, creating environments of *brigolage*[1] in which people not only pick and choose, but also tinker with the many religious/spiritual options available to them. All of these trends are expressed in Canada, a nation founded as a settler colony by the French and English on lands historically inhabited by First Nations peoples. Today the majority of newcomers to Canada arrive from Asian source countries, resulting in a substantial increase in the number of Canadians who report affiliations with religions such as Islam, Hinduism, Sikhism, and Buddhism. The number of Canadians who report "no religious affiliation" on census surveys is also on the rise[2] as typified by Canada's west coast, that has been described as expressing sacred ecologies rather than adhering to organized religions.[3] Of the English-speaking nations, the United States is generally deemed the most nonsecular and religious, with a flourishing religious market of both institutional religions and noninstitutional spiritualities.[4] Rapid growth of Pentecostalism in the Southern Hemisphere is adding to what were already diverse societies in South America and Africa. Noting that plurality and change are global phenomena, Amoah comments, "The reality of religious plurality can be seen everywhere in Africa."[5] Even European nations, sometimes referred to as the exception in regard to their secularity,[6] have seen some increase in religious diversity, especially as they have turned to immigrant sources to fill labor market needs. Here, as elsewhere, the rise in Islamic immigrants has more recently brought to the forefront the question of religious accommodation in the face of diversity.[7] Around the world, not only is there increased diversity, but also a strengthening or resurgence (sometimes with fundamentalist extremes)[8] of the salience and persuasiveness of religion to individual and public life.[9] These intersecting trends of global migration with increased religious pluralism, the resurgence of religion in some domains, continued secularism, and emergent spiritualities have raised questions about the role of religion/spirituality in the public realm. Whereas secular societies have traditionally held to neutrality of the public sphere and a relatively strict public–private divide, they are now considering moderate adjustments to account for the influence of religion.[10] These trends have also brought back into focus the political nature of religion and spirituality where social relations of power overlap across individual, institutional, and societal levels.[11]

By and large, nursing scholarship has not engaged with the implications of the relations of power mobilized through religion and spirituality. Nor has it accounted for the contingent nature of religion and spirituality as situated within particular sociopolitical contexts, shaped by intersecting social categories of gender, age, class, race, and so forth. Rather, the integration of religion and spirituality discourses in nursing scholarship has tended to: (a) culturalist readings of religion, where the focus typically centers on circumscribed cultural-religious practices; and (b) universalist readings of spirituality, emphasizing a presumed shared spiritual nature of humans with individualized spiritual interpretations. Gilliat-Ray observes that the way in which spirituality is understood in the nursing profession is "culturally and geographically bounded. It is a discussion taking place primarily in the Western, Anglophone world."[12] Given these tendencies to acontextual and apolitical approaches to religion and spirituality that risk exclusion rather than inclusion, our theoretical frameworks—as mechanisms for making particular phenomena visible—become crucial in moving nursing scholarship and ethical practice in pluralistic societies forward.

Postcolonial feminism and other critical perspectives can be helpful to clarify the social dynamics resulting from the contingent and political nature of spirituality and religion. Critical perspectives take as mandate the problematizing of normative approaches to study a given field, in this case the study of religion/spirituality—in its multiple social, political, literary, religious, and historical dimensions—pertaining to nursing and nursing ethics. Critical inquiry is sometimes discounted as ideological, with the criticism that scholars follow preconceived ideas to see oppression everywhere as advocates on behalf of "the oppressed." Importantly, from a postcolonial feminist perspective, the aim of scholarship is "not to serve particular 'interest groups;' rather the agenda is to unmask historically embedded taken-for-granted social structures that support the status quo, that position people in particular ways, and that are major determinants of health and well-being."[13] In this chapter, I consider the contributions of postcolonial theory, arguing that critical perspectives offer invaluable analytic tools in the critical analysis of religion, spirituality, and health/nursing. In so doing, I am urging a rethinking of nursing's typical de-emphasis on creedal religions in quest for a universal spiritual experience.[14] In order to make this argument, the chapter provides an overview of postcolonial theory as one form of critical inquiry particularly salient for the study of religion and spirituality, and highlights several methodological and practice implications for nursing ethics.

POSTCOLONIAL THEORY

The theoretical fields of postcolonialism, black feminism, cultural studies, and critical race theory have been invaluable to nursing scholarship in addressing health and health inequities,[15] and offering alternatives to apolitical conflations of religion and culture, and acontextual conceptions of generic spirituality. The applications of postcolonial theory to religion and spirituality—and to the intersections of race, gender, and class with religion—have been relatively unexplored until recently. Scholars writing within cultural studies and postcolonialism have offered cogent critiques of the damaging effects of race in the everyday with an account of intersecting and historical oppressions, and have tended to name religion as an instrument of colonialism, but have offered less conceptual depth around the intersections between nation, state, religion, and culture, and little explication of the ambivalences and contradictions that characterize social relations of power in the realm of religion and spirituality. A decade ago, Robert Young scolded his postcolonial colleagues for an

> unmediated secularism, opposed to and consistently excluding the religions that have taken on the political identity of providing alternative value-systems to those of the West. Postcolonial theory, despite its espousal of subaltern resistance, scarcely values subaltern resistance that does not operate according to its own secular terms.[16]

Since then, the nexus between religion and the postcolonial is beginning to be examined, to the extent that Ashcroft, Griffiths, and Tiffin assert "there has been no more dramatic shift in recent times in post-colonial studies."[17] "Religion" as a category has become the subject of critical analysis, with observations such as that by Fitzgerald (among others) who points out the processes of separation and reification that resulted historically in the construction of religion as a field of study and the assumption of the universality of religion. He throws doubt on

> modern uncritical reifications of religion as something that exists in and for itself, as something autonomous and essentially distinct from "politics" . . . religion is modern invention which authorizes and naturalises a form of Euro-American secular rationality. In turn, this supposed position of secular rationality constructs and authorises its "other," religion and religions.[18]

With this development came a series of oppositional binaries (e.g., natural/ supernatural; reason/faith; material/spiritual; inner/outer) that, although contested, continue to reinforce "religion" itself as an oppositional term to "nonreligious." Fitzgerald argues that by distinguishing between the material nature (the object of scientific study) and the immaterial or spiritual nature (the object of faith), the idea of religion as a special realm of inner experience separated from the rationality of the public space (the secular state and politics) resulted.[19] It is for such a project of questioning taken-for-granted assumptions about religion that postcolonial theory and other critical perspectives are well-employed.

A Synopsis of Postcolonialism

Postcolonialism, building on its central interest of the legacies of the colonial era, has developed into a body of scholarship that aims to shift the dominant ways in which "relations between western and non-western peoples and their worlds are viewed."[20] Many scholars have taken "post" to indicate the use of poststructural and postmodern forms of analysis.[21] The temporal meaning of "post" is also important in denoting the historical "end" of European colonialism and extends to the evolving configurations of power that circulate as residue of the colonial era.[22] Although "postcolonial" infers a literal transfer of government back into the hands of the colonized, scholars repeatedly remind us that the extent to which economic, cultural, and political influence remains means that in most situations of decolonization, there is not a truly "post" postcolonial.[23] Colonialism has been a recurrent feature stretching back across the millennia, of which modern European colonialism was the most widespread. Loomba details that by the 1930s, colonies and ex-colonies covered nearly 85% of the world's land surface. Remarkably, only parts of Arabia, Persia, Afghanistan, Mongolia, Tibet, China, Siam, and Japan have never been under formal European government. This worldwide sweep makes the colonial experience both universally shared and geographically distinct. Flows of profits and people from the colonies to the colonizers were shared, producing the economic imbalance necessary for the growth of an empire, and in the case of European colonialism, resulting in the birth of European capitalism.[24] The persistent, pervasive negation of indigenous peoples worldwide that continues to this day is rooted in colonialism.

The interrelated (and often interchanged) terms of "colonialism," "imperialism," and "neocolonial" all have to do with the postcolonial condition. Colonialism is defined by Loomba (2005) as "the conquest and control of other people's land and goods."[25] Imperialism is sometimes used in a temporal sense to refer to expansionism in the era of capitalism, and also has a spatial dimension to its meaning in that an imperial country is the center from which power flows. Neocolonialism is a term sometimes used to emphasize the ongoing and contemporary forms of colonialism whereby ex-colonial powers and more recent superpowers such as the United States continue to play a decisive role in nations that have achieved political independence. Insidious control may continue through the neoliberal[26] power of multinational corporations that artificially fix prices in world markets, and through a variety of other educational and cultural nongovernmental organizations.[27] Notably, postcolonialism signifies the possibilities for ongoing resistance to all forms of domination through theory, politics, and practice with a vision for societies built on respect.

The origins of the field of study are typically attributed to scholars and activists Aimé Césaire (with his 1950 *Discourse on Colonialism*), Franz Fanon (with his 1952 *Black Skin, White Masks* and 1961 *The Wretched of the Earth*), Albert Memmi (with his 1965 *The Colonizer and the Colonized*), and Edward Said (with his 1978 *Orientalism*);[28] and further built on by critics Gayatri Spivak[29] and Homi Bhabha.[30] From its inception, the field has been remarkably interdisciplinary in nature with uptake in the humanities and social sciences, especially in literary criticism, as well as in professional schools such as law and nursing. As postcolonial critique has been widely taken up in the "literary turn" and institutionalized in the Western academy, Parry[31] notes that the material consequences of power differentials rooted in colonizing relations have increasingly been de-emphasized. Yet, in the real worlds of illness and suffering, health and health services, these material consequences take form in social and health inequities of tremendous significance. The critique of essentialism has been levied against postcolonialism, drawing attention to the potentially homogenizing effect of grouping the colonial experience of many under one term. Ashcroft et al. explain, "every colonial encounter or 'contact zone' is different, and each 'post-colonial' occasion needs, against these general background principles, to be precisely located and analysed for its specific interplay."[32] The integration of feminist theories with postcolonialism[33] is one response to counter any homogenizing effect and to highlight intersecting forces of patriarchy and race-based colonizing that produce particular experiences of oppression for women, children, and other marginalized members of society.

Postcolonial analyses foreground certain conceptual themes that are salient for nursing scholarship at the juncture of religion, nursing, and ethics, but that have been largely absent from it. The range of key concepts explored under the umbrella of postcolonial studies is growing (indicative of the vibrancy of the field) and include: issues of slavery, migration, and diaspora formation; the effects of race, culture, class, and gender in postcolonial settings; the history of resistance and struggle against colonial and neocolonial domination; the complexities of identity formation and hybridity; language and language rights; and the ongoing struggles of indigenous peoples for recognition of their rights. More recent developments in postcolonial theory address globalization, environmentalism, speciesism, transnationalism, the sacred, economics, and the spread of neoliberalism.[34] Although the language of empire and colony may seem far removed from the day-to-day concerns of nurses, holding up for scrutiny taken-for-granted assumptions that can be traced back to some form of colonizing practices holds promise for nursing scholarship and practice.

CRITICAL CONTRIBUTIONS OF POSTCOLONIAL THEORY TO THE STUDY OF RELIGION, NURSING, AND NURSING ETHICS

For the purposes of this chapter, the postcolonial concepts of epistemic privilege and representation of Other; race and racialization; and hybridity and identity will be applied to the topic of religion and spirituality in nursing and nursing ethics. These three domains are interlaced with social relations of power, with both domination and resistance as operatives. Likewise, the dialectics of individual and society, the local and the global are relevant to each of these domains. Inherent in contemporary postcolonial theorizing is situating human experience (e.g., everyday reality) in the mediating contexts of social, economic, political, and historical force.[35]

Epistemic Privilege and Marginality

At the heart of postcolonial critique is the matter of epistemological privilege, epitomized by Eurocentrism that has taken on various historical and local forms but that consistently establish European (Western/Northern) systems and values as inherently superior to indigenous or "other" ways. Said's *Orientalism* laid the foundation for this type of critique, in which he drew attention to the ways in which the Orient (and other non-European societies) was not only influenced by the West, but was in effect produced by its relationship to Europe.[36] Postcolonial critics draw attention to the extent to which Enlightenment thinking (characterized by its rationalism, dualisms, individualism, objectivity, visions of development, and progress) has been taken as universal, whereby the experience of Western people (especially men) is taken as the norm for all people. Using the terminology of "provincializing Europe," Chakrabarty speaks to the decentering endeavor of finding out how and in what sense European ideas that were deemed "universal were also, at one and the same time, drawn from very particular intellectual and historical traditions that could not claim any universal validity."[37] This line of critique opens up the possibility for Spivak's question: "can the subaltern speak?"[38]

This question and the related problematic of the epistemological privilege of Eurocentrism carry particular relevance for the study of religion. Ammerman[39] critiques the secularization theories that have dominated the academy and Western societies as a type of Eurocentrism that ". . . like all such stories belongs to those who have the power to speak it. It has been crafted to make sense of the lives of those whose lives 'count' in ways that other lives do not."[40] Shani[41] similarly participates in decentering secularism narratives, pointing out that Islamic and Sikh communities reject the subordination of the religious to the political and thus challenge the Westphalian order (of separation of state and church). King[42] explicates how Orientalism and Western constructions of the "mystic east" as preeminently "otherworldly," private, and apolitical operate in conjunction to obfuscate the relations of power controlling the Orient. Similarly, indigenous peoples faced cultural and spiritual erasure through the colonizing efforts of the Europeans that constructed indigenous worldviews as "savage" and/or "exotic." By questioning epistemic privilege and marginalization, postcolonial theory prompts questions about how discourses of secularism can create spaces for open expression of values and beliefs, and when they function as a secular fundamentalism where only certain perspectives are counted as legitimate. Even where religion is considered as a legitimate focus for inclusion in academic study, McGuire and Maduro observe that "too often, the people whose meaningful religious practices have been redefined by the powerful as not properly 'religious' have been the poor, women, immigrants, indigenous peoples of a colonized land, the 'uneducated,' the dispossessed—in short, the Other among us."[43]

Thus, postcolonial theory alerts us to Westernized "lenses" through which we make sense of the world, and situations when these lenses are applied in an unquestioning, totalizing way, that places other ways of knowing and being on the periphery as Other. Jantzen, writing of the uneasy intersections of postcolonialism, feminism, and religion, suggests that Western study of religion should be less concerned with alterity (difference) and take a hard look instead "at our own investment in 'sameness,' and the technologies of power that we use to reinforce and impose our 'normativity.'"[44] To the extent that nursing scholarship portrays spirituality as a generic individualized phenomenon strategically distanced from religion, there is a risk of reinscribing Eurocentric epistemic privilege and Othering those expressions of religion and spirituality that do not neatly fit into a generic universal spirituality. Kwok suggests that "the appeal to universal human experience and the inability to respect diverse cultures are expressions of a colonizing motive: the incorporation of the Other into one's own culture or perspective."[45] Yet, the propensity toward universal constructions of spirituality in nursing can also be seen as gendered resistance to the dominant patriarchal voices of organized religion, and as mirroring the eclectic, creative expressions of contemporary "lived religion."[46]

In the mood of postmodern times, ethical theory—where it claims universalism—has increasingly been supplanted by contextualized ethical theories, and postcolonial voices echo this call. Yet, there remains a concern about moral imperialism and epistemic violence as bioethical theories are uncritically applied.[47] Western bioethics foreground principalism in ethical decision making, framing several principles (e.g., autonomy, distributive justice, beneficence, non-maleficence, fidelity) as universal, yet, as argued by Chattopadhyay and De Vries,[48] these principles are derived from Western secular belief systems that are not responsive to the cultural ethos and moral sensibilities of non-Western worldviews. Filipina ethicists Tan Alora and Lumitao articulate the results of these different worldviews,

> The very character of ethics in the West contrasts with ethics in the Philippines. . . . The focus of Western bioethics is individual; elsewhere it focuses on social units. Western bioethics often is oriented to principles; Filipino bioethics, on the other hand, is not articulated primarily in principles but in lived moral virtues. Whereas Western bioethics is almost always expressed in discursive terms, Filipino bioethics is part of the phenomenological world of living experience. For the West, bioethics is a framework for thought, a conceptual system. For the Philippines, it is a way of life, an embodied activity of virtue.[49]

Along similar lines, Myser[50] describes the "normativity of whiteness" present in mainstream bioethics discourse, a normativity that continues to propagate individualist emphases that are less likely to take seriously concerns regarding social justice and health inequities that fall along lines of class, gender, and race. A postcolonial lens takes seriously the charges of White normativity and moral imperialism, and requires the naming of these epistemological dominances, reflexivity regarding the complicity of us as academics in reinscribing a form of colonial relations, and shifts in power to welcome full participation of currently marginalized voices to revise mainstream ethical theories and practices.[51]

Disrupting Race-thought: Race, Religion, and the Racialization of Religion

Epistemic privilege and construction of marginalized Other is exemplified in the race-laden discourses of the colonial era that continue to reverberate through today's racialization of religion. Earlier the observation was made that nursing scholarship has, in conjunction with universalist portrayals of spirituality, tended toward culturalist approaches to religion as the common mode of exploring "difference" in nursing, reinforced by the frameworks of cultural competence and cultural sensitivity. A culturalist focus essentializes culture as a relatively static set of beliefs, values, norms, and practices attached to a discrete group sharing a common ethnic background. Likewise, a culturalist read of religion results in a conflation where religion is typically subsumed under ethnicity, again with enduring intrinsic beliefs and practices. Undoubtedly, the ties between religion and ethnicity are complicated and enmeshed. Asad[52] observes that anthropological readings of religion (often with a search for the essence of religion) served to separate it conceptually from the domain of power. Through a postcolonial lens, the politics of race are layered on to religion and spirituality to make visible how colonizing relationships were and continue to be enacted—and resisted—through religion.

Postcolonial theory invites the study of the complex interplay of colonialism and religion in the missionary movements that coincided with the era of European colonial expansion. Historically, the "discovery" of the New World in the 15th century with the subsequent centuries of expansion required dramatic revision to the Renaissance worldview that human beings were all descendants of the same family tree.[53] Race-thinking resulted, which classified human beings into physically, biologically, and genetically distinct groups that allowed colonialist powers to establish dominance over subject peoples and thereby justify the imperial enterprise.[54] A binary distinction was drawn between the "modern/civilized" and the "primitive/savage." Kwok explains,

> As colonial desire and imperialistic violence were masked and reconstituted in a blatant reversal as "civilizing mission," the Christian church played important roles through the sending of missionaries, establishing churches and schools, and propagating ideas of cleanliness and hygiene. Christianization and Westernization became almost a synonymous process in the colonial period[55]

(exemplified historically in the Spanish-Catholic colonization of South America). The history of slavery in the United States follows a similar story of religious rhetoric implicated in the degradation of people of Color and claims of White supremacy.[56] Recently, religious rhetoric mobilized a neo-conservative U.S. "warrior-state" in a move of imperial violence and expansionism with the apparent support of millions of nationalist evangelicals.[57]

The history of missions and the complicity of the church with colonizing state powers is clearly exemplified in the residential school system, operated by several religious groups including Anglican, Catholic, and United churches, which was widespread across Canada (as in other settler colonies such as New Zealand and Australia).[58] The Royal Commission on Aboriginal People[59] reports that from the mid-1800s to as recent as 1996, more than 100,000 children were taken into this version of state care, under the state policy of assimilation, that included the systematic suppression of language and culture, substandard living conditions, and second-rate education. The legacies of these schools—that saw First Nations children traumatized by enforced removal from their communities and some sexually, physically, spiritually, and emotionally brutalized—continue today as intergenerational trauma, and a key factor in Aboriginal Canadians' inequitable health status and access to health services.[60] Reflecting on the coexisting horrific oppression and benevolent efforts of these residential schools in her book *Victims of Benevolence: The Dark Legacy of the Williams Lake Residential School*, Furniss notes that

> Native people have responded to the forces of change brought in through colonialism with both resistance and accommodation. It is not surprising, therefore, that First Nations people today have different understandings of their residential school experiences. Some students strenuously resisted the system, others quietly made the best of their circumstances, while still others became dedicated members of the church.[61]

Although the story of Euro-American expansion and the story of missions are deeply intertwined, the relations between them are complex, filled with discontinuities and contradictions.[62] Decades ago, Memmi[63] notes that although colonizers and churches often worked together to maintain ruthless colonial relation, the conversionist agenda of the churches was often seen by colonial administrators as subversive of colonial hierarchical relations. Moreover, the role of missions in providing education and health care was construed as a dangerous act by many traders and settlers.[64] Mission presses were often the first places in which colonized people were able to find a voice, albeit under deeply constrained circumstances. Spiritual communities historically and presently have served as sites for generating anticolonialist resistance. For example, liberation theology (in which Paulo Freire's work is located),[65] originating in the Americas, fosters solidarity among groups from

Korea to Africa to South America to the Black Church in the United States. Young observes that important sites of anticolonial resistance lie in "movements of religious revivalism: anti-colonial discontent articulated through religious movements that assert a traditional indigenous culture in the name of a utopic decolonized future."[66]

With globalization, religion has reemerged as one of the key defining features of "difference."[67] Given the neocolonial configurations that continue to flow from earlier colonial dominance, it is not surprising that notions of "pagan," "primitive," and "infidel" are imbricated in today's racialization of religion. The racialization of religion occurs when one's national or ethnic heritage (real or imagined) is confounded with one's religion (and vice versa). Joshi[68] writes how South Asians (who may be a Hindu, a Sikh, or a Muslim) have been increasingly marginalized since the terrorist attacks in New York, deemed non-Christian Other. Racialization operates with a logic that makes the accompanying oppression invisible and/or acceptable by rendering non-Christian faiths as "theologically, socially and morally illegitimate in the public eye."[69]

In a recent study in Canada, Sikh patients and care providers recounted situations in which they were disadvantaged in hospital settings on account of their religion and ethnicity. Their concerns ranged from a lack of regard for religious prohibitions (such as cutting arm hair during preparation for intravenous infusion), a lack of accommodation for larger groups of visitors, to the comment that racism was an underlying attitude prevalent in hospitals.[70] The racialization of religion has real consequences for nurses at the level of social ethics, and my contention is that theoretical frameworks such as that offered by postcolonialism are vital to countering the discrimination and marginalization that accompanies the racialization of religion.

Hybridity and Identity

A postcolonial reading of religion and spirituality also draws attention to the complexities of identity and hybridity, particularly in how religion and spirituality are lived out in the everyday. Hybridity refers to the creation of new cultural forms within the contact zone produced by colonization.[71] Postcolonial critique has targeted modernist understandings of identity that rely on discrete categories such as same/other, rational/irrational, civilized/primitive, Christian/pagan, White/Black, male/female, rich/poor.[72] These categories have been supported with a range of exclusionary practices and resistant responses. Postcolonial theories examine the agendas that drive these polarizations, undermine the distinctions, and explore the in-between spaces in which people live in the everyday. According to Bhabha, "it is in the 'inter'—the cutting

edge of translation and negotiation, the *in-between space*—that carries
the burden of the meaning of culture."[73] Hybridity creates the space for
resistance to the hardened identities of colonialism, deconstructing essentialist notions of race and discrete cultural or—in the interest of this
volume—religious groups. Keller et al. explain ". . . in contexts where
boundaries are established to identify some as insiders, some as out,
the space collapses for this in-between existence of hybrid identities . . .
the systematic demand for fixed identities and absolute differences is
undermined . . ."[74]

Applied to religion, hybridity reflects the complex mixing of individual
(and institutional) religious/spiritual subjectivities in today's global societies.
Migration, gender, nationality, class, education, and age all factor into how
individuals live out religion. For example, Ramji notes that although the
Islamic diaspora in western countries is often viewed as a homogenous entity,
second generation Muslim women in Canada created their own *bricolages* of
religious identities within a wider Canadian context:

> These are not women who are just carrying out the traditions of their
> immigrant parents in a kind of exercise in religio-cultural preservation;
> nor are they women who are simply "assimilating" to the dominant cul-
> ture. . . . Their Islam is innovative rather than imitative, individual rather
> than communitarian, and covers . . . a vast spectrum of attitudes and
> behaviours. . . ."[75]

Employing the construct of hybridity as analytic lens thus compels reflexivity about the fluidity of the categories by which people, practices, and texts
are labeled as "Christian," "Muslim," "Jewish," "Buddhist," or "secular."[76]

Hybrid identities create ethical spaces for connections with alterity or
the Other, what has been referred to as an "ethics of hybridity."[77] At the
individual level, an ethics of hybridity is characterized by moral agency and
relational connections. By blurring the boundaries of Other, colonial identities are resisted and opportunities are created for strategic engagement
around shared aspects of one's identity. At the level of the social, Leela Gandhi
maps out how a postcolonial approach to an ethics of hybridity can result in a
"postnational utopia" of "an inter-civilizational alliance against institutional
suffering."[78] Here, the connections between postcolonial theorizing and
religious concerns are accentuated, to the extent that religions address
themes of suffering and utopian visions.

In summary, the analytic themes of postcolonial theory can shed new
light on how religion and spirituality might be taken up in nursing ethics.
Postcolonialism's attention to epistemic privilege uncovers the Eurocentric
tendencies of ethical theory and challenges us to "hear" and integrate marginalized ethical perspectives. We are challenged to critically examine the
locations from which we speak and how secularized versions of spirituality

and racialized religion might inadvertently silence those we provide health care to. Disrupting race-thought opens routes to social justice, whereby the racialization of religion is named and resisted. Finally, postcolonial conceptions of hybridity serve to counter essentializing tendencies in the realm of religion and spirituality, provide more accurate accounts for the ways individuals "live" religion, and open spaces for connection and moral agency. In the concluding section, I move from theory to application, discussing briefly the "methods" or strategies of postcolonialism.

ETHICAL IMPLICATIONS FOR CRITIQUE, REFLEXIVITY, AND PRAXIS

Critical inquiry, such as that enabled by postcolonial theory, encompasses three strategies; those of critique, reflexivity, and praxis. In the realm of religion, nursing, and ethics, these three strategies provide counterbalance to each. As elucidated in this essay, postcolonial theory offers cogent critique of the relations of power carried forward from the colonial era to continually circulate at the intersections of religion, race, and gender. Clearly, critique is needed of the culpability of religions—often together with the joint vices of patriarchy and racism—in oppressions, violence, and exclusions that result in social and health inequities. Critique also has us interrogate the universalist tendencies of secular spiritualities and the essentialist propensities of racialized religion; critique prompts us to question whether current nursing conceptions of a generic spirituality focused on meaning and purpose (at predominantly individual levels) represent dominant voices in nursing (White, Western, middle-class) that marginalize other expressions and practices (e.g., of creedal religion, particularly non-Christian religions). Yet, there is reason to proceed cautiously with our critique in the sacred sphere, recognizing, first, that one's faith-based values and beliefs are often held closely, definitional to one's identity[79] and, second, the indeterminacy of the mystical, transcendent realm.

The second strategy of critical inquiry, that of reflexivity, has us question: "How am I complicit in the colonizer/colonized dialectic?" and "From what epistemic location do I speak?" Spirituality discourses in nursing can be highly personalized with the implicit message that these are not open for critical scrutiny (the point made above), and yet what is required is a certain critical reflexivity that evaluates how the position one takes can unwittingly serve to advantage or disadvantage. Critical reflexivity goes far beyond "cultural awareness" to consider "otherness" within oneself. Critical reflexivity hinges self-knowledge to one's social location in the world as antidote to self-absorption. The call is thus for a "reflexive ethics" that interrogates relations of power that preclude social justice and human flourishing and, especially, one's complicity in these relations of power, thereby leading to praxis.

Postcolonialism's strategy of praxis reminds us of the transformative ideals of human flourishing and social justice that are possible at the juncture of religion, nursing, and ethics. To achieve these ends, there is a need to decolonize religion and spirituality by decoupling religious oppression and spiritual engagement. Restorative, liberatory themes need to be brought to our ethical discourses to counter violent histories and to decolonize religion. Enriching our ethical discourse with various religious and theological traditions will begin the project of decentering the moral imperialism of traditional Western bioethics. As our praxis-oriented interests in the hybrid between spaces of interdependence "shift from boundary protection to border crossings,"[80] inclusive moral communities will be established that focus on democratic, contextual, and respectful engagement. Inclusive moral communities not to foster sameness, but to inhabit meaningful spaces that foster "dialogical deliberation and symmetric participation."[81]

Here there is pause to consider the contributions of religious ethics. Are religious ethics—as ethical frameworks that derive explicitly from religious and/or theological traditions—capable of participating in the enterprise of decolonization through critique, reflexivity, and praxis, or are they too complicit (historically and/or currently) with colonialism? This edited volume offers glimpses of how ethics aligned with a faith tradition might take up the critical work represented by postcolonial theory and other forms of critical inquiry. Concerns shared by faith traditions[82] include theologies of liberation, feminism, ecology, and human rights. Cahill notes that certain features of religion make them particularly effective voices in the realm of ethics: "religions share a drive toward coherence, prophetic resistance to exploitation, and a transcendent framework for evaluating human projects . . . religion still remains a potent political force that can help to form social virtues of solidarity, commitment, and hope."[83] The role of religions in the public sphere is a contested matter, as many societies are increasingly seeing the inadequacy of distinctions between secular and sacred, public and private. The arguments against religious participation in the public realm commonly cite religiously motivated conflict, authoritarianism, faction and division, and the lack of common ground. Yet, Guinn[84] contends that such arguments miss the point because religion cannot be excluded; it has an "inevitable presence" on account of the relevance religion holds in the lives of many citizens. Although there is variation as to the extent to which secularism has taken hold (with European states as the most secular), for the most part, the "secular" sphere is not neutral, "since all participants inevitably come from communities of identity."[85] The challenge ahead is that of reintegrating religious perspectives into public discourse in a way that is representative and respectful of today's pluralistic societies, with the goal of providing a distinctive contribution to ethical discourses.

I have attempted to make a case for the contributions of postcolonial theory (as one type of critical inquiry) to the interplay of religion and nursing ethics. At the least, a postcolonial stance cautions against stereotyping and essentializing, calls for the giving of voice to marginalized groups, and brings attention to the social context and relations of power that serve as backdrop to the consideration of religion and nursing ethics. A fuller engagement with postcolonial theory calls into question the epistemic privilege that has dominated ethics in nursing and health care, disrupts race-based thinking that leads to social and health inequities, and opens hybrid spaces for social transformation.

> *"At its best the postcolonial embrace of complexity*
> *may stimulate not only analysis but action, not only*
> *the ironies of ambivalence but the conditions of hope."*[86]

NOTES

1. Hervieu-Léger, cited in Berger, Peter, Grace Davie, and Effie Fokas. *Religious America and Secular Europe? A Theme and Variations*. Surrey, UK: Ashgate, 2008.

2. Clarke, Warren, and Grant Schellenberg. *Who's Religious?* Statistics Canada, Ottawa, ON. Web. 3 Jan. 2011. http://www.statcan.gc.ca/pub/11-008-x/2006001/9181-eng.htm

3. Todd, Douglas. *Cascadia: The Elusive Utopia. Exploring the Spirit of the Pacific Northwest*. Vancouver, BC: Ronsdale Press, 2008.

4. Berger, Peter, Grace Davie, and Effie Fokas. *Religious America and Secular Europe? A Theme and Variations*. See also: Lynch, Gordon. *The New Spirituality: An Introduction to Progressive Belief in the Twenty-first Century*. London: I. B. Tauris, 2007. See also: Wuthnow, Robert. *America and the Challenges of Religious Diversity*. Princeton, NJ: Princeton University Press, 2005.

5. Amoah, Elizabeth. "African Spirituality, Religion and Innovation." *Religion: Empirical Studies*. Ed. Steven, Sutcliffe. Burlington: Ashgate, 2004. 219.

6. Berger, Peter, Grace Davie, and Effie Fokas. *Religious America and Secular Europe? A Theme and Variations*.

7. Casanova, José. "Immigration and the New Religious Pluralism: A European Union-United States Comparison." *Secularism, Religion and Multicultural Citizenship*. Ed. Goeffrey Levey and Tariq Modood. Cambridge, UK: Cambridge University Press, 2009. 139–163.

8. Moghadam, Assaf. *A Global Resurgence of Religion? Paper No. 03-03*. Cambridge, MA: Weatherhead Center for International Affairs, Harvard University, 2003. See also: Thomas, Scott. *The Global Resurgence of Religion and the Transformation of International Relations: The Struggle for the Soul of the Twenty-first Century*. New York: Palgrave Macmillan, 2005.

9. Thomas, Scott. *The Global Resurgence of Religion and the Transformation of International Relations: The Struggle for the Soul of the Twenty-first Century*.

10. Modood, Tariq. "Muslims, Religious Equality and Secularism." *Secularism, Religion and Multicultural Citizenship*. Ed. Geoffrey Levey and Modood Tariq. Cambridge, UK: Cambridge University Press, 2009. 164–185.

11. Ammerman, Nancy. "The Challenges of Pluralism: Locating Religion in a World of Diversity." *Social Compass* 57 (2010): 154–167. See also: Banchoff, Thomas, ed. *Religious Pluralism, Globalization, and World Politics*. Oxford: Oxford University Press, 2008.

12. Gilliat-Ray, Sophie. "Nursing, Professionalism and Spirituality." *Journal of Contemporary Religion* 18.3 (2003): 339.

13. Reimer-Kirkham, Sheryl, and Joan Anderson. "The Advocate-analyst Dialectic in Critical and Postcolonial Feminist Research: Reconciling Tensions around Scientific Integrity." *Advances in Nursing Science* 33.3 (2010): 204.

14. Pesut, Barbara, Marsha Fowler, Elizabeth Johnston Taylor, Sheryl Reimer-Kirkham, and Rick Sawatzky. "Conceptualizing Spirituality and Religion for Healthcare." *Journal of Clinical Nursing* 17.21 (2008): 2803–2810. See also: Reimer Kirkham, Sheryl, Barb Pesut, Heather Meyerhoff and Richard Sawatzky. "Spiritual Care-giving at the Juncture of Religion, Culture, and State." *Canadian Journal of Nursing Research* 36.4. (2004): 248–269.

15. See, for instance, Anderson, Joan. "Toward a Post-Colonial Feminist Methodology in Nursing Research: Exploring the Convergence of Post-Colonial and Black Feminist Scholarship." *Nurse Researcher: The International Journal of Research Methodology in Nursing and Health Care* 9.3 (2002):7–27. And: Browne, Annette J., Vicki Smye, and Colleen Varcoe. Postcolonial-Feminist Theoretical Perspectives and Women's Health. *Women's Health in Canada: Critical Perspectives on Theory and Policy*. Ed. Marina Morrow, Olena Hankivsky, and Colleen Varcoe. Toronto: University of Toronto Press, 2007. 124–142. See also: Mohammed, Selina. "Moving Beyond the 'Exotic': Applying Postcolonial Theory in Health Research." *Advances in Nursing Science* 29.2 (2006):98–109. See also: Racine, Louise. "Examining the Conflation of Multiculturalism, Sexism, and Religious Fundamentalism through Taylor and Bakhtin: Expanding Post-Colonial Feminist Epistemology." *Nursing Philosophy* 10 (2008): 14–25. See also: Reimer Kirkham, Sheryl, and Joan M. Anderson. "Postcolonial Nursing Scholarship: From Epistemology to Method." *Advances in Nursing Science* 25.1 (2002): 1–17.

16. Robert Young (2001) as cited in Taylor, Mark. "Spirit and Liberation. Achieving Postcolonial Theology in the United States." *Postcolonial Theologies: Divinity and Empire*. Ed. Catherine Keller, Michael Nausner, and Mayra Rivera. St. Louis: Chalice Press, 2004. 48.

17. Ashcroft, Bill, Gareth Griffiths, and Helen Tiffin. *Post-colonial Studies: The Key Concepts*. 2nd ed. London: Routledge, 2007. 188.

18. Fitzgerald, Timothy. *Discourse on Civility and Barbarity: A Critical History of Religion and Related Categories*. Oxford: Oxford University Press, 2007. 6.

19. Fitzgerald, Timothy. *Discourse on Civility and Barbarity: A Critical History of Religion and Related Categories*.

20. Young, Robert. *Postcolonialism: A Very Short Introduction*. New York: Oxford University Press, 2003. 2.

21. Crossley, Michael, and Leon Tikly. "Postcolonial Perspectives and Comparative and International Research in Education: A Critical Introduction." *Comparative Education* 40.2 (2004): 147–156.

22. Hall, Stuart. "Gramsci's Relevance for the Study of Race and Ethnicity." *Journal of Communicaion Inquiry* 10.2 (1986): 5–27. Rpt. in *Stuart Hall. Critical Dialogues in Cultural Studies*. Ed. Morley David, Kuan-Hsing Chen. London: Routledge, 1997.

23. McClintock, Anne. "The Angel of Progress: Pitfalls of the Term "Post-colonialism." *Social Text Spring* (1992): 1–15. Rpt in *Colonial Discourses and Post-Colonial Theory: A Reader.* Ed. Patrick Williams and Laura Chrisman. New York: Columbia University Press, 1994.
24. Loomba, Ania. *Colonialism/Postcoloniaism.* 2nd ed. London: Routledge, 2005.
25. Ibid., 4.
26. Neo-liberalism is a term used by many critics to describe the liberalization and globalization of market forces. This prevailing ideological paradigm leads to social, economic, and political approaches that emphasize individualism, individual freedom and responsibility; efficiency; egalitarianism; and free market economies that, in effect, shift risk from governments and corporations onto individuals. See: Ong, Aihwa. *Neoliberalism as Exception: Mutations in Citizenship and Sovereignty.* Durham, NC: Duke University Press, 2006. See also: Browne, Annette. "The Influence of Liberal Political Ideology on Nursing Science." *Nursing Inquiry* 8.2 (2001): 118–129. Ashcroft et al. assert that neo-liberalism is significant for postcolonial studies because it has become the most obvious medium of today's neo-colonial domination.
27. Ashcroft, Bill, Gareth Griffiths, and Helen Tiffin. *Post-colonial Studies: The Key Concepts.*
28. Césaire, Aimé. *Discours sur le colonialisme (Discourse on Colonialism),* 1955. See also: Fanon, Franz. *Black Skin, White Mask.* Trans. Charles Lam Markmann. New York: Grove Press, 1967. See also: Fanon, Franz. *The Wretched of the Earth.* Trans. Constance Farrington. New York: Grove Weidenfeld, 1963. See also: Memmi, Albert. *The Colonizer and the Colonized.* Boston: The Orion Press, 1965. See also: Said, Edward. *Orientalism.* New York: Vintage Books, 1978.
29. Spivak, Gayatri Chakravorty. "Can the Subaltern Speak?" *Marxism and the Interpretation of Culture.* Ed. Cary Nelson and Lawrence Grossberg. London: Macmillan, 1988. Rpt. in *Colonial Discourse and Post-Colonial Theory: A Reader.* Ed. Patrick Williams and Laura Chrisman. New York: Columbia University Press, 1994.
30. Bhabha, Homi, ed. *Nation and Narration.* Routledge, 1990. And also: Bhabha, Homi. *The Location of Culture.* Routledge, 1994.
31. Parry, Benita. *Postcolonial Studies: A Materialist Critique.* London: Routledge, 2004.
32. Ashcroft, Bill, Gareth Griffiths, and Helen Tiffin. *Post-colonial Studies: The Key Concepts.* 171.
33. Anderson, Joan. "Toward a Post-colonial Feminist Methodology in Nursing Research: Exploring the Convergence of Post-colonial and Black Feminist Scholarship." *Nurse Researcher: The International Journal of Research Methodology in Nursing and Health Care* 9.3 (2002):7–27. See also: Bahri, Deepika. "Feminism in/ and Postcolonialism." *The Cambridge Companion to Postcolonial Literary Studies.* Ed. Lazarus, Neil. Cambridge: Cambridge University Press, 2004. 199–220. See also: Lewis, Reina, and Sara Mills. ed. *Feminist Postcolonial Theory: A Reader.* London: Routledge, 2003.
34. Ashcroft, Bill, Gareth Griffiths, and Helen Tiffin. *Post-colonial Studies: The Key Concepts.*
35. Reimer Kirkham, Sheryl, and Joan M. Anderson. "Postcolonial Nursing Scholarship: From Epistemology to Method."
36. Ashcroft, Bill, Gareth Griffiths, and Helen Tiffin. *Post-colonial Studies: The Key Concepts.*

37. Chakrabarty, Dipesh. *Provincializing Europe: Postcolonial Thought and Historical Difference*. Princeton, NJ: Princeton University Press, 2000. xiii.

38. Spivak, Gayatri Chakravorty. Can the Subaltern Speak?

39. Ammerman, Nancy. "The Challenges of Pluralism: Locating Religion in a World of Diversity."

40. Maduro, Otto. "Religion" Under Imperial Duress: Postcolonial Reflections and Proposals." *Review of Religious Research* 45.3 (2004): 221–234.

41. Shani, Giorgio. "Religion, Politics and International Relations. 'Provincializing' Critical Theory: Islam, Sikhism and International Relations Theory." *Cambridge Review of International Affairs* 20.3 (2007): 417–433.

42. King, Richard. *Orientalism and Religion. Postcolonial Theory, India and 'The Mystic East'*. London: Routledge, 1999.

43. McGuire, Meredith, and Otto Maduro. "Introduction. Rethinking Religious Hybridity." *Social Compass* 52.4 (2005): 412.

44. Jantzen, Grace. "Uneasy Intersections: Postcolonialism, Feminism, and the Study of Religions." *Postcolonial Philosophy of Religion*. Ed. Purushottama, Bilimori and Andrew Irvine. Springer, 2009. 295–301.

45. Kwok, Pui-lan. *Postcolonial Imagination and Feminist Theology*. Louisville, KY: Westminster John Knox Press. 2005. 56.

46. McGuire, Meredith. *Lived Religion: Faith and Practice in Everyday Life*. New York: Oxford University Press, 2008.

47. Tan Alora, Angeles, and Josephine M. Lumitao, ed. *Beyond a Western Bioethics: Voices from the Developing World*. Washington: Georgetown University Press, 2001. See also: Arekapudi, Swathi, and Mathew K. Wynia. "The Unbearable Whiteness of the Mainstream: Should We Eliminate, or Celebrate, Bias in Bioethics?" *American Journal of Bioethics* 3 (2003): 18–19. See also: Chattopadhyay, Subrata, and Richard De Vries. "Bioethical Concerns are Global, Bioethics is Western." *Eubios Journal of Asian and International Bioethics* 18.4 (2008): 106–109.

48. Chattopadhyay, Subrata, and Richard De Vries. "Bioethical Concerns are Global, Bioethics is Western."

49. Tan Alora, Angeles, and Josephine M. Lumitao, ed. *Beyond a Western Bioethics: Voices from the Developing World*.

50. Myser, Catherine. "Differences from Somewhere: The Normativity of Whiteness in Bioethics in the United States." *The American Journal of Bioethics* 3.2 (2003): 1–11.

51. Myser, Catherine. "Differences from Somewhere: The Normativity of Whiteness in Bioethics in the United States."

52. Asad, Talal. *Genealogies of Religion: Discipline and Reasons of Power in Christianity and Islam*. Baltimore, MD: Johns Hopkins University Press, 1993.

53. Kwok, Pui-lan. *Postcolonial Imagination and Feminist Theology*.

54. Ashcroft, Bill, Gareth Griffiths, and Helen Tiffin. *Post-colonial Studies: The Key Concepts*.

55. Kwok, Pui-lan. *Postcolonial Imagination and Feminist Theology*. 17.

56. Burton, Olivette. "Why Bioethics Cannot Figure out What to do With Race." *The American Journal of Bioethics* 7.2 (2007): 6–12.

57. Taylor, Mark. "Spirit and Liberation. Achieving Postcolonial Theology in the United States." *Postcolonial Theologies: Divinity and Empire*. Ed. Catherine Keller, Michael Nausner, and Mayra Rivera. St. Louis: Chalice Press, 2004. 39–55.

58. Furniss, Elizabeth. *Victims of Benevolence: The Dark Legacy of the Williams Lake Residential School*. Vancouver, BC: Arsenal Pulp Press, 1995. See also: Fiske,

Joanne. "Pocahanta's Granddaughters: Spiritual Transition and Tradition of Carrier Women in British Columbia." *Ethnohistory* 43.3 (1996): 663–681.
59. Royal Commission on Aboriginal Peoples, 1996. Web. 15 Apr. 2011. http://www .ainc-inac.gc.ca/ap/rrc-eng.asp.
60. Smith, Dawn, Colleen Varcoe, and Nancy Edwards. "Turning Around the Inter-generational Impact of Residential Schools on Aboriginal Peoples: Implications for Health Policy and Practice." *Canadian Journal of Nursing Research* 37.4 (2005): 38–60.
61. Furniss, Elizabeth. *Victims of Benevolence: The Dark Legacy of the Williams Lake Residential School.* 34.
62. Ashcroft, Bill, Gareth Griffiths, and Helen Tiffin. *Post-colonial Studies: The Key Concepts.* See also: Rieger, Joerg. "Theology and Mission Between Neocolonialism and Postcolonialism. *Mission Studies* 21.2 (2004): 201–226.
63. Memmi, Albert. *The Colonizer and the Colonized.*
64. Ashcroft, Bill, Gareth Griffiths, and Helen Tiffin. *Post-colonial Studies: The Key Concepts.*
65. Lange, Elizabeth. "Fragmented Ethics of Justice: Freire, Liberation Theology and Pedagogies for the Non-Poor." *Convergence* 31.1–2 (1998): 81–94.
66. Young, Robert. *Postcolonialism: An Historical Introduction.* Oxford: Blackwell, 2001.
67. Ashcroft, Bill, Gareth Griffiths, and Helen Tiffin. *Post-colonial Studies: The Key Concepts.*
68. Joshi, Kyati. "The Racialization of Hinduism, Islam, and Sikhism in the United States." *Equity and Excellence in Education* 39.3 (2006): 211–26.
69. Joshi, Kyati. "The Racialization of Hinduism, Islam, and Sikhism in the United States." 211.
70. Reimer-Kirkham, Sheryl. "Lived Religion: Implications for Healthcare Ethics." *Nursing Ethics* 16.4 (2009): 406–17.
71. Ashcroft, Bill, Gareth Griffiths, and Helen Tiffin. *Post-colonial Studies: The Key Concepts.*
72. Keller, Catherine, Michael Nausner, and Mayra Rivera. ed. *Postcolonial Theologies: Divinity and Empire.* St. Louis, MO: Chalice Press. 2004.
73. Bhabha, Homi. *The Location of Culture.* 38.
74. Keller, Catherine, Michael Nausner, and Mayra Rivera. ed. *Postcolonial Theologies: Divinity and Empire.* 12.
75. Ramji, Rubina. "Being Muslim and Being Canadian: How Second Generation Muslim Women Create Religious Identities in two Worlds." *Women and Religion in the West: Challenging Secularization.* Ed. Kristin Aune, Sonya Sharma, and Giselle Vincett. Aldershot, Hampshire, England: Ashgate Publishing, 2008. 204.
76. Klassen, Pamela and Courtney Bender. "Introduction. Habits of Pluralism." *After Pluralism: Re-imagining Religious Engagement.* Ed. Courtney Bender and Klassen Pamela. New York: Columbia University Press. 2010. 1–28. 15.
77. Ghandi, Leela, *Postcolonial Theory: A Critical Introduction.* New York: Columbia University Press, 1998.
78. Ibid., 140.
79. Werbner, Pnina. "Religious Identity." *The Sage Handbook of Identities.* Ed. Margaret Wetherell and Chandra Talpade Mohanty. Los Angeles, CA: Sage, 2010. 233–257.

80. Keller, Catherine, Michael Nausner, and Mayra Rivera. ed. *Postcolonial Theologies: Divinity and Empire*. 14.
81. Deifelt, Wanda. "Intercultural Ethics: Sameness and Difference Re-visited." *Dialog: A Journal of Theology* 46.2 (2007): 118.
82. Referred to as 'interreligious global theological flows' by Robert Schreiter, cited in Cahill, Lisa Sowle. *Theological Bioethics: Participation, Justice, and Change*. Washington, DC: Georgetown University Press, 2005.
83. Cahill, Lisa Sowle. *Theological Bioethics: Participation, Justice, and Change*. 3.
84. Guinn, David. ed. *Handbook of Bioethics and Religion*. New York: Oxford University Press, 2006.
85. Cahill, Lisa Sowle. "Theology's Role in Public Bioethics." In: *Handbook of Bioethics and Religion*. Ed. Robert Guinn. Oxford: Oxford University Press, 2006. 37.
86. Keller, Catherine, Michael Nausner, and Mayra Rivera. ed. *Postcolonial Theologies: Divinity and Empire*. 10

6

Intersectional Analyses of Religion, Culture, Ethics, and Nursing

Sheryl Reimer-Kirkham and Sonya Sharma

INTRODUCTION

Today's global migration has resulted in societies with unprecedented diversity along multiple lines. Global cities are becoming increasingly cosmopolitan, as exemplified in Canada's largest cities reported to have "visible minority" populations nearing the majority.[1] At the same time, the global distribution of wealth is increasingly held in fewer hands[2] with the result that poverty (ranging from homelessness to working poor) is as widespread as ever. Other lines of social classification include (dis)abilities, sexual orientation, and as the focus in this volume, religion/spirituality. The landscape of religious/spiritual affiliation is a complex one with global trends and local specificities. Global migration is resulting in diverse religious profiles in many countries. Even those countries considered most secular (e.g., Europe[3]) are renewing attention to religion as a demographic feature with implications for public policy and social cohesion. Importantly, increased interest in the sacred is also occurring outside institutional religion with the postmodern age marked by personalized explorations of spirituality. Our thesis in this chapter is that in the context of this unprecedented diversity, religion and spirituality need to be understood as intertwined with other social categories such as gender, ethnicity, and class. Referred to as intersectionality, these interrelationships shape how identities are lived out and how social disadvantage and oppression operate in collective ways. The intersectionality of religion/spirituality

113

with other social classifications has, we suggest, not been adequately accounted for in the fields of nursing and nursing ethics. At the level of social ethics, religion and spirituality are implicated in the intersecting social determinants of health and health inequities. In the realm of clinical nursing ethics, a lens of intersectionality gives insight into the complexities of moral agency, ethical decision making, and relational practice.

We begin by providing an overview of intersectional theory. We argue that intersectional theorizing as it is typically employed today needs to be expanded to more intentionally incorporate religion and spirituality. Equally important, religion and spirituality must be understood as intersecting with other social classifications rather than studied as though they operate in isolation. That is, people rarely identify themselves by just religious affiliation or spiritual disposition, but rather understand their religious/spiritual selves in relation to gender, class, ethnicity, and so forth, and may well foreground different dimensions of these identities, depending on circumstance. Because religion and spirituality have been understudied in intersectional theorizing, their place as sites that exacerbate or mitigate disadvantage that ultimately lead to health inequities is not well understood.

A discussion of intersectionality itself illuminates the complex and varied ways in which the constructs of religion and spirituality are taken up.[4] As highlighted in this volume, considerable energy across the years has been put to defining both religion and spirituality, often with the aim of differentiating the two and distancing spirituality from religion. Spirituality, especially in the nursing literature, is commonly portrayed as the internal experience of things of immanent and transcendent nature, and religion as the external social organized pursuit of transcendence (whether named as God, Allah, or another ascription to deity). Rather than landing on a particular definition, an intersectional approach has us (for reasons we develop below) incorporating internal and external, immanent and transcendent dimensions in our conceptualization of religion and spirituality. Although spiritual experience is often intensely private, we caution against viewing it apart from social context (e.g., as purely transcendent), for, even though current discourse constructs spirituality as whatever an individual deems as "special."[5] a point we agree with, the influence of the social world on this individual construction, though not always recognized, is ultimately the interest of intersectionality. Also, in the spirit of intersectionality, less emphasis is put on defining the social constructs of interest (e.g., gender, race, class, sexuality, dis/ability, and—in this discussion—religion and spirituality) as to pin down the very essence of what one is examining, an endeavor that risks essentialism. Rather, these constructs are seen as loose abstractions to which people ascribe various meaning and that are laced with social significance and relations of power. In the case of religion/spirituality, the constellation of meaning hinges loosely on the sacred. A further factor that complicates attempts to define religion and spirituality and that also stands as a call for intersectional approaches to the topic is that of the power of religion and spirituality for inclusion and exclusion. Intersectionality prompts investigation of multiple axes of disadvantage, and the challenge in the case of religion and spirituality is to avoid essentialist constructions that would have them as only oppressor or oppressed.

A PRÉCIS OF INTERSECTIONALITY

Intersectional theorizing is not new, but has gained considerable profile in recent years,[6] popularized by Black feminists such as Crenshaw[7] and Collins.[8] Crenshaw, a legal scholar, uses the image of a road intersection where vehicles coming from different streets collide with a hapless victim. Fault cannot be easily attributed in this situation. By analogy, neither racism nor sexism (as vehicles) is ever held fully accountable for the harm they cause. Crenshaw lamented that the struggles of women of color "fell between the cracks of both feminist and anti-racist discourse."[9] Similarly, Collins argues that black women are uniquely situated at a focal point where two exceptionally powerful and prevalent systems of oppression come together: race and gender. With this foundation, she elucidate how matrices of domination operate; "oppression cannot be reduced to one fundamental type," but rather structural and interpersonal domains of power reappear in spaces of crosscutting interests. Importantly, intersectionality does not "trump" any one category of oppression over another, but rather understands them as a mutually constitutive matrix.[11] In fact, intersectionality's main contributions are fuller and more complex understandings of people's (a) identity formation, especially with an eye to multiple identities and (b) experiences of oppression, and the structural forces that perpetuate these oppressions. There are material consequences in people's lives from these intersecting categories. Intersectionality is premised on the conviction that understanding the social position occupied by black women compels us to see, and look for, other spaces where systems of inequality come together. By understanding the simultaneity and complexity of identities, advantage, and disadvantage (enmeshed in a broad spectrum of structural oppressions), solidarity is achieved, not in an essentialized view of "women's experience" but rather at strategic points in a "politics of solidarity."[12] Hence, intersectionality has, since its inception, been not only an analytic tool but also a political strategy to deconstruct social relations and promote more just alternatives.[13]

INTERSECTIONALITY, RELIGION, AND SPIRITUALITY

There is a mutual corrective that is much needed in bringing religion/ spirituality more overtly and intentionally into intersectionality discourse and praxis. On the one hand, scholars studying and practitioners practicing in relation to religion/spirituality desperately need to complicate their purview. Too often religion and spirituality (particularly in nursing and related health fields) are considered in isolation from the social contexts that unquestionably qualify how religion and spirituality are lived out. On the other hand, our contention is that religion and spirituality are often not taken seriously in intersectional analyses, resulting in incomplete analyses that leave invisible pathways to social inclusion and exclusion.

Complicating Conceptions of Religion/Spirituality With Intersectional Analyses

Increasingly, the emphasis on single categories of identity is seen as inadequate to represent the complexity of social life; for this reason, intersectionality counters one and two dimensional approaches.[14] Drawing on exemplars from a recent study on the negotiation of religious and spiritual plurality in health care, we have elsewhere[15] made a case for enriching the study of religion/spirituality in health care with intersectional analyses. We argue that "more nuanced readings of religion and spirituality are needed to account for how they are lived out in gendered, racialized, and classed ways."[16] Until very recently, religion and spirituality have been typically portrayed as "stand alone" phenomena or social categories, studied in isolation from ethnicity, race, gender, and class. This is particularly so in nursing. Nursing literature has tended to promote acontextual interpretations of spirituality and religion that holds spirituality as a highly personalized phenomenon that is either so transcendent that it is not contaminated with "earthly" realities such as race, class, and gender or so immanent that it is everywhere and everything, making other social categories essentially meaningless. As for religion, many nursing texts, for example, subsume religion under culture or spirituality. When deemed a subcategory of culture, religion is essentialized as a set of static cultural practices. When subsumed within spirituality, religion is often made invisible. In contrast, intersectional analyses foreground social operations of power, making acontextual interpretations of religion and spirituality improbable. By illuminating the complexity of multiple social locations influencing identity, intersectional theorizing guards against reifying or essentializing religion and spirituality. Intersectionality also contends that social categories matter equally, with the relationship between categories open to empirical investigation (specific to each situation).[17] For such reasons, we contend that intersectional frameworks are needed to enrich the study of religion and spirituality in nursing and nursing ethics.

Nursing literature has shown some consideration of feminist interpretations of spirituality (including how gender and spirituality are mutually constitutive), indicative of an interest in intersecting social classifications. However, one could well imagine that the Black feminists who so convincingly argued for intersectional analyses—in part as a mechanism to bring the experience of women of color to the attention of the predominantly White feminist discourse—would offer a heavy critique to feminist studies of spirituality and religion that do not take into account race and class. Indeed, Reuther,[18] noted feminist theologian, observes the criticism in the 1970s and 1980s by women of color of the racial tendencies in an effort to create an "essential" woman within feminism more broadly, and feminist theology in particular.

Religion and Spirituality as More Than "etc."

From another angle, we observe that intersectional analyses have often been deficient in accounting for religion/spirituality as intersecting categories. Shifting trends in regard to religion and spirituality, with the accompanying recognition of the widespread relevance of "lived religion," religion as embodied and experienced in everyday life for many individuals,[19] as well as the relations of power mobilized through religion and spirituality, have led us to make a case for the inclusion of religion and spirituality more routinely in intersectional analyses.[20] Although acknowledging that many scholars have been wary of conservative religion that has sought to colonize political and social organizations and perpetuate patriarchy, there is a need to account for how religion and spirituality are an intricate part of many people's lives, complicating intersections of gender, race, and class.[21] In short, religion and spirituality need more than a perfunctory nod in the position of "etc." at the end of a string of "race, class, and gender."

Sojourner Truth's widely cited speech punctuated with the question "And ain't I a woman?" is described by Brah and Pheonix as deconstructing

> every single major truth-claim about gender in a patriarchal slave social formation. . . . The discourse offers a devastating critique of socio-political, economic and cultural processes of 'othering' while drawing attention to the simultaneous importance of subjectivity—of subjective pain and violence that the inflictors do not often wish to hear about or acknowledge.[22]

Sojourner Truth's words drive to the heart of her spiritual beliefs: "I have borne children and seen most of them sold into slavery, and when

I cried out with a mother's grief, none but Jesus heard me. And ain't I a woman?" Pheonix and Brah acknowledge the foregrounding of the importance of spirituality to this type of activism. Collins, a contemporary Black feminist, often noted as one of the originators of intersectionality, observes that African Americans have long relied on religion and faith-based sources as sites of resistance to racism.[23] She compares the use of religion by immigrant groups as an avenue to maintain group identity to African Americans for whom their religion (Christianity in particular) evolved in response to their suffering under American historical slavery and ongoing racism. She points out that African American spirituality can take on recursive secular or sacred dimensions, contributing powerfully to ethnic identity. From these excerpts, we see that Sojourner Truth and Patricia Hill Collins clearly understand religion and spirituality as integral aspects of identity and resistance, signaling them as integral to intersectional analyses.

Religion and spirituality thus need to be understood as powerful social forces for inclusion and exclusion, particularly as they intersect with other social influences. Because of the intersection with other social influences, inclusion and exclusion do not operate as binaries but often overlap, creating a tension between the two. For example, in recent interviews conducted with women about their experiences of church life,[24] a Black Nigerian woman named Faraa spoke about an experience she had at her church. One day her son was asked to do a Bible reading. After this, people from the congregation whom she identified as White English remarked on how well he read. They went on to say that they could understand her son, but not her husband when he preached. Her husband's position as a university lecturer and a deacon at their church, a mark of esteem and social status, did not alter their viewpoint. Faraa explained that they understood her child because he was raised with an English accent, but when they heard her husband they heard Africa. In North America and Western Europe, Christianity and Whiteness are intimately linked and generate social norms and expectations.[25] Racializing religions such as Christianity, Hinduism, or Sikhism, "results in essentialism; it reduces people to one aspect of their identity and thereby presents a homogeneous, undifferentiated, and static view of an ethnoreligious community."[26] Faraa later said that she disliked being critical of her church because it was a place of belonging and she had close friends there. Her religiosity gave her a place where she experienced a sense of inclusion. However, when religion is overlapped onto culture, ethnicity, and race, it can invoke colonial images of the racialized other, positioning those who are not White Christians or whom do not "fit" the host society's perceptions on the margins, thereby reinscribing longstanding patterns of exclusion and inclusion.[27] Faraa's story demonstrates the contradictions that abound in her church—Christianity seeks universal membership, but can enforce partial norms—and the underlying intersections between religion, race, class, and power.

In summary, intersectional analyses are needed to move beyond singular analyses of religion and spirituality that risk essentializing and/or incomplete analyses. Regardless of methodology or theoretical framework, our goal as scholars is to understand phenomena accurately. Intersectionality can offer a theoretical grid toward this end. Although scholars employing intersectional analyses have tended to shy away from religion/spirituality, examples from Black feminists, immigrant, and indigenous scholars demonstrate how lived experiences of oppression and resistance are often intertwined with religious/spiritual meanings, practices, and structures.[28] In the next section, we focus on a particular dimension of nursing—that of nursing ethics—with the aim of elucidating how intersectional analyses that intentionally incorporate religion and spirituality enhance ethical nursing practice.

INTERSECTIONAL APPLICATIONS TO NURSING ETHICS

Intersectionality in general has not been widely taken up in nursing to-date, although it is emerging as a very helpful analytic framework for nurse scholars working in the field of population health and health disparities.[29] Our discussion here articulates with this emerging discourse, focusing on the nexus of religion and spirituality with other intersecting social differences that contribute to the social determinants of health and health disparities, and nursing ethics. Intersectionality, as a method of inquiry and praxis with its focus on matters of identity and intersecting oppressions, brings particular angles of investigation to the field of nursing ethics, especially with the incorporation of religion and spirituality. We focus on several interrelated domains in which this type of inquiry can especially enrich nursing ethics: social justice and health inequities; and identity and moral agency. In these interdependent domains, intersectionality reminds us of the embeddedness of ethics in the everyday—of "lived ethics" as not only a system of formal theory, but also the mutual shaping of ideas and real life.[30]

Social Pathways to Health Inequities

At the heart of intersectional theorizing is concern for oppression, or those social relations that systematically disadvantage groups of people and act as social pathways to economic, social, and health inequities. Hankivsky and colleagues explain,

> those who engage in intersectionality research or policy are committed to social justice and seek significant shifts in power. Because intersectionality

recognizes relational constructs of social inequality, it is an effective tool for examining how power and power relations are maintained and reproduced.[31]

The moral end (or social good), then, of intersectional praxis is social justice, and for nursing ethics specifically, this end involves addressing social determinants of health and eradicating health inequities. Importantly, here we follow Whitehead's conception of health inequities as "differences in health which are not only unnecessary and avoidable, but in addition are considered unfair and unjust."[32] At this point in time, little research has been conducted that uncovers how religion intersects with other social categories as a determinant of health and health inequities; however, as scholars increasingly document the racializing of religion,[33] and as we understand more about racialization as a determinant of health inequities,[34] this social pathway of intersecting oppressions merits attention. Experts in population health have gathered convincing evidence from studies that repeatedly demonstrate health inequities along the lines of race/ethnicity and gender, although there is still some debate about the exact mechanisms of this differentiation.[35] Here we focus on racialized religion and religious patriarchy as two illustrations of how religion and spirituality can intersect with other social categories to contribute to health inequities.

First, racialization results in essentialism; it reduces people to one aspect of their identity and thereby presents a homogeneous, undifferentiated, and static view of an ethnoreligious community.[36] For example, by phenotypical and cultural markers, South Asian adherents of religions such as Islam, Hinduism, and Sikhism are deemed "other" in societies such as Canada, the USA, Australia, and Britain where Whiteness and Christianity continue to be normative. Joshi points out that the racialization of religion locates certain religious populations within lower social strata of these societies by applying ideological forces in conjunction with social and political relations of domination. In studying the effects of racialization of religion, Joshi found that although South Asians tend to be lumped together as "other," religious identities are also racialized in particular ways. She note that in the current sociopolitical and cultural context, Hinduism tends to be exoticized, Islam demonized, and Sikhism vilified. The sense of danger historically associated with the West's post-Crusades view of the Muslim world, again heightened after terrorist attacks in the United States and Europe, feeds into ideological notions of the other that result in systematic oppression. For example, cleanliness before prayers and eating is very important to practicing Sikhs. Yet, the significance of these practices can be sometimes overlooked within systems of care, whether due to workload of health care professionals or a lack of knowledge about religious rituals within different ethnic communities. It may also be the case, however, that when race and religion are conflated in association with certain ethnic groups, religious practices important to specific communities are ignored or deemed different, resulting in the racialization of religion, and the treatment of health and wellbeing as it relates to the religion and/or spirituality of particular groups as inequitable.

Second, by another angle of analysis, religion as an identity category can lead to further discrimination of women[37] and thus exacerbate social and health inequities. In many societies, religion operating as one of the major social institutions of control by which women and men are treated differently[38] affects worldviews on women's roles and is an element of patriarchal systems.[39] Patriarchal systems of doctrine and practice carry a range of effects, from perpetuating gendered domestic roles to systematically disadvantaging life opportunities (such as education, adequate housing, and income) and negatively and directly impacting health outcomes for women (e.g., in regard to reproductive rights). With the rise of fundamental, politicized forms of religion, and rising global awareness of women's human rights, more attention is being given to oppressive conditions at the intersection of religion and gender. Okin observes "It has become clear, from evidence from many parts of the world and many religions, that fundamentalism of various kinds—many of which are clearly growing in power—is harsh on women and imposes rules irreconcilable with women's rights."[40] For example, within contemporary East Asian Confucian cultures, women have progressed and evolved with modernization and globalization. However, as Nyitray[41] contends, a parallel and digressive fundamentalism is occurring within these societies, resulting in oppression and resistance to women's changing identities and increased opportunities. As such, for many women in fundamentalist contexts, including those in the West, there is a tension between oppression and liberation, accommodation and resistance. Even as women recognize the ways in which fundamentalism can limit their roles, there are many elements within fundamentalist contexts that they negotiate and embrace.[42]

We have highlighted these two examples—racialized religion and religious patriarchy—pertaining to how religion may operate within a "matrix of domination"[43] to differentially impact health outcomes. However, important these oppressions are as determinants of health and health inequities, they are never fully determinate of that experience.[44] Resistance to oppression—at social and individual levels—are expressions of moral agency, often rooted in, taking strength from, or coalescing around the multiple dimensions of identities also made visible through intersectional theory. The personal and the social are intertwined, and in the realm of ethics where moral decisions carry personal consequences, these touch points must be kept in mind.

Identity and Moral Agency

Nursing ethics is increasingly taking an expanded view of moral agency, moving beyond traditional conceptions of agency that emphasize rationality and deliberate choice to contextual views that understand agency as "enacted through relationships and in particular contexts."[45] Moral agency is then "inclusive of rational and self-expressive choice, notions of identity, social and historical relational influences, autonomous action, and embodied engagement."[46] In these ways, we understand moral agency as situated and inevitably shaped by multiple intersecting sources of social identity constituted by race, class, gender, religion/spirituality, and other contextually relevant social classifications.[47]

As with intersecting forms of oppression that demand the attention of nursing ethics, so too do intersecting formations of identity. Taking an intersectional approach to identity provides an invaluable guard against essentialist and oversimplified interpretations of moral agency and "lived ethics." Inhorn, in her exemplary summation of ethnographic research on women's health, points out that moral decisions are inextricably linked to women's health experiences, and that women are "moral pioneers" who negotiate between their own religious belief systems and the moral possibilities arising from the worlds of science, technology, and biomedicine.[48] When shifting identities are recognized, multiple avenues arise whereby to make the connections between individuals characteristic of relational ethics. Relational ethics is grounded in commitment to each other and hence expressed through intersubjective or human-to-human connection.[49] In our empirical work, we have witnessed how religious/spiritual identities may provide these avenues for connection—sometimes via shared views, other times not the shared beliefs per se, but rather a shared valuing of religious/spiritual dimensions.[50] With an emphasis on the multiple dimensions of self, health care providers become more reflexive about their own religiously/spiritually informed values and beliefs that might well shape their views on various ethical issues[51] and their propensity to engage (or not engage) with patients and families deemed "other." The same connections through multiple identities can also provide the foundation for strategic alliances. Collins underscores the importance of situated knowledge for the formation of coalitions:

> Each group speaks from its own standpoint and shares its own partial, situated knowledge. But because each group perceives its own truth as partial, its knowledge is unfinished. Each group becomes better able to consider other groups' standpoints without relinquishing the uniqueness of its own standpoint or suppressing other groups' partial perspectives.[52]

Relational ethics, thus, benefit from an intersectional approach, in making visible how the specific social location of individuals can affect their moral agency,[53] creating intentional opportunities for connections through various facets of identity, and leveraging these same types of connections for strategic alliances. In these ways, intersectionality elucidates the interplay of identity, morality, and relationality which, in turn, influence health and health inequities and thus provide the stage for approaches that begin to shift those nursing practices and health care services that reinscribe advantage and disadvantage.

CONCLUDING COMMENTS AND CAUTIONS

Bringing an intersectional approach to ethics—one that incorporates religion/spirituality with intentionality—is not straightforward. Sherwin observes that bioethics has tended to focus on "modest, familiar [problems] with a well-defined scope"[54] when more complex approaches are needed to address the nature of problems facing humanity. A challenge, then, is that of countering dominant circumscribed ethical approaches. Yet, the complexity of intersectional analyses can pose challenges to the scientific integrity (e.g., rigor) of one's work—there are limits to how many "variables" one considers concurrently.[55] Although a fundamental principle of intersectional theorizing is that no single category is preeminent, the tendency is to focus on "master categories" such as gender or race rather than "emergent categories" such as Dossa's work on disabled immigrant Muslim women.[56] Another disincentive to intersectional approaches is that of our propensity—particularly in the study of religion and spirituality—to focus on either individual or social levels. In the realm of the individual, one finds a focus on spirituality with its internal personalized, privatized dimensions anchored in intersectionality's study of identify formation (multiple identities). At the social level, emphases on religion—with its affiliations with patriarchy, colonization, and other structures of power that result in oppression and disadvantage for some, and dominance/privilege for others—too often lack linkages to "lived religion"[57]

Despite these cautions, we call for nursing ethics to embrace integrative, interdisciplinary, and intersectional approaches, bringing the individual and group together for the most effective way of making visible pathways to social inclusion and exclusion. As we understand intersectional influences on moral agency (for all stakeholders involved in health care) and relational ethics, we gain increased explanatory capacity in our analyses, and greater compassion and social justice in enacting ethical practice. Intersectionality applies to everyone. Where the social level may infer that intersectionality is most relevant to those "marginalized" within society's matrices of domination, the individual level (multiple identities) reminds us that all are implicated in one way or another in the social relations that result in health inequities, and conversely, in creating opportunities for human flourishing.

NOTES

1. "Minorities to Rise Significantly by 2031: Stats Can." *CBC.ca* CBC, 9 Mar. 2010 Web. 4 Apr. 2011.
2. Raphael, Dennis. "Social Determinants of Health: Canadian Perspective." *Social Determinants of Health: Canadian Perspectives*. Ed. Dennis Raphael. Toronto: Canadian Scholars Press, 2009.
3. Berger, Peter, Grace Davie, and Effie Fokas. *Religious America, Secular Europe? A Theme and Variations*. Ashgate, 2008.
4. Reimer-Kirkham, Sheryl, and Sonya Sharma. "Adding Religion to Gender, Race, and Class: Seeking New Insights on Intersectionality in Health Care Contexts." *Intersectionality-Type Health Research in Canada*. Ed. O. Hankivsky. Vancouver, BC: University of British Columbia Press.
5. Taves, Ann. *Religious Experience Reconsidered: A Building-Block Approach to the Study of Religion and Other Special Things*. Princeton, NJ: Princeton University Press, 2009.
6. McCall, Linda. "The Complexity of Intersectionality." *Signs: A Journal of Women in Culture and Society* 30.3 (2005):1771–1800. See also: Yuval-Davis, Nira. "Intersectionality and Feminist Politics." *European Journal of Women's Studies* 13.3 (2006): 193–209.
7. Crenshaw, Kimberlé. "Mapping the Margins: Intersectionality, Identity Politics, and Violence against Women of Color." *Stanford Law Review* 43.6 (1991):1241–1299.
8. Hill Collins, Patricia. *Black Feminist Thought*. Boston: Unwin Hyam, 1990.
9. Davis, Kathy. "Intersectionality as Buzzword. A Sociology of Science Perspective on What Makes a Feminist Theory Successful." *Feminist Theory* 9.1 (2008): 68.
10. Hill Collins, Patricia. *Black Feminist Thought: Knowledge, Consciousness, and the Politics of Empowerment*. New York: Routledge, 2000. 18.
11. Hill Collins, Patricia. *Black Feminist Thought*. See also: Yuval-Davis, Nira. "Intersectionality and feminist politics." *European Journal of Women's Studies* 13.3 (2006): 193–209.
12. Carastathis, Anna "The Invisibility of Privilege: A Critique of Intersectional Models of Identity." *CRÉUM - Revue Les Ateliers de l'Ethique* 3.2 (2008): 23–38.
13. Luft, Rachel, and Jane Ward. "Toward an Intersectionality Just out of Reach: Confronting Challenges to Intersectoral Practice." *Perceiving Gender Locally, Globally, and Intersectionally*. Eds. Vasilike Demos and Marcia Segal. Bingley, UK: Emerald House Publishing. 2009. 9–38.
14. Hankivsky, Olena, and Renée Cormier. "Intersectionality: Moving Women's Health Research and Policy Forward." *whrn.ca*. Women's Health Research Network, 31 Mar. 2010. Web. 4 Apr. 2011.
15. Reimer-Kirkham, Sheryl, and Sonya Sharma. "Adding Religion to Gender, Race, and Class: Seeking New Insights on Intersectionality in Health Care Contexts."

16. Ibid.
17. Hancock, Ange-Marie. "When Multiplication Doesn't Equal Quick Addition: Examining Intersectionality as Research paradigm." *Perspectives on Politics* 5.1 (2007): 63–80.
18. Radford Reuther, Rosemary. *Movements in Feminist Theology*. Keynote address, *Gender, Religion, and the Third Wave Symposium, Gender Studies Institute*, Langley, B.C.: Trinity Western University, 2009.
19. McGuire, Meredith B. *Lived Religion: Faith and Practice in Everyday Life*. Oxford: Oxford University Press, 2008. See also: Orsi, Robert B. "Is the Study of Lived Religion Irrelevant to the World we live in? Special Presidential Plenary Address, Society for the Scientific Study of Religion, Salt Lake City, November 2, 2002." *Journal for the Scientific Study of Religion* 42.2 (2003): 169–174.
20. Reimer-Kirkham, Sheryl, and Sonya Sharma. "Adding Religion to Gender, Race, and Class: Seeking New Insights on Intersectionality in Health Care Contexts."
21. Klassen, Chris. "Confronting the Gap: Why Religion Needs to be Given More Attention in Women's Studies." *Thirdspace: A Journal of Feminist Theory & Culture* 3.1 (2003): n.p.
22. Brah, Avtar, and Ann Pheonix. "Ain't I a Woman? Revisiting Intersectionality." *Journal of International Women's Studies* 5.3 (2004): 77.
23. Hill Collins, Patricia. *From Black Power to Hip Hop: Racism, Nationalism, and Feminism*. Philadelphia: Temple University Press. 2006. 84.
24. Sharma, Sonya. *The Impact of Protestant Church Involvement on Young Women's Sexual Identities*. Unpublished dissertation Lancaster University, Lancaster, UK. 2007.
25. Joshi, Khyati Y. "The Racialization of Hinduism, Islam, and Sikhism in the United States." *Equity and Excellence in Education* 39.3 (2006.): 211–226.
26. Ibid., 212.
27. Reimer-Kirkham, Sheryl, and Sonya Sharma. "Adding Religion to Gender, Race, and Class: Seeking New Insights on Intersectionality in Health Care Contexts."
28. Bilge, Sirma. "Beyond Subordination vs. Resistance: An Intersectional Approach to the Agency of Veiled Muslim Women." *Journal of Intercultural Studies* 31.1 (2010): 9–28. See also: Dossa, Parin. *Racialized Bodies, Disabled Worlds: Storied Lives of Immigrant Women*. Toronto: University of Toronto Press, 2009. See also: Kuokkanen, Rauna. "Globalization as Racialized, Sexualized Violence: The Case of Indigenous Women." *International Feminist Journal of Politics* 1468–4470, 10.2 (2008): 216–233. See also: Williams, Toni. "Intersectionality Analysis in the Sentencing of Aboriginal Women in Canada: What Difference Does it Make?" *Intersectionality and Beyond: Law, Power and the Politics of Location*. Eds. Davina Cooper, Emily Grabham, Didi Herman, and Jane Krishnadas. London: Routledge, 2008.
29. Varcoe, Colleen, Olena Hankivsky, and Marina Morrow. "Introduction: Beyond Gender Matters." *Women's Health in Canada: Critical Perspectives on Theory and Policy*. Eds. Marina Marrow, Olena Hankivsky, and Colleen Varcoe. Toronto: University of Toronto Press. 2007. 3–32. See also: Guruge, Sepali, and Nazilla Khanlou. "Researching the Health of Immigrant and Refugee Women." *Canadian Journal of Nursing Research* 36.3 (2004): 32–47.
30. Peterson, Anna. *Being Human: Ethics, Environment and Our Place in the World*. Berkeley, CA: University of California Press, 2001.

31. Hankivsky, Olena, Colleen Reid, Renee Cormier, Colleen Varcoe, Natalie Clark, Cecilia Benoit, and Shari Brotman. "Exploring the Promises of Intersectionality for Advancing Women's Health Research." *International Journal for Equity in Health* 9.5 (2010). 3.

32. Whitehead, Margaret. "The Concepts and Principles of Equity and Health." *Health Promotion International* 6.3 (1991): 220.

33. Dunn, Kevin, Natascha Klocker, and Tanya Salabay. "Contemporary Racism and Islamaphobia in Australia." *Ethnicities* 7.4 (2007): 564–589. See also: Joshi, Khyati Y. "The Racialization of Hinduism, Islam, and Sikhism in the United States." 211–226.

34. Tang, Sannie Y., and Annette J. Browne. "Race Matters: Racialization and Egalitarian Discourses Involving Aboriginal People in the Canadian Health Care Context." *Ethnicity and Health* 13.2 (2008): 109–127. See also: Weber, Lynn and Elizabeth Fore. "Race, Ethnicity, and Health: An Intersectoral Approach." *Handbook of the Sociology of Racial and Ethnic Relations.* Eds. Hernán Vera and Joe Feagin. Springer. 2007. 191–218.

35. Krieger, Nancy. "Does Racism Harm Health? Did Child Abuse Exist Before 1962? On Explicit Questions, Critical Science, and Current Controversies: An Ecosocial Perspective." *American Journal of Public Health* 93.2 (2003): 194–199; See also: Nazroo, James. "The Structuring of Ethnic Inequalities in Health: Economic Position, Racial Discrimination, and Racism." *American Journal of Public Health* 93.2 (2003): 277–284. And: Paradies, Yin C. "Defining, Conceptualizing and Characterizing Racism in Health Research." *Critical Public Health* 16.2 (2006):143–157. See also: Williams, David A., and Selina A. Mohammed. "Discrimination and Racial Disparities in Health: Evidence and Needed Research." *Journal of Behavioural Medicine* 32.1(2009): 20–47.

36. Joshi, Khyati Y. "The Racialization of Hinduism, Islam, and Sikhism in the United States."

37. Sticker, Maja. "Considering Intersectionality." *Governing Difference* 22 January 2008.

38. See Johnson, Joy, Lorraine Greaves, and Robin Repta. "Better Science with Sex and Gender: Facilitating the Use of a Sex and Gender-based Analysis in Health Research" *International Journal for Equity in Health* 8.14 (2009).

39. Klassen, Chris. "Confronting the Gap: Why Religion Needs to be Given More Attention in Women's Studies."

40. Okin, Susan. "Feminism, Women's Human Rights, and Cultural Differences." *Hypatia* 13.2 (1998): 32–52.

41. Nyitray, Vivian-Lee. "Confucianism and Chinese Religion." *Fundamentalism and Women in World Religions.* Eds. Arvind Sharma and Katherine K. Young. New York: Continuum. 2007.

42. Sharma, Arvind, and Katherine K. Young. *Fundamentalism and Women in World Religions.* New York: Continuum, 2007.

43. Hill Collins, Patricia. *Black Feminist Thought: Knowledge, Consciousness, and the Politics of Empowerment.*

44. Sherwin, Susan. *The Politics of Women's Health: Exploring Agency and Autonomy.* Philadelphia: Temple University Press, 1999. 3.

45. Rodney, Paddy, Helen Brown, and Joan Liaschenko. "Moral Agency: Relational Connections and Trust." *Toward a Moral Horizon: Nursing Ethics for Leadership and Practice.* Eds. Janet Storch, Paddy Rodney, and Rosalie Starzomski. Toronto, ON: Pearson. 2004. 155.

46. Ibid., 157.

47. Appelbaum, Barbara. "Why Situated Moral Agency Matters." *Philosophy of Education Society*. 2002. Web. 2002. http://ojs.ed.uiuc.edu/index.php/pes/article/viewFile/1841/552.

48. Inhorn, Marcia. "Defining Women's Health: A Dozen Messages from More than 150 Ethnographies." *Medical Anthropology Quarterly* 20.3(2006): 345–378.

49. Bergum, Vangie, and John Dossetor. *Relational Ethics: The Full Meaning of Respect.* Hagerstown, MD: University Publishing Group, 2005.

50. Reimer Kirkham, Sheryl, Barb Pesut, Heather Meyerhoff, and Richard Sawatzky. "Spiritual Care-giving at the Juncture of Religion, Culture, and State." *Canadian Journal of Nursing Research* 36.4 (2004): 248–269. See also: Pesut, Barb, and Sheryl Reimer-Kirkham. "Situated Clinical Encounters in the Negotiation of Religious and Spiritual Plurality: A Critical Ethnography." *International Journal of Nursing Studies* 47.7 (2010): 815–825.

51. Pesut, Barb, and Sheryl Reimer-Kirkham. "Situated Clinical Encounters in the Negotiation of Religious and Spiritual Plurality: A Critical Ethnography."

52. Hill Collins, Patricia. *Black Feminist Thought: Knowledge, Consciousness, and the Politics of Empowerment.* 270.

53. Sherwin, Susan. *The Politics of Women's Health: Exploring Agency and Autonomy.*

54. Sherwin, Susan. "Whither bioethics? How Feminism can help Reorient Bioethics." *International Journal of Feminist Approaches to Bioethics* 1.1 (2008): 8.

55. Warner, Leah R. "A Best Practices Guide to Intersectional Approaches in Psychological Research." *Sex Roles* 59 (2008): 454–463.

56. Dossa, Parin. *Racialized Bodies, Disabled Worlds: Storied Lives of Immigrant Women.* Toronto: University of Toronto Press, 2009.

57. McGuire, Meredith B. *Lived Religion: Faith and Practice in Everyday Life.* See also: Orsi, Robert B. "Is the Study of Lived Religion Irrelevant to the World We Live In?" Special Presidential Plenary Address, Society for the Scientific Study of Religion, Salt Lake City, November 2, 2002.

7

Missionary Nursing: Internationalizing Religious Ideals

Sonya Grypma

The founding of the nursing profession [in China] by Christians was an even greater achievement than the introduction of modern medicine (…) young women would not have taken up nursing without the example set them by Christian women of the West.

Margaret H. Brown, Canadian missionary[1]

The modern Chinese nurse was named into being in 1914 when American missionary nurses in the newly established Nurses Association of China (NAC) adopted the term *hu shih* (literally, "caring scholar") to describe the new professional role being taken up by their Chinese *protégés*. Thirty years earlier, when Philadelphia Woman's Hospital graduate Elizabeth McKechnie arrived in China as the first "trained" nurse in 1884, there was no equivalent in Chinese culture to the conceptualization of nursing popularized by Florence Nightingale—that is, as a noble profession suitable for unmarried, God-fearing ladies. In late 19th century China, it was inconceivable that Chinese ladies "of good family" would care for the sick, other than their own relatives.[2] Nor was there an equivalent of "the Christian ethic in which caring could be lifted onto a plane of moral obligation" to become a "respected profession in which the most unpleasant work could be ennobled."[3] The missionary ideal of nursing as an honorable profession was "so novel" that "the Chinese had no word in their language to express the concepts "nobly" and "properly" for the nursing pioneers."[4] Yet by 1914, there was a small but growing cadre of Chinese women and men poised to enter missionary-sponsored nurses training.[5] In 1922, 8 years after its inception, the NAC joined the International Council of Nurses, bringing China into the growing imagined community of women from around the world with a shared identity of woman-as-nurse.[6] By the 1930s, mission-trained Chinese nurses had replaced many of the foreign missionary nurses as leaders in the mission hospitals, training schools, and the NAC itself. The expulsion of all foreigners from China after Mao Zedong's 1949 victory marked the end of missionary nursing in China, making way for a secular version of the modern nursing it introduced.

An exploration of the history of missionary nursing offers valuable insight into an expression of religion in nursing. This chapter will focus on the origins and development of missionary nursing in China as an offshoot of the broader Protestant missionary movement in the late 1800s. Using a critical approach informed by postcolonial and feminist theories, it will examine how the evangelizing mission of the Protestant church in North America contributed to the internationalization of modern nursing, particularly in China. Drawing particular attention to the influencing factors of religion, race, and gender, it will explore some of the tensions inherent in the global-ization of nursing as a hospital-based profession for unmarried, middle-class Christian women.

LAYING THE GROUNDWORK FOR MISSIONARY NURSING

The political, economic and social questions, which cause so much agita-tion in every land are, fundamentally, spiritual problems, and they will only be solved aright when the majority of the people learn to love and serve Jesus Christ.
                    -Dr. James Frazer Smith, Pioneer missionary to Henan[7]*

Perhaps nowhere is the link between religion and health care more readily seen than in the historic role of the missionary nurse. And nowhere were overseas missions more ambitious than in turn-of-the-20th-century China. Although Catholic sisterhoods from Quebec had been sending missionary nurses to the West since 1844,[8] a unique set of socio-political factors con-verged in the 1880s to set the stage for a new Anglo-Protestant brand of missionary nursing. That is, China's defeat in the Opium Wars, the women's suffrage movement, the establishment of professional nursing education, ad-vances in transportation, and the evangelistic student missionary movement of the late 1880s together provided an unprecedented opportunity for unmar-ried, ambitious, bright women looking for a way to express their religion in practical terms—as missionary nurses and physicians.

---

*The pinyin system of spelling is used here for easier recognition of places by contemporary readers.

The earliest factor to influence the eventual development of missionary nursing was China's defeat in the Opium Wars (1842, 1860). These events led to the removal of political barriers to China through the establishment of unequal treaties by which Westerners gained access to most regions of China. By the late 1800s, Chinese were required by law not only to tolerate missionaries, but also to protect them. Missionary nurses would not have been allowed into China had it not been for the imperialistic aims of their own nations.

The women's suffrage movement (1860s and 1870s) inspired a generation of women to recognize and resist existing social barriers to meaningful work outside of marriage and motherhood, and was a second factor to influence the development of missionary nursing. When Dr. Elizabeth Shattuck, a graduate of the Woman's Medical College of Pennsylvania, was barred from entering the foreign missionary field in 1858 because she was an unmarried woman, a group of Christian women banded together to form the "Woman's Union Missionary Society of America for Heathen Lands" (commonly referred to as the Woman's Union Missionary Society, WUMS), in 1860.[9] Founded to provide a way for single women to be sent to Asia "to address the physical, educational, and spiritual needs of the women there," the WUMS exemplified the mission phenomenon referred to as "woman's work for women."[10] In 1884, the WUMS sponsored the first missionary nurse, Elizabeth McKechnie, to China. In 1888, the first Canadian missionary nurse, Harriet Sutherland, was sponsored by the newly formed Women's Foreign Missionary Society (later Woman's Missionary Society, WMS) of the Presbyterian Church in Canada.[11]

A third influencing factor in the laying of the foundation for missionary nursing was the development of professional training schools for nurses (1870s and 1880s). The Philadelphia Woman's Hospital, from which Elizabeth McKechnie graduated in 1883, was the first institution in the United States to offer organized training to nurses.[12] The Toronto General Hospital (TGH) Training School for Nurses was the second English-language program for nurses in Canada. Opened in 1881, the TGH graduated most of the Canadian Protestant missionary nurses sent to China, including its first, Harriet Sutherland, and its longest serving, Margaret McIntosh.[13] In 1894, the TGH was the largest nursing program in Canada, having graduated 210 nurses, with room to accept only 53 of the 647 applications for admission.[14] In 1889, the year McIntosh graduated from TGH, the term "trained nurse" had come to epitomize the best in nursing care. According to the inaugural address at the opening of the Johns Hopkins Training School for Nurses in 1889 by Miss Isabel A. Hampton (later Robb), of all the professions open to women, none met with more public favor than the trained nurse: "The trained nurse is acknowledged superior (...) [because] technical skill can only be acquired by a systematic course of practical and theoretical study under competent teachers."[15]

Nurses were expected to "morally recognize the sacredness of the work they engage in," to be "fairly intellectual" and "strong and enduring physically."[16] State-of-the-art nursing practice in 1889 was considered an extension of physician care, where "the hands of a nurse are a physician's hands *lengthened out* to minister to the sick."[17] For their part, missionary physicians, who had been in China since 1835, began to see the potential in having the support of a trained nurse. Harriet Sutherland went to China to support Dr. James Frazer Smith in Henan province; Elizabeth McKechnie, to support Dr. Elizabeth Reifsnyder in Shanghai.[18]

The 1881 minutes of the Woman's Hospital of Philadelphia expounded the view that the female physician–nurse relationship was a sacred alternative to the traditional woman's role in a family, and a high moral calling in itself. "It will be observed" the secretary wrote, "that not until in the order of time the true status of women in medicine was recognized and granted in the community, was the want fully met of a band of thoroughly trained nurses filled with a high sense of the moral responsibility of their profession."[19] The McKechnie-Reifsnyder missionary dyad represented well the high aims of Reifsnyder's alma mater, where it was deemed in 1881 that "now and henceforth through a century of progress, the trained woman-nurse may complement the educated woman-physician, and in each find her own field the fulfillment of a lofty ambition, and the realization of the triest [sic] ministry of women outside the family relation."[20] For the earliest missionary nurses, accompanying missionary physicians to China was a socially sanctioned way to exercise their independence, assert their authority, and plumb their intellectual, emotional, and spiritual capacities.

A fourth influencing factor—the advancement of transportation technologies—is not typically recognized as a factor in health care development (1880s). The internationalization of nursing in general and of missionary nursing in particular was dependent on middle-class women having access to affordable means of transportation. Although China became politically accessible to Westerners in the late 1800s, it was halfway around the globe from nurses in eastern Canada and the United States. The significance of the newly built transnational railways and steamships to the development of missionary nursing cannot be overstated. In 1887, for example, for the first time in history, Canadians in Toronto could travel west across the country to Vancouver, via the Canadian Pacific Railway (CPR), and then board a CPR passenger steamship to China. It is no coincidence that the first three groups of Canadian missionaries set off to China within 4 years of the CPR steamship's launch: the Presbyterian Church in Canada and the China Inland Mission (CIM) in 1888, and the Methodist Church of Canada in 1891. Many of these earliest missionaries were from the Toronto area; China was suddenly within reach of "Toronto the Good."

Toronto's reputation as "the Good" emerged in 1885, the year that William Howland was elected mayor. Known for his dedication to the poor and disadvantaged, Howland reportedly put a 12-foot banner on his office wall: Except the Lord keep the city, the watchman waketh but in vain (Psalm 127:1).[21] Howland's conversion to "a vibrant evangelical faith" came on a wave of religious revival that had spread to Canada from England and the United States on the strength of preachers like Charles Spurgeon and Dwight L. Moody.[22] This movement provided the greatest impetus for the missionary enterprise, which in turn launched missionary nursing. If political, economic, and social factors provided the opportunity to work in China, religious factors provided the motivation. Through the missionary movement (1880s), missionary nurses would join evangelists, teachers, and physicians as purveyors of the Christian faith, first to Asia, and then around the world.

MISSIONARY NURSING: A RESPONSE TO THE CALL

Bringing in Chinese,
Bringing in Chinese,
We shall come rejoicing,
Bringing in Chinese.
-Sung to George Minor's tune for "Bringing in the Sheaves," 1880[23]

Canadian historian Alvyn Austin's germinal study of Canadian missionaries in China begins with a description of an unusual event in Toronto in late September 1888. "One thousand enthusiastic young people marched down the main street of Toronto in a torch-lit parade," he writes, "singing hymns to escort 'the first Canadian party' of missionaries bound for China to the train station."[24] Hudson Taylor, founder of the CIM—300 strong and serving in 15 of the 18 provinces of China by 1888—arrived in Canada that summer from England en route to China. Taylor, the most famous missionary in the world since the death of Dr. David Livingstone 12 years earlier in Africa, discovered an evangelistic fervor in Toronto. He recruited 13 Canadians to the CIM. This group of young, unmarried men and women had little formal education, but shared a great enthusiasm for the Scriptures. The new recruits sailed for China with Taylor almost immediately. As part of his "faith mission," CIM missionaries had no guarantee of a regular salary, just a mandate to preach the gospel to the "million a month" who were "dying without God."[25]

The CIM recruits were not the first Canadians to arrive in China. Two months previous, on July 27, 1888, graduate nurse Harriet Sutherland boarded a ship in Vancouver with the newly married James and Minnie Frazer Smith as part of the first group of Canadian Presbyterian missionaries to China. Considering themselves "adventurers going out in faith," they were on their way to the treaty port of Zhifu to meet up with fellow-Canadians Jonathan and Rosalind Goforth, who had arrived a few months earlier, in March.[26] Bachelors Dr. William McClure and Donald McGillivray soon added to their number, bringing the total to seven. Dubbing themselves "the Honan Seven," this small band of Canadians was to take up the daunting task assigned of establishing a Christian mission in Henan, the "second most hostile province in the whole of China."[27]

Nurses were not part of the original plan for missionary work in Henan. When the General Assembly of the Presbyterian Church in Canada appointed the first two Canadian missionaries to Henan, Reverend Jonathan Goforth and Dr. James Frazer Smith, in June 1887, the option of sending single missionary women to China had not been considered.[28] Having learned from local missionaries upon arriving in China in 1888 that Chinese mores would not allow missionary men to have contact with Chinese women, Goforth wrote to the Foreign Mission Committee (later Foreign Mission Board, FMB), requesting "single lady missionaries" because "I am told that without the latter the women can scarcely be reached."[29] Dr. Frazer Smith, seeing an opportunity to procure assistance with his own medical work, pressed the FMB to appoint a nurse.[30] On May 25, 1888 the FMB appointed Harriet Sutherland. Her salary was paid by the newly formed Woman's Foreign Missionary Society. During the next 3 years, while the expanding group of "North Honan" missionaries made unsuccessful attempts to acquire property on Henan soil, Dr. Frazer Smith engaged the services of two additional nurses, Jennie Graham and Margaret McIntosh, with the idea that they would assist him in his growing work of treating the illnesses of rural Chinese. By 1891, Sutherland and Graham had resigned due to marriage and illness, respectively, leaving Margaret McIntosh as the sole nurse at the mission for the next quarter century.

Missionary nursing, like other forms of missionary work, came to China on the wave of evangelistic fervor taken up by college students in the late 1800s. The Student Volunteer Movement for Foreign Missions (later Student Volunteer Movement, SVM) was a powerful catalyst in the development of missions and missionary nursing. In fact, Austin considers the birth of the SVM to be the "birth of the modern missionary movement."[31] Founded in 1886 as a grassroots organization to recruit students for foreign missions, the SVM emerged from the new missionary zeal of the 1880s—the earnest 80s—where the complacent mid-Victorian church was increasingly being taken over by aggressive young people. Describing this shift from "the church sentimental" to "the church militant," Austin notes, "It was the difference between saying 'Oh, isn't it wonderful what those missionaries are doing to civilize the heathen?' and the young people's response: 'As a Christian, you are personally responsible for the salvation of the world. Think about it. Pray about it. Then give or go.'"[32] The catchphrase of the SVM became, "Evangelization of the world in this generation."[33] Newly graduated nurses were among the first to respond to the call.

AN ARM OF THE (MALE-DOMINATED) CHURCH

Woman's work in the foreign field must be careful to recognize the headship of man in ordering of affairs in the kingdom of God. . . . 'the head of woman is the man.'
-American Baptist Missionary Union, 1888[34]

Between 1888 and 1949, the Canadian presence in China as a whole was most recognizable through six main missions: The Presbyterian Church in Canada mission in Taiwan (est. 1871), the Presbyterian mission in North Henan (est. 1888), the Methodist Church of Canada mission in Sichuan (est. 1891), the Presbyterian mission in Guangdong (est. 1902), the Catholic Scarboro Foreign Mission Society in Zhejiang (est. 1902), and the Anglican Church of Canada mission south of the Yellow River in Henan (est. 1910).[35] The Presbyterian mission in Taiwan was the first overseas field of the Canadian Presbyterian Church, but the eccentricity of its founder George Leslie McKay, its remoteness from Mainland China, and its continuance with the Presbyterian Church after "Union" kept Taiwan on the fringe of Canadian missions.[36] The union of all Methodists, Congregationalists, and most Presbyterians into one United Church of Canada in 1925 set the United Church apart as the largest Canadian mission in China, with the North China Mission in Henan, the West China Mission in Sichuan, and the South China Mission in Guangdong. The United Church was the largest employer of Canadian missionary nurses.[37] An estimated 100 or more Canadian nurses worked in at least 9 provinces of China during this period.[38]

The revivals of the 1880s gained momentum in Canada and the United States through the message of preachers and missionaries traveling back and forth across the Atlantic between England and North America whose message caught the imagination of a generation of college students. One aim of the revivals was to reimagine the church as a social setting; to make people feel at home in their churches. Turn of the 20th century churches became communal centers where one could spend every night of the week, and where missions was the topic of the day.[39] Unlike the CIM, the Presbyterian and Methodist missions preferred to sponsor missionary candidates with advanced education, including ministers, physicians, and nurses. And, also unlike the CIM, Presbyterian and Methodist missions developed and provided a formalized method of financial support for missionaries. Individual congregations would pledge support for "their" missionaries, raising funds through donations by church members, regular collections, and fund-raising activities like women's teas and information evenings. This commitment to funding missions made the 1920s shift from evangelism to service possible, even if not sustainable. For example, when the Canadians determined to build a modern 250-bed hospital and training school for nurses at Weihui, Henan in the 1920s, church members provided funding. The total cost of the hospital project to the Mission was $58,614.52, of which the Woman's Missionary Society paid $17,697.00. Other funding came from the Forward Movement Peace "Thank offering Fund," and gifts from the Chinese. In addition to the cost of the hospital was the cost of a nurses' residence; Mrs. Geo Bingham donated the requisite $4,000.00 in memory of her late husband.[40]

Missionary nursing for Canadians was, from the beginning, intrinsically linked with specific church institutions—particularly the Methodist and Presbyterian churches, later joined as the United Church of Canada. Financially and ideologically dependent on the church at home, Canadian missionary nurses both benefitted from and felt constrained by their sponsoring denominations. Individual missionary nurses could count on the financial support of their local congregations for their outfit, travel, language training, and housing for their 7-year terms. However, as will be seen, early Canadian nurses were also bound to the evangelistic priorities of the church and mission boards.

One of the most intriguing differences between early Canadian and American missionary nursing in China relates to the timing and extent of missionary nurse involvement in the training of Chinese nurses. Whereas nurses training in Shanghai began only 2 years after the 1884 arrival of Elizabeth McKechnie, it took almost four decades for Canadians to start nurses training in Henan. A closer look at the Canadian situation in Henan reveals some reasons why. First, Canadian missionaries did not actually secure property in Henan until 6 years after their arrival, in 1894, whereas the Americans had secured land within months of their arrival in Shanghai. By the time the Canadians had a property, the first two missionary nurses, Harriet Sutherland and her replacement Jennie Graham had resigned. The third Canadian nurse, Margaret McIntosh, did some work with Dr. James Frazer Smith, but she preferred evangelistic work over nursing. McIntosh spent considerable time with other female evangelistic workers, bringing the Christian gospel message to Chinese women and children at fairs, Sunday school classes, and in their homes. In 1894, Dr. Frazer Smith was invalided back to Canada; he had become sick with typhus, pneumonia, and thrombosis in quick succession; he did not recover sufficiently to return to China. Because none of the remaining physicians perceived a need for the assistance of a nurse, McIntosh removed herself from nursing—earning the criticism of the next generation of nurses: "How different the story might have been," wrote Canadian missionary nurse Preston, "if Miss Margaret McIntosh, our first nurse, had used her gifts, with her courage and consecration in pioneering our nursing work instead of the evangelistic work."[41]

In fairness to McIntosh, the Canadian mission at Henan was hardly supportive of the advancement of nursing. In May of 1909, Dr. William J. Scott, a Henan missionary for 3 years, reported to the Henan Presbytery on some of the medical work, stating that he "deplored" the deficiency of nursing facilities there.[42] According to Dr. Scott's son, both Dr. Scott and his colleague Dr. O. Shirley McMurtry were "shocked" to discover "what was called a hospital in Henan," and to find that the hospital was "totally lacking in nursing service."[43] Their request to improve medical facilities—in part via a financial grant from McMurtry's father—was favorably received at first. However, Rev. Jonathan Goforth and other elders later objected to the scheme on the basis that it would undermine the evangelistic priority of the mission. The Henan Presbytery turned down the money, stating that it could not accept a grant that would be meant for materialist and non-religious purposes. Nurses were not consulted in the decision. It was not until the 1920s and 1930s, after Rev. Goforth quit the mission in protest of the Presbyterian amalgamation with the United Church that the vision of nursing education caught on.

Once the aims shifted from evangelism to social service, missionary nurses found their grounding, particularly as nurse educators, and nursing enjoyed a decade of unprecedented growth and productivity in Henan. However, it was short lived. Japan's 1937 invasion struck a devastating blow to China and indirectly to the development of nursing. In 1939, Canadian mission sites in occupied China were evacuated; its nurses scattered throughout free areas of China.[44] In 1941, missionary nurses, who remained occupied in China when Japan's attack on Pearl Harbor brought the United States and Britain into the war, were imprisoned in civilian internment camps.[45] By the time the 13,500 internees in China and Hong Kong were liberated in August 1945, missionary nursing had lost both momentum and motivation. Postwar attempts to rehabilitate the Henan mission were quickly abandoned in the face of a renewed civil war in 1947, rendering the last few months of Canada's 60 year mission in China as a mere epilogue to the epoch of internment. Mao Zedong's 1949 expulsion of foreigners from China spelled the end of missionary nursing there. The sense of failure that accompanied the end of the missionary era in China cast a shadow over missionary nursing from which it has never completely recovered.[46]

AN ARM OF THE (FEMALE-DOMINATED) PROFESSION

As a profession, we are beginning to feel an increasing necessity for some such definite moral force or laws that shall bind us more closely together in this work of nursing.

-Isabel Hampton Robb[47]

The study of missionary nursing is an emerging field. In most mission scholarship, missionary nursing has been subsumed under the rubric of missionary medicine. While helpful in providing the context for nursing, this nonetheless leaves gaps in terms of understanding how nursing developed as its own entity and overlooks the connection of missionary nurses to the broader community of professional nurses. Still, while to date there are no comprehensive studies of American missionary nurses in China, an originative article by Kaiyi Chen makes it clear that American missionary nurses wielded significant influence in the development of modern nursing in China.[48] Missionaries are credited with the development of numerous, if not the majority, of nursing schools across China between 1886 and 1914.[49] As nursing education burgeoned across China, American missionary nurses organized themselves as the NAC in 1909. The main thrust of the NAC was to raise the standard of nurses' training in China by the adoption of a "uniform course of study and examination."[50] In the absence of uniform governmental authority on nursing education, the NAC took responsibility for setting the standard for all nursing schools in the country, formulating a model curriculum and holding certification examinations.[51] At the national NAC convention in Shanghai in 1914, Miss Elsie Mawfung Chung (later Mrs. Bayard Lyon), a graduate of the Guys Hospital in London and the first Chinese nurse to be trained abroad, introduced the Chinese term *hu shih* (caring scholar) to represent the emerging role for Chinese women.[52] First and foremost a missionary organization, the NAC expressed its "theology" in seven words: "For God so loved that He gave."[53]

Compared with the Canadians in Henan, a preliminary review of early American missionary nurses suggests that these women enjoyed a fair amount of autonomy and agency. This is reflected in part by their role in establishing the first training schools for nurses in China. In 1886, Elizabeth McKechnie started a school in Shanghai with Dr. Elizabeth Reifsnyder. In 1888, Esther H. Butler, a missionary of the American Friends Mission ("Quaker") and a graduate of the Chicago Training School started a nursing school in Nanjing. That same year, Ella Johnson started a training class in Fuzhou.[54] Gage "supplemented" Johnson at Fuzhou in 1908, and then established a nurse training program in Hunan as part of the Yale University mission.[55] Gage later became President of the NAC. By 1920, before the Canadians in Henan started nurses training programs, 48 Chinese graduate nurses had joined the NAC, 52 training schools had been registered, and 150 Chinese nurses had successfully passed the NAC examinations and received the NAC diploma.[56]

The achievements of the missionary nurses won praise from their medical colleagues. In 1914, the Medical Missionary Association of China declared, "Nothing in medical mission work in China of the past few years has been more marked in its development than the growth in training schools for both male and female nurses."[57] The remarkable progress of nursing under the NAC continued for two more decades. In 1920, the NAC commenced its own quarterly journal, the *Nursing Journal of China*, which carried each article in English and Chinese. In 1922, it formed the Committee on Nursing Education and was admitted into the International Council of Nurses—the first Asian country to do so. By 1926, there were 112 schools of nursing registered under the NAC, with 2,000 students enrolled. Most schools were associated with American mission organizations; five were Canadian.[58] That same year, the NAC membership had shifted from predominantly Western to two thirds Chinese. By the late 1930s, there were 6,000 nurses in the NAC.[59] In recognition of her status as the first graduate nurse in China, Elizabeth McKechnie was granted a lifetime membership to the NAC.[60] Although she resigned from the WUMS in 1896 to marry Archdeacon E. H. Thompson [Thomson], McKechnie remained in Shanghai for 38 years, until her husband's death in 1921.[61]

Elizabeth McKechnie and other early American missionary nurses seem to have been less burdened with church or mission board bureaucracy than Canadians. The emphasis on social justice that came later for the Canadian missionaries in North China was an integral part of the American understanding of mission work early on. Whereas the turn-of-the-20th-century Canadian mission in North China resisted the development of hospitals and nursing care as distracting from the primary evangelical aim of missions, American missions approached the establishment of nursing schools *as* mission itself. Rather than perceiving themselves as agents of their sponsoring church denomination, adapting their work to church priorities without protest, American missionary nurses seem to have developed early on a sense of solidarity with other professional nurses—from a variety of mission organizations, but also from nursing leaders in the United States. The notion of Christian duty was not reserved for the mission field; it was a central aspect of nursing education and practice as a whole. Tomes and Boschma note that, in the late 1800s, the language of Anglo-American Protestantism suffused science, domestic politics, and international affairs.[62] At the same time, church life became a more exclusively female domain, with women outnumbering men as converts and church members. A shared sense of Christian purpose "became a powerful force unifying women from different regional and social backgrounds," including nursing.[63] The growing assumption that educated and refined women had a special obligation to strengthen their less privileged sisters carried over into what Tome and Boschma call "the crusade for international nursing uplift."[64] The missionary movement and the women's suffrage crusade shared a sense of women's work for women as a moral obligation, domestically and overseas. By 1900, 41 American women's boards of varying size had come into existence, stimulating and reflecting a shift from American missions as a predominantly male enterprise to a female one.[65]

The same impetus that gave rise to the development of woman's missionary societies also stimulated the development of the International Council of Women (ICW). And it was the ICW that birthed the International Council of Nurses, in 1900.[66] Nursing leaders caught the vision of the ICN as an imagined community around the shared identity of woman-as-nurse. The seed of the international nursing movement was sown in conversations between British nurse leader Ethel Fenwick and American leaders Isabel Hampton (later Robb) and Lavinia L. Dock, at the Johns Hopkins School of Nursing where Hampton was superintendent. They continued to champion the cause of nursing as an international profession; it is no coincidence that Isabel Hampton's foundational textbook *Nursing: Its Principles and Practice* was among the earliest textbooks used in China, available in Guangdong as early as 1896.[67] Nursing leaders envisioned the development of nursing into a standardized, moral vocation for intelligent women; missionary nurses enacted that vision.

In contrast to denominational mission boards that tended to view missionary nurses as minor—even unnecessary—players in the evangelical enterprise, the ICN viewed missionary nurses as key to its professionalizing aims. Missionary nurses were also a natural fit with the ICW, whose ultimate aim was cast in unmistakeably Christian terms—to apply "the Golden Rule to society, custom and law [which is to] do unto others as ye would that they should do unto you."[68] In China, as elsewhere, nursing leaders perceived it as their role to pave the way for a strong profession. From a professional nursing perspective, the gospel of intelligent caring was not at odds with the gospel of Christ; it was a natural extension of it.

ELIZABETH MCKECHNIE: PROXIMITY WITH WOMEN OF INFLUENCE

Founder of this hospital; a pioneer missionary; a skilled surgeon and physician; an understanding loving friend of the Chinese; a devoted, untiring, self-sacrificing worker; a resourceful, strong, capable character; a loyal follower of The Great Physician.

-In memoriam for Dr. Elizabeth Reifsnyder[69]

It is doubtful that Elizabeth McKechnie would have had the opportunity to work in China had it not been for her association with two women of influence, Dr. Elizabeth Reifsnyder and philanthropist Mrs. Margaret Williamson. Indeed, were it not for the renown of Dr. Reifsnyder, who came to early fame in Shanghai following the successful removal of a patient's massive (50 lb) ovarian tumor, the archival record of Elizabeth McKechnie may well have been confined to two lines—the record of her graduation on December 19, 1883 from the Philadelphia Woman's Hospital, and a note in a 1925 hospital history celebration that McKechnie ("now Thompson") was "first graduate nurse in China."[70] As it is, the fame of Elizabeth Reifsnyder allows us to trace the movements of Elizabeth McKechnie and gain at least a superficial sense of her work as a missionary nurse.

Elizabeth Reifsnyder and Elizabeth McKechnie were both appointed to China by the WUMS, sailing to China in September 1883 and March 1884, respectively.[71] They likely met in Philadelphia in 1883 when both were at the Philadelphia Woman's Hospital—Reifsnyder as a resident physician, McKechnie as a nursing student.[72] Although Reifsnyder had originally been rejected by the WUMS in 1881 because of her young age (21), she seemed the perfect candidate the following year. That year, in 1882, two young women "laid before the [Women's Union Missionary] society a need of a Hospital for Women and Children" in Shanghai.[73] Chinese women were reportedly subject to a "great number of misfortunes and calamities," which took the form of disease that was "intensified by their lives of seclusion, and the want of exercise and air resulting from the impossibility of their moving around much on their cramped [bound] feet."[74] Mrs. Margaret Williamson, a founding member of the WUMS, "responded most generously" to the news by offering a donation of $5,000 to build the hospital.[75] Sadly—though fortuitously for Reifsnyder and McKechnie—Mrs. Williamson died the following year, leaving in her will the provisions to build and furnish the new hospital and provide "the salary of a physician and nurse for seven years, at an expense of $35,000."[76] Dr. Reifsnyder was selected to oversee the construction and work of the new hospital. It was a perfect situation for a bright young doctor and nurse: financial security with minimal accountability to, or interference from, one's benefactor.

Armed with the ideological and practical support of the sisterhood back home, Elizabeth McKechnie and Dr. Elizabeth Reifsnyder were well positioned to take up their new role in China. Although ultimately it would be their acceptance among the Chinese population that would determine their success, the point here is that these women could not have even attempted this new work in China had it not been for the initial support from home. The two women secured a two-room house in Shanghai that they used as a dispensary, reportedly treating as many as a 100 daily.[77] "I shall need nurses," reported Reifsnyder in 1885 as soon as the hospital was under construction, "as well as other helpers in connection with the hospital and dispensary service, and can find Chinese girls who wish to study. One such I am now teaching at night."[78]

Within an astonishingly short period, the new hospital was opened on June 4, 1885 "exclusively for relieving the suffering of Chinese women."[79] Initially, the hospital was promoted as a foreign enterprise, part of the Protestant ideal of women's work for women—"for suffering women, who would otherwise be untouched by the means provided for the relief of suffering among men."[80] Very quickly, however, Reifsnyder established the importance of Chinese involvement and financial support. Perhaps recognizing that the Williamson endowment would eventually run out, she deemed it best "to have the wealthy Chinese pay for services rendered while the poor were being cared for at no cost."[81] By 1905, "over *half a million patients have received attention*" [emphasis in original].[82] Considering that the hospital was run by two physicians and one head nurse for the first 20 years, the statistics from 1905 are remarkable: patients treated in the wards and hospital, 839; patients treated in the dispensary, 45,700; home visits, 321; prescriptions filled, 623,119; money received from Chinese patients, $8,105.27.[83]

Although it is clear that religious values acted as an impetus for missionary medicine and nursing in China, what is less clear is how individual missionary women viewed the intersection between faith and practice. Formal mission reports, geared toward an audience of mission supporters at home, emphasize evangelical strategies like Bible studies, "hymn sings," and the distribution of religious tracts to patients—the implicit intention being the conversion of patients to Christianity. The 1905 Margaret Williamson Hospital report reassured readers that through "Preaching every day to the dispensary patients, bedside talks and instructions, distribution of tracts to those who come daily (…) it can be readily seen that the object for which the hospital was built, namely, the spread of the Gospel, is being aided very greatly."[84] Whether or not the evangelizing efforts were effective, it is important to note that the religious activities reported in missionary reports may not have been an accurate reflection of the actual evangelistic efforts of medical staff, some of whom may have either subordinated emphasis on saving the soul to healing the body or who may have seen healing the body as necessarily prior to evangelism, or who may have embraced healing-as-evangelism.[85] As I have noted elsewhere, reports of "preaching to patients" from Canada, for example, seem to have been more of a reflection of mission board expectations than actual practice.[86] Scholars must be cautious, therefore, about drawing conclusions about the intimate aspects of missionary nurses' religious faith from public records meant for an audience of religious supporters.

Although public records provide a sense of the socio-religious context within which nurses were acculturated, without personal documents such as diaries or letters home, one cannot examine in any depth how individuals like Elizabeth McKechnie understood and expressed their

Christian faith. What is clear is that McKechnie did not have to choose between nursing and evangelism; providing nursing care was accepted as a religious expression in itself. "These women [at the Williamson Hospital] give their lives," the American Consul-General in Shanghai later commented, "not for money, but for love for these people, which they get from Christ. It is the spirit of Jesus."[87]

"WORTHY OF THE NAME": INTERNATIONALIZING A RELIGIOUS IDEAL

A nurse worthy of the name must have education and refinement, and a character above reproach. Go forth with love, faith and purity of heart; your hope for the future is bright.
-Surgeon-General Ch'uan, Army Medical College, to NAC delegates, 1915[88]

In 1922, the School of Nursing at the Margaret Williamson Hospital in Shanghai was registered with the NAC.[89] Thirty-eight years after Elizabeth McKechnie sailed for China, the nursing program she founded was 1 of 50-some schools of nursing registered in China, with similar structures and purpose. Applicants to the Margaret Williamson training school for Chinese nurses were to be 20 and 30 years of age and had to bring certificates from two people as to their "mental and moral fitness."[90] The course of study was 3 years, with board, laundry, and textbooks furnished. There were 55 students enrolled in 1922, the majority of whom received their high school educations from mission schools. Those who were graduates of approved high schools could gain entrance upon a letter of recommendation from the principal. Other applicants were subject to an examination. In terms of the religious underpinnings of the school, the recorded composition of the student population is telling: "Christians on entering, 39, Non-Christians on entering, 16. During the past year since entering 12 have become Christians and four who are not Christians are interested in Christianity."[91]

Perhaps one of the most remarkable aspects of missionary nursing was not its lack of focus on direct evangelism—United Church of Canada missionary nurses, after all, did not see it as their role to evangelize patients— but its unapologetic expectation that Chinese nurses themselves be Christian.[92] In the educational milieu in which North American-born missionary nurses were acculturated, nursing and Christianity were inextricably linked; Christian discourse and traditions were part of the larger social fabric. And yet, for the Chinese people, to be a professing Christian was relatively rare. As such, Chinese nursing students and staff were part of a small Chinese subculture comprised mostly of those connected to foreign missionaries— either directly, as graduates of mission schools, or indirectly, as members of the Church of Christ in China. This was the main pool from which potential students were drawn. Thus, although Canadian missionary nurses in Henan criticized the early emphasis on evangelism, they also benefited from it. To missionary nurses, nursing personified Christian service. They believed that Christianity, with its emphasis on moral responsibility toward the sick, poor and dying, provided the foundation upon which successful nursing services could be built. There seems to have been little debate among missionary nurse educators as to the intended outcome of nursing education: Chinese nursing was meant to be a sinified offshoot of missionary nursing.[93]

Religious activities in the Margaret Williamson School of Nursing in 1922 included chapel services every morning, "twilight prayers" every evening, church services on Sunday, and Bible study classes.[94] Across China, the NAC encouraged schools of nursing to "instill the highest ideals of nursing ethics throughout the profession" and to "encourage Chinese nurses to regard their work as a true act of service to God and to their countrymen."[95] Following the Nightingale ideal, missionary nurses in China perceived a virtuous character as central to good nursing care. Although a detailed discussion about the extent to which Chinese nurses came to embody and express Christian ideals in their nursing practice is beyond the scope of this chapter, it is important to note that the development of nursing in China required significant changes in social mores there. For centuries, Chinese women had been denied the opportunity to obtain any schooling.[96] As Chen notes, although Protestant missionaries began to establish boarding schools for girls in the mid-19th century, it was not until after the 1911 revolution that the republican government recommended that middle schools for girls be included in the national educational system.[97] Furthermore, the Christian ethos of caring for strangers contrasted with traditional approaches to caregiving in China, where ill family members were cared for by family, or by servants of the same gender as the patient. Similarly, traditional gender mores prohibited Chinese women from serving men they did not know. Mission hospital schools of nursing responded by taking in male nursing students and having separate wards or hospitals for male and female patients and staff. "How long this necessity will continue," Harold Balme wrote, "is, of course, impossible to predict, but there are already signs of changing sentiment in the more progressive cities."[98] The hope was that one day it would be possible to employ female nurses in any of the hospitals in the larger cities. Canadian superintendent Ratcliffe's comments capture this attitude well: "Women," she wrote, "naturally possess more aptitude for the work than the men."[99]

As nursing education gained traction in China in the 1920s, missionaries began to recognize the potential of the ambitious project being undertaken by missionary nurses as a collective. Dr. Harold Balme, Dean of Medicine at the Shandong Christian University in Jinan, expressed with astonished pride that "at the present time the molding of the new nursing profession in China is almost entirely in the hands of missionary nurses from Great Britain and North America, and of Christian Chinese who have had their nursing training abroad."[100] It was an "extraordinary opportunity" to shape the Chinese nurse of the future, "and thus to inspire the whole profession with the loftiest ideals."[101] Balme also expressed a hope that western nursing, with its Christian underpinnings, would be well rooted in China "within the next ten or twenty years." However, it was not to be. Nursing education was stalled, even halted altogether, when Japanese forces invaded China in 1937.

Between 1937 and 1949, China faced a barrage of calamities that brought it to the brink of disaster, and undermined the work of missionary nurses to the point of collapse. The 8-year war with Japan was compounded by catastrophes like famine, flooding, and widespread outbreak of communicable diseases like cholera and typhoid. Mission compounds and hospitals were evacuated. Missionaries who refused to leave areas of occupied China were placed under house arrest by the Japanese the day after the successful attacks on Pearl Harbor, in December 1941. Japan held 13,500 civilian "enemy aliens" captive in China and Hong Kong between 1941 and 1945, missionary nurses among them.[102] Nurses who returned to China after 1945 with plans to rehabilitate the hospitals and schools of nursing found themselves in the middle of the civil war between Nationalist and Communist forces.[103] By the time missionaries were forced to leave China in 1949, some of the missions had already been closed permanently. The missionary era in China came to an abrupt and unceremonious end.

CONCLUSION

From this standpoint the nurse's work is a ministry; it should represent a consecrated service, performed in the spirit of Christ, who made himself of no account but went about doing good.

-Isabel Hampton Robb[104]

Missionary nursing as a lifelong career has all but disappeared from the landscape of professional nursing preparation and practice in 21st century North America. In the current lexicon, the term "missionary nursing" tends to connote short-term (2 weeks to 2 years) volunteer missions to poor, devastated, or disaster regions of the world. Ideologically, it is differentiated from international or cross-cultural nursing by explicitly Christian aims, whether service or evangelistic. Practically speaking, however, the distinctions between "international nursing" and "missionary nursing" are not clear. Individual nurses, for example, may consider themselves as missionaries (or not), regardless of the mandate of their employer or sponsoring organization. The point is that missionary nursing, understood today as having a core aim of "sharing your faith" or "reaching out in Jesus Christ's name" has been long relegated to the margins of contemporary nursing practice. But then again, so has Christianity.

Elsewhere I have argued that the silencing of missionary nursing occurred after the abrupt closure of the mission field in China in the late 1940s.[105] I identified three factors that helped shift missionary nursing from the center to the margins of nursing discourse: self-censorship of repatriated missionaries, the mission identity crisis catalyzed by the "failure" of the missionary enterprise in China, and the equation of the missionary movement with the devastating policies of colonialism and imperialism. Here I offer a fourth influencing factor—the shift of religious (Christian) discourse itself from the center to the margins of nursing preparation and practice.

As we have seen, Protestant missionary nursing emerged at a unique period in history. China's defeat in the Opium Wars, the women's suffrage movement, the establishment of professional nursing education, advances in transportation, and the evangelistic student missionary movement converged in the late 1800s to create a favorable climate for the development of missionary nursing. The central tenets of missionary nursing, however, were not unique to overseas work. The notions of nursing as a lifelong ministry and "a consecrated service performed in the spirit of Christ" were not sectarian ideals meant for a fragment of the nursing populace, missionary or otherwise. Instead, they were central to the professional nursing envisioned, developed, and propagated by a string of capable nursing leaders, starting with—but hardly limited to—Florence Nightingale. Missionary nursing, in other words, was neither unique in its religious impulse, nor in its propagating tendencies. Those who led the professional nursing movement at the turn of the 20th century were as relentless in their pursuit of new opportunities to advance the profession on North American soil as missionaries were in their pursuits overseas. The profession that leaders envisioned was rooted in Christian perspectives on suffering as a symptom of a broken world, with nursing as an enactment of Christ's care for the poor, sick, and weak. Missionary nursing was not an outlier. It was simply the furthest extreme of a profession already suffused with internationalizing, religious ideals.

ACKNOWLEDGMENTS

Research funding was provided by The Social Sciences and Humanities Research Council of Canada and The Isobel Sholtis Brunner Fellowship for Historical Research in Nursing, Barbara Bates Center for the Study of the History of Nursing, University of Pennsylvania.

NOTES

1. Brown, Margaret H. *History of the Honan (North China) Mission of the United Church of Canada, Originally a Mission of the Presbyterian Church in Canada.* Toronto: United Church Archives. LXVI:8. Print.
2. Chung-tung, Liu. "From San Gu Liu to 'Caring Scholar': The Chinese Nurse in Perspective." *International Journal of Nursing Studies* 28.4 (1991): 315–24. Print.
3. Ibid., 320.
4. Ibid., 322.
5. Chan, Sally and Frances Wong. "Development of Basic Nursing Education in China and Hong Kong." *Journal of Advanced Nursing* 29.6 (1999): 1300–07. Print.
6. Brush, Barbara L., Joan E. Lynaugh, Geertje Boschma, Anne Marie Rafferty, Meryn Stuart, and Nancy J. Tomes. *Nurses of All Nations: A History of the International Council of Nurses, 1899–1999.* Philadelphia: Lippincott, 1999. Print.
7. Frazer Smith, James. *Life's Waking Part: Being the Autobiography of Reverend James Frazer Smith, Pioneer Medical Missionary to Honan, China and Missionary to Central India.* Toronto: Thomas Nelson and Sons, 1937. Print.
8. Paul, Pauline. "Religious Orders of Canada: A Presence on All Frontiers." *On All Frontiers: Four Centuries of Canadian Nursing.* Eds. Christina Bates, Dianne Dodd and Nicole Rousseau. Ottawa: University of Ottawa Press & Canadian Museum of Civilization: 125–138, 2005. Print.
9. Marshall, Clara. *The Woman's Medical College of Pennsylvania: An Historical Outline.* Philadelphia: P. Blakiston, Son & Co., 1897. Print.
10. Foster, Arnold. *Christian Progress in China: Gleanings from the Writings and Speeches of Many Workers.* Hankow: The Religious Tract Society, 1889. Print.
11. Grypma, Sonya. *Healing Henan: Canadian Nurses at the North China Mission, 1888–1947.* Vancouver: University of British Columbia Press, 2008. Print.
12. Letter from Dora Ruland, Medical Director, to Miss Ella Best, Executive Secretary, American Nurses Association, New York. 8 November 1948. BBC.
13. Kirkwood, Lynn. "Enough But Not Too Much: Nursing Education in English Language Canada (1874–2000)." *On All Frontiers: Four Centuries of Canadian Nursing.* Eds. Christina Bates, Dianne Dodd and Nicole Rousseau. Ottawa: University of Ottawa Press & Canadian Museum of Civilization: 183–96. Print.
14. Celebrating Our History: The Toronto General Hospital School for Nurses. Web. 5 Mar. 2010.
15. Hampton, Isabel. "The Aims of the Johns Hopkins Hospital Training School for Nurses." *The Hopkins Hospital Bulletin* 1 (December 1889): 2. UBC WLA.
16. Hampton Robb, Isabel. *Nursing Ethics: for Hospital and Private Use.* Cleveland: JB Savage, 1901. Print.
17. Hurd, Henry. "The Relation of the Training School for Nurses to the Johns Hopkins Hospital." *The Johns Hopkins Hospital Bulletin* 1 (December 1889): 7. UBC WLA (emphasis in original).
18. Frazer, Smith, Kaiyi Chen. 129–149.
19. Woman's Hospital of Philadelphia, Minutes (1863–1881). Drexel University College of Medicine, The Legacy Center, Archives and Special Collections (Philadelphia), hereafter DUCM.
20. Ibid.
21. Bus, Peter. Toronto the Good: William Howland, 1844–1893. Web. 24 Apr. 2010.

22. Ibid.
23. Austin, Alvyn. *Saving China: Canadian Missionaries in the Middle Kingdom, 1888–1959*. Toronto: University of Toronto Press, 1986. Print.
24. Ibid., 4.
25. Ibid., 6–8.
26. Brown 3:8.
27. Frazer Smith 74.
28. Lawrie, Bruce R. Summary of the Honan Mission. FA 186. United Church Archives (Toronto), hereafter UCA.
29. Letter from Jonathan Goforth to FMB in 1888. Cited in Brown 4: 8.
30. Frazer Smith 75.
31. Austin 26.
32. Austin 5.
33. Mott, John R. *The Evangelization of the World in This Generation*. New York: Student Volunteer Movement for Foreign Missions, 1905. Print.
34. Hunter, Jane. *The Gospel of Gentility: American Women Missionaries in Turn of the Century China*. New Haven: Yale University Press, 1984. Print.
35. Cheung, Yuet-wah. Missionary Medicine in China: A Study of Two Canadian Protestant Missions in China before 1937. Lanhan, MD: University Press of America, 1988; Austin, Alvyn. Saving China: Canadian Missionaries in the Middle Kingdom, 1888–1959. Toronto: University of Toronto Press, 1986; Maxwell, Grant. "Partners in Mission: The Grey Sisters," in Assignment in Chekiang: Seventy-one Canadians in China, 1902–1954. Scarborough, ON: Scarboro Foreign Mission Society, 1984.
36. Austin 32–35. See also MacKay.
37. Beaton, Kenneth. *Serving with the Sons of Shuh: Fifty Fateful Years in West China, 1891–1941*. Toronto: United Church of Canada, 1941. Print.
38. This estimate includes married nurses.
39. Austin.
40. Grypma. *Healing Henan*.
41. Preston, Louise Clara. *Flowers Amongst the Debris: A Canadian Nurse in War Torn China*. Brockville, ON: Preston Robb, n.d. Print.
42. Brown 57:11.
43. Stursberg, Peter. *The Golden Hope: Christians in China*. Toronto: United Church Publishing House, 1987. Print.
44. Grypma. Withdrawal from Weihui, 306–319.
45. Grypma. (Almost) Chinese.
46. Grypma. Withdrawal from Weihui.
47. Hampton Robb 11.
48. Grypma. *Healing Hena;* Chen; Simpson.
49. Chen, Kaiyi. "Missionaries and the Early Development of Nursing in China." *Nursing History Review* 4 (1996): 129–49. Print.
50. Chen 133.
51. Chen 134.
52. Simpson, Cora. *A Joy Ride through China for the NAC*. Shanghai: Kwang Hsueh, 1922. Print.
53. Simpson 11.
54. Chen.
55. Gage, Nina D. "Stages of Nursing in China." *American Journal of Nursing* 20.2 (1919): 115–21. Print.

56. Balme, Harold. *China and Modern Medicine: A Study in Medical Missionary Development.* London: United Council for Missionary Education, 1921. Print.
57. Chen.
58. Simpson.
59. Chen.
60. Simpson.
61. McGillivray, Donald. Ed. *A Century of Protestant Missions in China (1807–1907) Being the Centenary Conference Historical Volume.* New York: American Tract Society, 1907. Print.
62. Tomes, Nancy J. and Geertje Boschma. "Above All Other Things – Unity." *Nurses of All Nations: A History of the International Council of Nurses, 1899–1999.* Eds. Barbara L. Brush, Joan E. Lynaugh, Geertje Boschma, Anne Marie Rafferty, Meryn Stuart and Nancy J. Tomes. Philadelphia: Lippincott, 1999. 1–38. Print.
63. Ibid., 5.
64. Ibid., 5.
65. Hunter 14.
66. Tomes and Boschma.
67. Chen 130.
68. Tomes and Boschma 11.
69. Report of the Margaret Williamson Hospital, Shanghai, China, 1922. Women's Co-operating Foreign Mission Boards. DUCM.
70. Tyng, Anita E. Report of the Training School for Nurses for the Year 1883. Woman's Hospital of Philadelphia Annual Reports 1–25; BBC.
71. McGillivray 470.
72. Twenty-first Annual Report of the Board of Managers of the Woman's Hospital of Philadelphia January 1882, DUMC.
73. McGillivray; Margaret Williamson Hospital, 1885–1935. Acc 69 Missionaries, Box 1, Folder 24. China: Margaret Williamson Hospital, Shanghai, 50th Anniversary Pamphlet. DUCM.
74. Foster 192.
75. McGillivray 470.
76. Selmon, Bertha. "Women in Medicine Early Service in Missions (Continued)." *Medical Woman's Journal* 54.6 (1947): 44–6. Print.
77. Fiftieth anniversary booklet of the Margaret Williamson Hospital, 1885–1935. DUCM.
78. Ibid.
79. Foster, Arnold. Christian Progress in China: Gleanings from the Writings and Speeches of Many Workers. Hankow: The Religious Tract Society, 1889. Print.
80. Foster 192–193.
81. McGillivray 471.
82. McGillivray 471.
83. McGillivray 472.
84. McGillivray 472.
85. Grypma. *Healing Henan.*
86. Grypma, Sonya. "James R. Menzies: Preaching and Healing in Early 20th Century China." *Canadian Medical Association Journal* 170.1 (2004): 84–5. Print.
87. Margaret Williamson Hospital 18. DUMC.
88. Balme 149.

89. School of Nursing. Margaret Williamson Hospital. DUMC.
90. Ibid.
91. Ibid.
92. Grypma. *Healing Henan.*
93. Grypma. *Healing Henan.*
94. School of Nursing. Margaret Williamson Hospital. DUMC.
95. Balme 150.
96. Chen 135.
97. Chen 135.
98. Balme 150.
99. Jeanette, Ratcliffe. "Weihwei Hospital." *Honan Messenger* 13.4: 14–15. 83.058C Box 57 File 16 Series 3. UCA, n.d.
100. Balme 153.
101. Balme 153.
102. Leck, Greg. *Captives of Empire: the Japanese Internment of Allied Civilians in China, 1941–1945.* Bangor, PA: Shandy Press, 2006. Print.
103. Grypma. (Almost) Chinese.
104. Hampton Robb 11.
105. Grypma. Withdrawal from Weihui.

8

A History of Roman Catholic Nursing in the United States

Barbra Mann Wall

INTRODUCTION

This chapter explores the history of Roman Catholic religious women in nursing in the United States by focusing on Catholic sisters, or nuns, who are part of the official Catholic Church structure. They profess public vows of poverty, chastity, and obedience; commit themselves to live communally; and follow constitutions, or rules, of their particular religious order.[1] A focus on these women allows us to rethink religious roles in nursing by seeing sisters' power within religious institutions, such as Catholic hospitals. They exerted a significant influence on professional nursing in public and private facilities, in times of epidemics and wars, in cities, in mining and railroad centers, and on the frontier. This history is divided into three chronological periods: Catholic nursing and caretaking up to 1800, Catholic hospitals and nursing in the United States in the 19th and 20th centuries, and transitions in church and society after 1950.

History is important to nurses, especially today when issues of health care policy and practice are becoming prominent in the public arena. History provides a critical place to explore "the contingent relationships among the social, political, and economic forces that shaped nursing practice and modern health policy."[2] Although many understand the history of nursing as only that of powerlessness, of women who cannot gain control over their profession, there are alternative histories that show otherwise. Religion plays an important part in these alternative histories. One way to conceptualize power is through the experiences of Catholic nursing sisters, often invisible in the history of nursing, who did not see themselves as powerless[3] and whose religious identities created a special space for them to nurse.

The Catholic Church owns the nation's largest group of not-for-profit health care systems and facilities; thus, it is a major stakeholder in the health care field. As of 2009, more than 85 million patients were assisted in 636 Catholic hospitals. Furthermore, more than 4,500,000 fulltime employees work in Catholic hospitals, many of whom are nurses.[4] Only 14.6% of nurses employed in Catholic hospitals are Catholics.[5] In the United States, then, Catholic health care institutions are significant conduits for religious ideas about health and healing to both Catholics and non-Catholics. It is important to note that it was sister-nurses who were the leaders, developers, nurses, supervisors, and administrators of these Catholic hospitals. An examination of their work can create new knowledge about nursing's origins and its actual power and work in hospitals and policy.

In the 19th and 20th centuries, Catholic sister-nurses, more than most women of the day, wielded significant power and authority as hospital owners and administrators. They shared power in their hospitals with physicians, with whom nuns often battled over who should control access to care. In Catholic hospitals, sister-nurses created a space in the United States where a specific, socially beneficial type of care could be provided and purchased.[6] These sisters, while clearly mission-driven, were nevertheless skillful business managers who learned to fully understand and work within the often perilous hospital marketplace.

Catholic sisters also had an influence on Florence Nightingale. Even though Nightingale had a significant effect on modern nursing, in the 1850s she worked with both Protestant and Catholic sister-nurses in England, Germany, and France. Her experience as a nurse was relatively slight before the Crimean War, and Nightingale's work with nuns during that war significantly influenced her conception of nursing as a religious duty and as a disciplined and organized practice under a female hierarchy.[7]

Catholic hospitals began as individual, stand-alone institutions, and the majority of the ones in the United States were established and managed by sisters. An exception to female-based institutions was the Alexian Brothers from Aachen, Germany, who also were founded to care for the sick and dying. These women and men established their hospitals in the United States with religious missions to care for both Catholics and non-Catholics. In the last 50 years, however, all hospitals have experienced massive transformations as modern medicine made new demands and the number of Catholic women and men in religious orders plummeted.

CATHOLIC NURSING AND CARETAKING UP TO 1800

A nursing tradition developed during the beginning years of Christianity when church members cared for the sick, helped widows and children, and offered hospitality to strangers. Charity continued with the growth of monastic orders in the 5th and 6th centuries and extended into the 1500s as monasteries added hospital wards to their buildings. Caring meant giving comfort and spiritual sustenance, and it provided the rationale for nursing the sick to become part of the work of Catholic men and women's religious orders. Yet, just because nursing was done, it did not mean that women became nuns specifically to nurse. Indeed, many factors influenced women to join religious orders. Until the 17th century, nursing was irrelevant to their primary goal of spiritual perfection. Thus, whatever nursing they did, it was not a ministry but a means to obtain grace from God.[8,9]

The Alexian Brothers organized in Germany and the Low Countries in the early 14th century to bury the dead during the Black Death, or bubonic plague. By the 17th century, they had expanded their care to a variety of social outsiders, such as criminals and the mentally ill. Although many religious orders of men nursed in the medieval period, in the 17th century St. Vincent de Paul and St. Louise de Marillac made women more prevalent in nursing when they established the Daughters of Charity in France in 1633.[10] This was an active community of unmarried women and widows who lived together and dedicated themselves specifically to charitable works, including serving the sick poor.[11] Unlike the cloistered women's communities that participated primarily in contemplative prayer, the Daughters of Charity cared for the sick by living among the people that society had abandoned. They joined humility, obedience, and simplicity to good works, and they practiced nursing as an imitation of Christ's charitable qualities.

CATHOLIC HOSPITALS AND NURSING:
THE 19TH AND 20TH CENTURIES IN THE UNITED STATES

Expansion of Nursing Orders

Sisters framed their hospital roles after Vincent de Paul's model as they expanded to other countries. In 1728, the Ursuline sisters opened the first Catholic hospital in the North American continent in New Orleans, but the settlement was not part of the United States at that time. In 1809, Elizabeth Ann Seton founded the first American congregation, the Sisters of Charity of St. Joseph in Emmitsburg, Maryland. The sister-nurses linked charity and market activities as they expanded in the United States in the

19th century. In 1823, university officials at the Baltimore Infirmary asked them to staff their facility, where the nuns charged a small fee for admission. In 1828, Mullanphy Hospital, the first Catholic hospital in the United States, was founded, and the local bishop invited the Sisters of Charity to staff it. Between 1828 and 1860, this congregation established 18 hospitals in 10 states and the District of Columbia. These 18 hospitals constituted more than half of the Catholic hospitals founded before 1860. They cared for medical and surgical cases, patients with mental disorders, and those affected by epidemics.[12] In 1850, the Emmitsburg community joined with the international Daughters of Charity based in Paris, thus beginning the first American community of the Daughters of Charity of St. Vincent de Paul.[13]

It was in the 1840s and 1850s that the unprecedented immigration enlarged the possibilities for nursing by religious orders of women. Between 1820 and 1840, over 260,000 Irish came to the United States, fueled by the Great Famine that struck Ireland between 1846 and 1851. Germans were another Catholic immigrant group that settled in the United States before 1860, and larger increases in immigration occurred after 1890 when southern and eastern Europeans emigrated.[14] A primary reason for establishing Catholic hospitals was that Catholics could not enter non-Catholic facilities without being proselytized by Protestants. Urbanization and industrialization also contributed to hospital establishments as labor unrest and a breakdown of traditional sources of moral authority occurred. Church leaders sensed that significant Catholic populations existed with inadequate spiritual institutions. To tap this growing group, the Catholic Church created separate hospitals, orphanages, and schools, and staffed them with sisters who could preserve the Catholic identity.[15]

The epidemic-stricken cities of the mid-19th century needed hospitals immediately, and the Sisters of Charity of Nazareth was another congregation that responded quickly. After the cholera epidemic of 1832, they began caring for the sick in Louisville, Kentucky, under the direction of Mother Catherine Spalding. In 1842, they started a hospital in Nashville, Tennessee. The cholera and yellow fever epidemics between 1830 and 1840 brought other sisters into health care. For example, the Sisters of Charity of Our Lady of Mercy worked in a hospital in Charleston, South Carolina.[16,17] Racial discrimination limited African Americans' institutional development, but two communities of African American women cared for the sick during epidemics: the Oblate Sisters of Providence, founded in Baltimore in 1828, and the Sisters of the Holy Family, founded in New Orleans in 1842. During the 1832 cholera epidemic, the Oblate Sisters nursed over 200 patients in the Baltimore Almshouse; and in New Orleans in the 1850s, the Sisters of the Holy Family cared for victims of cholera and yellow fever.[18]

The daily arrival of immigrants, the church's fear of Protestant proselytizing, and the social problems brought on by urban growth all provided the impetus for nuns to establish hospitals in the United States. Although Protestant growth occurred particularly in the southern regions of the country, Catholic enclaves of European immigrants predominated in eastern cities such as New York, Boston, and Philadelphia, and midwestern cities such as St. Paul, St. Louis, and Chicago. The Catholic Church was in the minority in Texas and Utah, but these areas attracted many immigrant miners and railroad workers from Catholic countries who were potential American Catholics.[19,20] Thus, sisters went there, as well.

From 1840 to 1870, nuns from 34 different congregations either established or took charge of more than 70 acute hospitals in the United States.[21] Many sisters came from Europe, including the French Congregation of the Sisters of St. Joseph, who arrived in the United States in 1836. From 1849 to 1859, they staffed St. Joseph's Hospital in Philadelphia, largely to care for Irish immigrants. They also opened a hospital in Wheeling, Virginia (now West Virginia) in 1853 and St. Joseph's Hospital in St. Paul, Minnesota, in 1854.[22]

Irish women were particularly active in nursing. A prominent community that augmented nursing in the United States after 1840 was the Sisters of Mercy, founded by Catherine McAuley in Dublin in 1831. They arrived in the United States in 1843 with a history of caring for the sick poor in homes and in hospitals. They established a hospital in Pittsburgh in 1847 and in Chicago in 1852.[23] The Sisters of Mercy also went to Vicksburg, Mississippi, where they nursed victims of war and epidemics.[24]

Catholic women's congregations followed the immigrant into new industrial, railroad, and mining centers in the Trans-Mississippi West. For example, led by Mother Joseph Pariseau, the Sisters of Providence came from Montreal in 1856 to open a hospital in Vancouver, Washington, and eventually they established many hospitals in the Northwest. Another group of Irish Sisters of Mercy (now of Burlingame) under the direction of Mother Baptist Russell arrived in San Francisco in 1854. Mother Baptist, an immigrant from Ireland, and her sisters took charge of the county hospital during a cholera epidemic, but the county did not pay them for their care of 140 patients. Mother Baptist told the county supervisors to assume responsibility for payment or she would open her own hospital. She did so in 1857 when she established St. Mary's Hospital.[25,26]

Sisters' images as nurses improved during wars, such as when they nursed both Union and Confederate soldiers during the Civil War. The Sisters of the Holy Cross were not nurses until they volunteered their services during this period. Sister Paula Casey had left her family in Ireland and entered the Congregation of the Sisters of the Holy Cross at the age of 19. She had only been in the convent 3 years before she was sent to work as a nurse at

St. Johns' Hospital in Cairo, Illinois, in 1861. The initial task of the nurses was to clean the hospitals because no sanitary regulations were observed. Upon her arrival at St. Johns', Sister Paula recalled the filth of the hospital and the amputated arms and legs that piled up. She and another young sister were distressed, but their superior provided guidance. Sister Paula wrote, "Mother looked at us both in a kind, pitying look, and said now stop, you are here and must put your heart and Soul to the work. Pin up your habits, we will get three brooms, three buckets of water and we will first begin by wash- ing the walls and then the floors."[27] Nursing care included giving supportive care through nutritional diets, providing hygienic care, administering non- specific medications, and carrying out doctors' orders for dressing wounds. In addition to working in U.S. Army hospitals, the Sisters of the Holy Cross staffed the first U.S. Navy hospital ship, the USS Red Rover, thus becoming the first Navy nurses. As a result of good nursing care, the public's percep- tions of nuns and the Catholic Church itself improved dramatically after the Civil War.[28]

Because of religious persecution in Germany under Bismarck, addi- tional German women's communities sought refuge in the United States and opened hospitals across the Midwest. In 1869, the Poor Handmaids of Jesus Christ established hospitals in Fort Wayne and Mishawaka, Indiana, and in Chicago, Illinois.[29] The Sisters of the Third Order of St. Francis ex- panded their work in Illinois, which included the founding of St. John's Hos- pital in Springfield in 1875. That same year, the Poor Sisters of St. Francis Seraph of the Perpetual Adoration opened St. Elizabeth's Hospital in Lafay- ette, Indiana, one of 20 health care institutions they established across the Midwest in the late 19th and early 20th centuries. Many of these hospitals were founded to strengthen group cohesion for German immigrants, par- ticularly in the areas of language and devotional life.[30]

Sisters and brothers from Germany also opened health care institutions in areas with especially large numbers of German immigrants. Between 1866 and 1894, the first community of nursing brothers in the United States, the Alexian Brothers, opened hospitals in Chicago; St. Louis; Elizabeth, New Jersey; and Oshkosh, Wisconsin. Established in 1866 in a German neigh- borhood in Chicago, the Alexian Brothers Hospital drew patients mostly of German origin, along with men from dozens of other ethnic groups.[31] As the Chicago Tribune noted in August 1880, the institution wore the "stamp of decided German character"; patients could eat German food and obtain German Nauheim baths.[32] Admission demographics changed over time, however, as more U.S.-born patients were admitted, second-generation German Americans moved to the suburbs, and U.S.-born men joined the congregation.[33]

From 1870 to 1920, 189 different Catholic religious congregations established 275 Catholic acute care hospitals.[34] The Daughters of Charity continued their hospital expansion, opening St. Vincent's Hospital in Indianapolis in 1881 and many others across the United States. The Sisters of the Sorrowful Mother came from Rome in 1889 and opened 10 hospitals in the Midwest and Southwest. Beginning in 1891, Mother Frances Cabrini and the Missionary Sisters of the Sacred Heart established hospitals in New York, Chicago, and Seattle to care for Italian Americans. Also in 1891, Katherine Drexel, an heiress from Philadelphia and convert to Catholicism, founded the Sisters of the Blessed Sacrament for Indians and Colored People, and this community staffed nine different hospitals.[35-37]

Sisters also nursed in 1898 during The Spanish–American War, and eventually 282 nuns either volunteered their services or were asked to serve by the government and military officials. At Camp Hamilton in Lexington, Kentucky, 12 Sisters of the Holy Cross worked with both secular and religious sisters. Holy Cross Sister Lydia Clifford, a Civil War nurse who had experience in several hospitals, was "Chief Nurse" to: 50 Daughters of Charity from Emmitsburg, Maryland; 11 Sisters of St. Joseph of Carondelet; and 50 lay nurses.[38] The Sisters of St. Joseph of Carondelet went on to different camps in Georgia and Cuba. Most of the nursing care in the camps involved comfort measures and help with feeding and bathing for men suffering with typhoid fever. In her letters to her superior, Sister Lydia described long hours of hard work and the sisters' on-the-job training. In asking for more sister-nurses, she wrote, "There is so much *walking* . . . Sr. DeSales could give [the new sister nurses] some lessons on taking pulse, temperature, and respiration—for a day or two, and practice here will soon make them proficient."[39]

Significantly, sister-nurses' religious congregations offered some of the earliest health insurance policies. In 1875, for example, the Sisters of the Holy Cross established a scheme whereby miners in Salt Lake City, Utah, could receive care whenever they needed it if they donated $1.00 from their salaries.[40] During the 1890s, the Sisters of St. Joseph in Minneapolis generated funds to care for the needy during an economic depression. They issued "Sisters' Tickets" to those who would donate $100. These tickets allowed the donor to send a needy person to the hospital, where the ill person could have care free of charge.[41]

Expansion of Catholic Nursing Education

Years before the first nurse training schools were established in America in the 1870s, Catholic sisters were receiving nursing instruction in an apprentice-like system. Most women's religious communities had a period of training either during or after the novitiate, when young sisters trained for their future work. Teaching included not only nursing skills but also instructions on prayer, the Catholic Mass, and other religious practices. Congregations' constitutions articulated how the sick were to be treated, what daily schedule nurses should follow, how they should relate to physicians, how they were to prepare food and medicines, and most important, by what means the nuns should prepare a person for death.[42]

One of the earliest Catholic texts for sister-nurses is a handwritten one in two parts for the Daughters of Charity. The first section was written in French by a priest that included rules for religious nurses in France. Composed in 1796 during the French Revolution, it was particularly important for the Daughters of Charity, because priests could not exercise their clerical functions and the Daughters carried out much of the religious instruction of the sick during their work as nurses. This first section was recycled in 1841 when Mother Xavier Clark, superior of Elizabeth Seton's Daughters of Charity in the United States from 1839 to 1845, wrote a second section, in English, entitled *Instructions on the Care of the Sick*.[43] She wrote her *Instructions* to sister-nurses so they could carry the text in their pockets as a supplement to directions of doctors and experienced sister-nurses. For example, she instructed the sisters how to pray with a patient while not ignoring physical problems. Indeed, they were to care for them first because "the union between the soul and the body is so close that when the latter is suffering a great deal, the other, attentive to its wants, cannot think of anything else." She insisted, "But remember one thing—never begin to speak of religion before you have afforded them all the little relief and comforts you can to the poor body. By these you will find your way to the soul."[44]

In their evangelical work, sisters' rules and constitutions also provided guidelines. The 1888 *Manual of Decrees* of the Sisters of St. Joseph stated that they were to attend to a patient's bodily wants while being "very solicitous for the welfare of his soul." They were to avoid actively seeking Protestant converts, though, and to respect their religious convictions.[45] Yet, sisters' very work was a powerful form of evangelization. They proselytized by the virtue of their deeds and accomplished conversions in this way. Upon going to Utah in 1875, Sister Augusta Anderson remarked that the best way to do any good with the Mormons was "to have little to say, and give them good example."[46]

Sioban Nelson contextually situates sister-nurses in North America before the Civil War, in contrast to those in France, as being subject to Protestant hostility and part of a financially poor Catholic Church. Thus, they had to construct a new kind of nursing that focused on accountability, innovation, skill, and flexibility.[47] Mother Xavier's text reflects these concerns. She reminded sister-nurses that they would be in charge. The experienced sisters should "know everything," so that they could guide the less experienced sisters and also teach the men who were caring for male patients. Although the sister's model emphasized self-abnegation, respect, and devotion, the nurse also was to seek knowledge and ask questions. Sister-nurses were to be concerned with practical nursing care as well. They were to speak softly and to work gently, quietly, and unhurriedly. Nurses were to keep medicines covered to prevent evaporation, avoid mixing them, know the correct doses, and use clean utensils and clean water in all the preparations.[48]

Soon after the training school movement started, sisters of the various nursing congregations began providing official hospital training for their own nurses and eventually for non-Catholic nurses.[49] Few Catholic schools of nursing were in existence before the Spanish–American War; however, although the Sisters of Mercy's Mercy Training School for Nurses opened in Chicago in 1889. The war catalyzed the formation of other Catholic nursing programs, such that, between 1903 and 1913, following the trend of secular schools of nursing, Catholic sisters opened 203 training schools.[50] Nursing leaders' crusade to separate the trained from the untrained nurse was especially influential on nuns. Nursing was evolving from a service to a trained practice, and scientific and technological advances were developing. Hence, a good nurse came to be measured not only by her character but also by her technical competencies, knowledge of disease prevention, discipline, and organization.[51] Nuns responded to these challenges and updated their nursing practice by establishing their own nursing schools.

In 1915, the Catholic Hospital Association (later the Catholic Health Association [CHA]) was formed in response to technological advances and the hospital standardization movement that was changing health care delivery in the United States. At that time, more than 30 women's religious congregations sponsored 220 schools of nursing. By 1925, there were 581 Catholic acute and specialty hospitals in the United States, mainly under the care and administration of nuns; and most had their own nurse training programs.[52] Lectures typically included anatomy and physiology, medical and surgical problems, infection and contagion, orthopedics, bacteriology, surgical cases, sterilization and preparation of dressings, gynecology, obstetrics, and pediatrics. Sisters used textbooks, which secular training schools adopted.[53] Nurses worked 12-hour shifts, usually 6 days a week, and while physicians gave most of the early lectures, sisters provided the clinical instruction on hospital units. Yet there was little time to teach ethical and religious instruction. It was not until the 1920s that many Catholic schools of nursing introduced history and ethics courses.[54] In the mid-20th century, nursing education began to move from 3-year hospital-based diploma programs to 4-year baccalaureate schools in U.S. colleges and universities, and Catholic schools followed this path. Sisters eventually relocated their programs from hospital-owned to private and public baccalaureate schools.[55]

Nuns also worked to raise the standards of nursing education. In the 1930s, Sister John Gabriel Ryan, a Sister of Providence in Seattle, Washington, lobbied the state legislature against exploitation of nursing students. One judge said, "She took a man's name in religion, and I said of her that she was the ablest man in Olympia."[56] Her masculine name helped her transcend the usual female stereotype, and this minimized gender limitations. This was particularly helpful in the male-dominated realm of education policy.

As sisters adapted to changes in modern medicine and nursing, their training schools legitimized their nursing practice and increased their influence with student nurses and physicians. Nuns opened their schools to both sisters and lay women. As they updated their scientific training, sisters also could impress upon their students that nursing was a ministry to suffering humanity and in this way influenced secular nursing education.[57,58]

Specific Nursing Practices

Writings by 19th- and early 20th-century theologians as well as sisters reveal a range of interpretations of illness and suffering that affected nursing practice. According to Catholic beliefs, both religious and non-religious explanations prevailed when one became ill. Disease could be a deviation from normal health, caused and potentially correctable by natural means, or it could be caused by supernatural means, with healing by religious measures. Often, natural causes were subsumed under ultimate supernatural causes that only divine intervention could ameliorate.[59,60] Sisters of the 19th and 20th centuries adhered to all of these beliefs.

The 1888 *Manual of Decrees* of the Sisters of St. Joseph of Carondelet recorded a statement on sickness as a guide for sister-nurses. Indicating God's hand in illness, it stated: "God's fatherly providence frequently visits negligent Christians with sickness, in order to lead them back to the fold from which they unfortunately strayed."[61] It followed that Catholic sisters viewed illness not only in biological terms but also within a spiritual framework. Yet sisters' care differed from priests, who provided patients with messages that they should endure suffering as a means of strengthening faith. Rather, nuns placed greater emphasis on alleviating pain and suffering.[62,63]

In addition, records make it clear that sisters were concerned about making their patients well. In 1847, Sister Matilda Coskery, a Daughter of Charity, taught nursing to young sisters in the United States. Her notes, assembled in *A Manual for the Care of the Sick*, included a long section of care for patients with mental conditions such as alcoholism. She provided information on how to minister to physical and spiritual needs, how to interview a relative or friend of the patient, and the questions to ask when taking a history of the patient's past conditions.[64]

The *Manual of Decrees* for the Sisters of St. Joseph of Carondelet prescribed practical nursing tips: "She tries to be exact in carrying out the directions with regard to the remedies ordered, either by the physician or by Superiors, and does not, except by the doctor's advice, give any but ordinary remedies."[65] Prescriptions also focused on caring and compassion as necessary attitudes for sister-nurses. The Incarnate Word Sisters were to "serve [patients] with a tireless zeal," and entertain for the sick, not only a compassion, kindness and devotedness, but likewise a great respect.[66] The Sisters of the Holy Cross were to be mild, vigilant, patient yet firm, and compassionate for the suffering of others.[67]

By the latter decades of the 19th century, in addition to taking temperatures, pulses, and respirations, sister-nurses prepared and applied dressings and used hot and cold body packs for fever cases. They administered medications such as laudanum (opium in its liquid form), ointments, and poultices for pain relief; bathed patients; changed their linen; and prepared and administered food for special diets. They kept the sick room clean and well ventilated, protected the patient against contagious diseases, and prepared the dead for burial. They also observed patients for signs and symptoms of disease and its complications, recorded them in some form of clinical record, and reported them to the physician.[68] During one particularly hectic week in 1889, the Sisters of Charity of the Incarnate Word at St. Joseph's Infirmary in Fort Worth, Texas, admitted 19 patients, discharged 6, transferred 1 to another room, and cared for 24 others, prompting the annalist to remark, "Our heels are praying very hard all day."[69]

The experiences of the Sisters of St. Francis of Our Lady of Lourdes in Rochester, Minnesota, provide a case study of nursing in the late 19th and early 20th centuries. They cared for persons after a tornado struck that city in 1883. Afterward, Mother Mary Alfred Moes proposed to build and staff a hospital in that city if Dr. William Worrall Mayo and his sons would agree to provide the medical care. This collaboration resulted in the development of St. Mary's Hospital and what is now known as the Mayo Clinic. The first sister-nurses were trained by Edith Graham, the only trained nurse in Rochester and an employee of the Mayo physicians. No other formal training was available for the sisters, and nursing was extremely challenging. Their duties included preparing and serving meals, bathing patients and keeping them comfortable, dressing wounds, and giving medications. They used thermometers and gave enemas. Nurses particularly had to rely on their powers of observation, and they learned how to distinguish between pallor from anemia and pallor from internal bleeding. St. Mary's Hospital and the Mayo Clinic excelled not only because of the skill of the Mayo brothers as surgeons but also because of the excellent nursing care by the sisters. Patients found that the hospital was a place where people could go to be healed. Within five years of St. Marys' opening, the sisters treated more than 500 patients annually.[70] Sisters carried the major responsibility for nursing and other departments as they headed different floors, X-ray departments, kitchens, and the like.

In 1913 at Mercy Hospital in Chicago, the Sisters of Mercy had various specialties in addition to nursing, including operating room care, X-ray technology, and pharmacy. Three sisters were anesthetists. A sister-nurse was in charge of the obstetrical department, and each floor was supervised by a nursing sister.[71]

After 1900, religious congregations' successes in the United States improved their financial standings. Hospitals installed electricity and other conveniences, while at the same time, chapels were built that included beautiful religious icons. Sisters marketed their health care institutions as including "sacred" space within the "medical" space of the hospital. Hospital art and architecture were important to Catholics, and they accepted paintings, sculptures, and other religious icons that distinguished them from the Protestant tradition, which emphasized preaching. To Catholics, artworks were signs that mediated religious meanings. Because Catholic sisters viewed illness in both biological terms and within a spiritual framework, they supplemented their nursing care with prayer cards, rosary beads, and other religious symbols designed to provide comfort and healing. They also accompanied patients to Mass in hospital chapels.[72]

Catholic sisters also held devotions to the saints with their Catholic patients to remind them of their faith. In the 19th to the mid-20th century, devotions were an important aspect of Catholic spirituality. As McDannell asserts: "Catholics learned and accepted the reality of a supernatural community because they were taught how to interact with it through their devotional practices."[73] Devotions were a form of popular religion that bridged the Church's intellectual teachings and expressed one's personal piety. Sisters helped patients with exercises such as the rosary, a private prayer consisting of stating 150 "Hail Mary's" and devotions to the Sacred Heart of Jesus, which focused on His divine love for mankind and encouraged humility. Devotions to the saints and the Virgin Mary were especially popular,[74] making the hospital's Catholicism unmistakable. At the same time, by caring, serving, and treating the poor, the sick, and the dying, sisters were involved in important religious experiences. Indeed, nursing the sick and dying placed religious sisters in situations that linked the worldly and the divine. They could participate in important and dramatic religious experiences such as baptism and helping a Catholic to confess their sins before dying; this conferred on them a special mission. In their hospitals, sister-nurses could do spiritually important work for their patients.[75–77]

Prayers for the sick and dying had a long history in the Catholic Church, and references were particularly prominent in nuns' writings. Rather than representing a single action, however, prayer was integrated into sister-nurses' work. Their prayers served as invitations to religious encounters.[78] To Catholics, prayer and the sacraments could bring grace and favors from Jesus and Mary, including healing the sick. Lay Catholics often asked sisters to pray for them, believing that nuns' prayers were more powerful than their own. For example, in 1897 a patient at Santa Rosa Infirmary in San Antonio requested that his remaining salary go to the Incarnate Word Sisters so that they would pray for him after he died. A few months later, family members transferred a woman's remains from one cemetery to another that was in closer proximity to Santa Rosa so the Incarnate Word Sisters could pray for her when they visited the site.[79] In addition to healing the sick, one of the corporal works of mercy, according to Catholic tradition, was to bury the dead.[80] The Incarnate Word Sisters kept a "dead house" behind Santa Rosa Infirmary, which held bodies of the deceased until relatives arrived. Sisters frequently held wakes in their hospital parlors, and families often asked nuns to attend to burial services.[81]

Catholic sisters participated in all of these activities in their traditional dress. They maintained their authority in the Catholic community partly through their vow of chastity, which marked a boundary between them and members of the laity. They underscored their asexual identities not only by their vow of chastity but also through their religious clothing that covered their physical bodies.[82] Sisters' religious clothing was a physical representation of religion. In the early 20th century, however, they adapted their clothing to meet newer scientific standards by wearing washable white habits instead of the traditional black ones, considered by some medical authorities to harbor germs.[83]

As late as 1945, Catholic nursing texts continued to call for compassion for the suffering patient and prayers for deathbed conversions.[84] In her book, *The Nurse: Handmaid of the Divine Physician*, Sister Mary Berenice Beck, RN, PhD in nursing education, wrote about the Catholic nurse's obligations for the spiritual care of patients. She included lessons for the care of dying Catholic patients and specific prayers to use. She also had a chapter on care of the non-Catholic patient. Catholic nurses, either lay or sisters, were to emphasize common beliefs and practices and to encourage patients to seek ministrations from their own churches. Although the nurse could use indirect methods such as prayers and the exercise of good example, she may more directly leave reading materials conveniently at hand for the patient to pick up and read. Yet, she should never engage in heated arguments or belittle others' religions.[85]

By examining sisters' writings, including those of both Mother Xavier Clark and Sister Mary Berenice Beck, one can see continuity of instruction in the religious meaning of sickness and dying and a religious understanding of nursing. Indeed, care was an essential component of Catholic sisters' nursing, and it included tending the sick physically, psychologically, and spiritually. In the late 19th to the mid-20th century, everything about the design and ambiance of the Catholic hospital reflected that it was both a medical facility and a sacred place.[86]

TRANSITIONS IN CHURCH AND SOCIETY: AFTER 1950

Changes in Education, Hospitals, and the Catholic Church

Much changed for American Catholics after World War II as their affluence and education rose. In the 1950s, the Sister Formation Conference led to better education for sisters, including nurses, and prepared them for their professional roles. By 1966, for example, 65% of the nation's 175,000 sisters had college degrees, and many of them were nurses working and administering hospitals.[87]

Paralleling educational changes were transformations within the Catholic Church. Between 1962 and 1965, the Second Vatican Council (Vatican II) met, which, begun by Pope John XXIII, attempted to bring the church up-to-date. *Aggiornamento*, or change and adaptation to meet the needs of the times, was a key term used during the Council. The Council document most often linked with aggiornamento is *Gaudium et Spes* ("Joy and Hope," or the Pastoral Constitution on the Church in the Modern World), which for the first time saw all people, including laymen and women, as having distinctive missions in the church rather than being mere "helpers of the hierarchy." As a result, more leadership roles in Catholic institutions became open to the laity.[88] After Vatican II, religious congregations of women renewed their commitment to the poor and oppressed.

Changes in health care also occurred as all American hospitals had to face rising hospital costs; consequently, hospitals had to balance their responsibilities to the public with economic realities. Medicare and Medicaid expanded coverage for the elderly and poor, investor-owned hospitals entered the hospital marketplace, and not-for-profit hospital systems grew. For the sisters, in particular, social justice issues began taking priority as they worked to expand care for minorities and the uninsured. Thus, in the 1960s, they took social causes of disease, such as unemployment, racism, and poverty, into account as significant factors in disease causation.[89] This was a distinct change.

Nurse Activists for Social Justice

Social justice has been a fundamental part of Catholic social teaching, beginning in 1891 when Pope Leo XIII issued his encyclical, *Rerum Novarum*, which offered a program of reform for labor based on the concept of social justice. In 1963, Pope John XXIII addressed the world in his encyclical, *Pacem in Terris* (Peace on Earth), which included the right to health care as part of his list of individual human rights. It was at this time that sisters came to believe that charity alone was only part of their mission. Many became active in the civil rights movement.[90] Events in the 1960s provide examples of how Catholic sister-nurses, in particular the Sisters of St. Joseph from Rochester, New York, and the Daughters of Charity in Chicago, expanded their work for racial justice.[91]

The Sisters of St. Joseph participated in the southern civil rights movement that culminated on March 7, 1965, or "Bloody Sunday," when Selma authorities attacked 600 marchers who were crossing the Edmund Pettus Bridge in route from Selma to Montgomery as a protest against voting restrictions. The Sisters of St. Joseph cared for the injured marchers in their Good Samaritan Hospital throughout the afternoon, and the workers tended more than 100 people.[92,93] On March 10, a group of priests and nuns from the Midwest chartered a plane and arrived in Selma to stand in solidarity with the marchers. Two of the sisters were nurses: Sister Ann Benedict from St. Joseph's Hospital in Kansas City, the first African American to enter the Sisters of St. Joseph of Carondelet; and Sister Mary Antona Ebo, one of the first African American members of the Franciscan Sisters of Mary. When the protest march began on March 10, the sister-nurses walked in the front lines.[94]

Three months after "Bloody Sunday," some of the Daughters of Charity of St. Vincent de Paul became involved in racial protests in Chicago. Since 1947, they had operated a settlement house, Marillac House, in an African American section of the city. The Daughters were especially aware of the poverty and racial discrepancies that handicapped their neighbors, having lived in the same neighborhood with them. Sister Jane Breidenback, for example, was a nurse and was also known as "the Alley Sister" because she organized neighborhood cleanups to make playgrounds safe for children.[95]

On June 12, 1965, Sister Jane heard about a civil rights gathering that would be held that afternoon to protest public school segregation. She decided to participate in the march because she wanted to represent the people in her neighborhood who were unable to attend, "and because I myself believe that the Negro children are not given equally good educational advantages in this city . . . And I believe there is a need for religious to support their cause."[96] The march soon turned acrimonious when a policeman told them that unless they got back on the sidewalk, they would be arrested. At the instruction of the leaders of the march, Sister Jane knelt and promptly was arrested. She and the others went to police headquarters and were fined $200. She considered the demonstration and the fine to be a small price to pay for the privilege of representing the needs of the poor.[97]

Increasing Influence of the Vatican

It was also in the post-Vatican II period that the Vatican had greater influence in medical ethics documents for Catholic hospitals in the United States. The *Ethical and Religious Directives for Catholic Health Care Services* affirm certain ethical standards of behavior based on the church's teaching on the dignity of the human person; as such, they provide direction on moral issues. In 1920, the Archdiocese of Detroit published the first written set of medical ethical norms for Catholic hospitals, which most Catholic facilities followed. In the 1950s, Catholic theologians took a leading role in bioethical discussions, such as those concerning abortion and reproductive issues that were becoming matters of public policy.

In the last decades of the 20th century, ethical issues continued to develop over the growth of biotechnology. For-profit hospitals also were expanding, and many Catholic hospitals began to merge or partner with non-Catholic facilities. As these hybrid organizations emerged, tensions developed that challenged Catholic identity. To counter these threats, bishops and the Vatican became more influential in hospital decisions.[98] In 1971, the bishops came out with a new version of *Ethical and Religious Directives*, which more clearly banned tubal ligations, artificial insemination, and artificial birth control. In 1975, the Vatican barred sterilizations that might be performed when necessary to avoid diseases arising from pregnancy.[99] In 1994 and 2001, the National Conference of Catholic Bishops again revised the *Ethical and Religious Directives*, this time to be more specific about partnerships between Catholic and non-Catholic hospitals, especially in banning reproductive services such as sterilization and in vitro fertilization. Today, supporting the Catholic Church's teachings on abortion and reproductive services has become a distinct mark of Catholic hospitals' identity. Nurses who work in these facilities were (and still are) expected to keep these *Ethical and Religious Directives*.

At the beginning of the 1970s, as the Vatican reasserted the Catholic Church's traditional male supremacy, sisters' decreasing numbers in congregations were also occurring, as many sisters left and fewer entered religious communities. Other roles in the church opened up to women who did not require taking vows. Thus, nuns' influence in the overall hospital market declined as the laity, usually men, took over administrative positions. In some parts of the country, however, individual sisters maintained power over their institutions, whereas in others they lost control over hospital operations but gained influence as members of boards of directors and officers in the CHA.[100] Many sisters have now moved into new areas of care. Just as they formerly nursed patients during cholera epidemics, they now work with patients with HIV/AIDS and care for the elderly, people whose needs are not being met by other groups.

Catholic hospitals' public identities as institutions that originated largely through religious movements and values dimmed over time. Yet religion still has an important role in the American health care system and nursing. Today, pastoral care is emphasized with participation by laity, sisters, brothers, Protestant ministers, and Catholic priests.[101] Although sisters are not as readily visible in their hospitals, they mentor pastoral care ministers who are charged with the role of carrying out the hospital's original missions. Furthermore, some Catholic hospitals still have sister-nurses as administrators who understand that it is people themselves that ultimately matter most—not dollars and cents, but individuals' needs.[102]

Finally, the health care crisis beginning in the 1990s saw greater participation of Catholic sister-nurses as leaders of the CHA. Most significant is their support for universal health care insurance. In July of 2009, the CHA published a statement calling upon legislators to enact health care reform that would provide access to care for all Americans. Yet abortion was the key negotiating issue that held up passage of any bill, pitting bishops, who feared the bill would support abortion, against sisters, who did not. Rather, they saw the legislation as supporting health care for the poor and marginalized. The historic legislation (HR 3590, the Patient Protection and Affordable Care Act) passed on March 21, 2010, and sisters' support was definitely influential, although some bishops and conservative laity have criticized the sisters in public and private. Abortion issues reveal the conflicts within the church over how much to pit opposition to abortion and other procedures against concerns for social justice.[103]

CONCLUSION

In closing, Catholic hospitals have historically recognized the importance of nursing. In the early 20th century, sisters' nursing roles gave them influence and prestige with physicians and their patients. Although they could not administer the sacraments, they still could influence nursing education for both Catholics and non-Catholics while also functioning as spiritual agents of care.[104] The sisters' historical construction of nursing in the 19th century and the obstacles they faced later, such as the Vatican's greater attempt to control hospitals through the *Ethical and Religious Directives*, indicate a distinct approach to Catholic nursing.

Today, as they move away from the bedside into administrative and corporate roles, sister-nurses use skills they learned as nurses.[105] Most important, as Catholic sister-nurses worked with non-Catholics in public arenas such as hospitals and military facilities, admitted laywomen into their nurse training programs, hired more lay people for their hospitals, and worked toward accepted standards of education, they also stamped their own understanding of nursing onto society.

NOTES

1. McBrien, Richard. *Encyclopedia of Catholicism*. San Francisco: HarperCollins Publishers, 1995.
2. D'Antonio, Patricia, Cynthia Connolly, Barbra M. Wall, et al. "Histories of Nursing: The Power and the Possibilities." *Nursing Outlook* 58.4 (2010): 208.
3. Ibid., 207–213.
4. Nicholson, Sumitra, ed. *Official Catholic Directory 2009*. New York: National Register Publishing, 2009.
5. American Hospital Association. *American Hospital Association Annual Survey 2009*. Chicago: American Hospital Association, 2009.
6. Wall, Barbra M. *Unlikely Entrepreneurs: Catholic Sisters and the Hospital Marketplace, 1865–1925*. Columbus, OH: Ohio State University Press, 2005.
7. Wall, Barbra M. "Textual Analysis as a Method for Historians of Nursing." *Nursing History Review* 14 (2006): 227–242.
8. Wittberg, Patricia. *The Rise and Fall of Catholic Religious Orders: A Social Movement Perspective*. Albany, NY: SUNY Press, 1994.
9. Wall, 2005, *op. cit.*
10. Rapley, Elizabeth. *The Devotes: Women & Church in Seventeenth-Century France*. Montreal: McGill-Queen's University Press, 1990.
11. Nelson, Sioban. *Say Little, do much: Nursing, Nuns, and Hospitals in the Nineteenth Century*. Philadelphia: University of Pennsylvania Press, 2001.
12. Farren, Suzy. *A Call to Care: The Women Who Built Catholic Healthcare in America*. St. Louis: The Catholic Health Association of the United States, 1996.
13. Hannefin, Daniel. *Daughters of the Church: A Popular History of the Daughters of Charity in the United States, 1809–1987*. Brooklyn, NY: New City Press, 1989.
14. Dolan, Jay. *The American Catholic Experience: A History from Colonial Times to the Present*. Notre Dame and London: University of Notre Dame Press, 1992.
15. Wall, 2005, op. cit.
16. Stepsis, Ursula, and Doris Liptak, eds. *Pioneer Healers: The History of Women Religious in American Health Care*. New York: Crossroad, 1989.
17. Kauffman, C. *Ministry and Meaning: A Religious History of Catholic Health Care in the United States*. New York: Crossroad, 1995.
18. Morrow, Diane. *Persons of Color and Religious at the Same Time: The Oblate Sisters of Providence, 1828–1860*. Chapel Hill: University of North Carolina Press, 2002.
19. Dolan, op. cit.
20. Wall, 2005, op. cit.
21. Stepsis and Liptak, op. cit.
22. Coburn, Carol, and Martha Smith. *Spirited Lives: How Nuns Shaped Catholic Culture and American Life, 1836–1920*. Chapel Hill: University of North Carolina Press, 1999.
23. Clough, Joy. "Chicago's Sisters of Mercy." *Chicago History* 32.1. (Summer 2003): 42–55.

24. Oakes, Mary. *Angels of Mercy: An Eyewitness Account of the Civil War and Yellow Fever by a Sister of Mercy.* Baltimore: Cathedral Foundation Press, 1998.

25. Stepsis and Liptak, op. cit.

26. Kauffman, op. cit.

27. Casey, M. P. *Letter to Mother M. Augusta Anderson.* Bertram Hall, Saint Mary's, Notre Dame, IN: Archives, Congregation of the Sisters of the Holy Cross, 1894.

28. Wall, Barbra. "Grace Under Pressure: The Nursing Sisters of the Holy Cross, 1861–1865." *Nursing History Review* 1 (1993): 71–87.

29. Specht, A. "The Power of Ethnicity in a Community of Women Religious: The Poor Handmaids of Jesus Christ in the United States, 1868–1930." *U. S. Catholic Historian* 19 (Winter 2001): 53–64.

30. Ibid.

31. Alexian Brothers' Hospital. *74th Annual Report.* Elk Grove Village, IL: Alexian Brothers of America, 1939.

32. *Chicago Tribune.* August 25, 1880.

33. Alexian Brothers Archives. *Hospital Statistics.* Alexian Brothers Archives, Arlington Heights, IL: 1942.

34. Stepsis and Liptak, op. cit.

35. Stepsis and Liptak, op. cit.

36. Kauffman, op. cit.

37. Wall, 2005, op. cit.

38. Wall, Barbra. "Courage to Care: The Sisters of the Holy Cross in the Spanish-American War." *Nursing History Review* 3 (1995): 55–77.

39. Clifford, Mary Lydia. *Letter to Mother M. Annunciata McSheffery.* Bertram Hall, Saint Mary's, Notre Dame, IN: Archives, Congregation of the Sisters of the Holy Cross, 1898, September 21.

40. Wall, 2005, op. cit.

41. Sampson, A. T. *Care with Prayer: A History of St. Mary's Hospital and Rehabilitation Center.* Minneapolis: St. Mary's Hospital and Rehabilitation Center, 1987.

42. Wall, Barbra. "Science and Ritual: The Hospital as Medical and Sacred Space, 1865–1920." *Nursing History Review* 11 (2003): 51–68.

43. Clark, Mother X. *Instructions on the Care of the Sick.* St. Louis, MO: Marillac Provincial House, Daughters of Charity of St. Vincent de Paul, 1841.

44. Ibid.

45. Sisters of St. Joseph of Carondelet. *Manual of Decrees, Customs and Observances, for the use of the Congregation of the Religious of St. Joseph of Carondelet.* St. Louis, MO: Ev. E. Carreras, Steam Printer and Binder. Archives of the Congregation of the Sisters of St. Joseph of Carondelet, 1888: 114.

46. Sisters of the Holy Cross. *Sister Augusta Anderson Letter to Father Sorin.* Saint Mary's, Notre Dame, IN: Congregation of the Sisters of the Holy Cross, 1875, July 13.

47. Nelson, Sioban. *Say Little, Do Much: Nursing, Nuns, and Hospitals in the Nineteenth Century.* Philadelphia: University of Pennsylvania Press, 2001.

48. Clark.

49. Wall, 1995, op. cit.

50. Kauffman, op. cit.

51. Reverby, Susan. *Ordered to Care: The Dilemma of American Nursing, 1850–1945.* Cambridge: Cambridge University Press, 1987.

52. O'Grady, John. *Catholic Charities in the United States.* New York: Arno Press, 1971.

53. Wall, Barbra. "Definite Lines of Influence: Catholic Sisters and Nurse Training Schools. *Nursing Research* 50.5 (2001): 314–321.
54. Kauffman, op. cit.
55. Wall, Barbra. *American Catholic Hospitals: A Century of Changing Markets and Missions*. Piscataway, NJ: Rutgers University Press, 2011.
56. Geraghty, James. Letter to Sister John [of the Cross], 7 Jul. 1939. (1257) RPP, Box 2, Biography, Miscellaneous Correspondence, Sisters of Providence Archives, Seattle, WA.
57. Richardson, Jean. "Sisterhood is Powerful: Sister-Nurses Confront the Moderniza-tion of Nursing." *Florence Nightingale and her Era: A Collection of New Scholarship*. Ed. Vern Bullough et al. New York and London: Garland Publishing, Inc., 1990. 261–273.
58. Wall, 2001, op. cit.
59. Amundsen, Darrel. *Medicine, Society, and Faith in the Ancient and Medieval Worlds*. Baltimore: Johns Hopkins University Press, 1996.
60. Ferngren, Gary. *Medicine and Health Care in Early Christianity*. Baltimore: Johns Hopkins University Press, 2009.
61. *Manual of Decrees, op. cit.*
62. Wall, 2001, op. cit.
63. Wall, Barbra. "Textual Analysis as a Method for Historians of Nursing." *Nursing History Review* 14 (2006): 227–242.
64. Kauffman, op. cit.
65. *Manual of Decrees*, op. cit.
66. Sisters of Charity of the Incarnate Word. *Directory of the Sisters of Charity of the Incarnate Word*. Archives of the Motherhouse, Sisters of Charity of the Incarnate Word, 1906. 207.
67. Sisters of the Holy Cross. *Rules of the Congregation of the Sisters of the Holy Cross*. Bertram Hall, Saint Mary's, Notre Dame, IN: Archives, Congregation of the Sisters of the Holy Cross, 1895. 142.
68. Hinssen, L. *The Nursing Sister: A Manual for Candidates and Novices of Hospital Communities*. Springfield, IL: H. W. Rokker Co., 1899.
69. Sisters of Charity of the Incarnate Word. *Remark Book, St. Joseph's Infirmary.*, San Antonio, TX: Archives of the Motherhouse, Sisters of Charity of the Incarnate Word, 1889.
70. Whelan, Ellen. *The Sisters' Story; Saint Mary's Hospital – Mayo Clinic 1889–1939*. Rochester, NY: Mayo Foundation for Medical Education and Research, 2002.
71. Sisters of Mercy. "Training School Methods and Organization Under Religious Orders." *American Journal of Nursing* 13.1 (1913): 260–263.
72. Wall, 2005, op. cit.
73. McDannell, Colleen. *Material Christianity: Religion and Popular Culture in America*. New Haven: Yale University Press, 1995. 142.
74. Wall, 2005, op. cit.
75. Wall, 2003, op. cit.
76. Wall, 2005, op. cit.
77. Wall, 2011, op. cit.
78. Wall, Barbra, and Sioban Nelson. "Our Heels are Praying Very Hard all Day: The Working Prayer of the 19th-century Religious Nurse." *Holistic Nursing Practice* 17.6 (2003): 320–328.

79. Sisters of Charity of the Incarnate Word. *Remark Book, Santa Rosa Infirmary*. San Antonio, TX: Archives of the Motherhouse, Sisters of Charity of the Incarnate Word, 1896. Web. Jan. 6 and Oct. 27.
80. McBrien, op. cit.
81. *Remark Book Santa Rosa Infirmary.* 24 Oct. 1896; 6 Jan. and 27 Oct. 1897.
82. Wall, 2003, op. cit.
83. Kauffman, op. cit.
84. Kauffman, op. cit.
85. Sister Mary B. Beck. *The Nurse: Handmaid of the Divine Physician*. Philadelphia: Lippincott, 1945.
86. Wall, 2005, op. cit.
87. Kennelly, Karen. *The Religious Formation Conference, 1954–2004*. Silver Spring, MD: Religious Formation Conference, 2009.
88. Sullivan, Maureen. *The Road to Vatican II: Key Changes in Theology*. New York: Paulist Press, 2007, 120.
89. Wall, 2011, op. cit.
90. Ibid.
91. Wall, Barbra. "Catholic Sister Nurses in Selma, Alabama, 1940–1972," *Advances in Nursing Science* 32.1 (2009): 91–102.
92. Wall, 2011, op. cit.
93. Ibid.
94. Stepsis and Liptak, op. cit.
95. *Chicago Sun Times.* 20 March 1966.
96. Jane B. *Personal Statement Regarding June 12, 1965 Demonstration*. Marillac House Papers, Box 2, June 1965 folder. Chicago, IL: Chicago History Museum, June 13, 1965.
97. Wall, 2011, op. cit.
98. Pellegrino, Edmund. "Catholic Health Care Ministry and Contemporary Culture: The Growing Divide." *Urged on by Christ: Catholic Health Care in Tension with Contemporary Culture*. Ed. E. J. Furton. Philadelphia: National Catholic Bioethics Center, 2007, 13–30.
99. Wall, 2011, op. cit.
100. Kauffman, op. cit.
101. Wall, 2011, op. cit.
102. Wall, 2011, op. cit.
103. Wall, 2005, op. cit.
104. Wall, 2011, op. cit.
105. Wall, 2011, op. cit.

9

Hinduism and Nursing

Rani Srivastava, Bhartendu Srivastava, and Raman Srivastava

INTRODUCTION

Hinduism is a way of life, as well as a highly organized social and religious system. As the world's third largest religion, Hinduism is practiced by people primarily from the Indian subcontinent. It is difficult to ascertain the origin of Hinduism, as it can neither be linked to any one individual nor associated with a definitive time. Widely regarded as the world's oldest religion, Hinduism is a reflection of combined cultural, religious, and philosophical ideas that originated in India during the Vedic age (3000–1500 BCE).[1]

The word Hindu refers to the geographical origins of the river Indus in the north of India. In the Indian language, the river was called *Sindhu*, but was mistakenly identified as Hindu by foreigners. Thus the region became known as Hindustan (place of Hindus), its inhabitants were referred to as Hindus, and their religion was called Hinduism. To this day, the relationship between religion and the culture of the region is intertwined. Interestingly, the scriptures do not refer to the religion as Hinduism; rather, they refer to *Sanatan Dharma* (eternal duties or path). Other religions that are also considered as *Sanatan Dharma* include Jainism, Sikhism, and Buddhism. While each of these religions has unique characteristics, collectively they are seen as "branches of the same tree" and can trace their roots back to Hinduism.

This chapter begins with an overview of the core tenets of Hinduism. An extensive discussion of the religion is beyond the scope of this chapter; however, we have highlighted key concepts and principles that provide the foundation required to understand Hinduism's impact on health care. The overview is followed by discussion of how Hindu perspectives view the concepts and constructs central to nursing, such as person, health, environment, nurse, and ethics. The notion of spirituality, as it is implicated in the religious tradition, will be highlighted throughout. We conclude with a discussion of how the religion and philosophy of Hinduism may influence the response to illness, for both patients and nurses.

It is important to state that the content of this chapter describes the most traditional views of the religion. Individuals of the Hindu faith differ tremendously in their understanding, interpretation, belief, and adherence to the concepts described. Our intention is to provide a deeper understanding of the religious concepts as a way of exploring the potential influence of religion on individuals. However, such information must be thoughtfully considered and applied and must not be used as a definitive guide from which to make assumptions about people's beliefs, values, or thought processes.

OVERVIEW OF HINDUISM

The Hindu religion and way of life are traditionally characterized by five prominent themes. These include a belief in: one absolute being (*Brahman*); rebirth or reincarnation (*Sansara* or *Samsara*); law of cause and effect leading to a desire for right action (*Karma*); doctrine of religious and moral duties, conduct, and virtue (*Dharma*); and an ultimate goal of *Moksha* or liberation from the cycle of birth and rebirth. Although Hindus believe in one eternal, omniscient (all knowing), omnipresent (all pervading), omnipotent (unlimited) supreme being called Brahman or *Ishwar*, there are many manifestations of Brahman and the religion is characterized by a multiplicity of Gods and Goddesses among whom individuals are free to choose to worship. Each deity, in fact, represents an aspect of Brahman and these multiple manifestations should not be misunderstood as polytheism. Brahman is formless, infinite, eternal and beyond anything that we can conceive. Neither male nor female, Brahman can manifest itself in multiple forms, including Gods and Goddesses. The relationship between the many manifest deities and the unmanifest Brahman has been compared to the relationship between the sun and its rays. We cannot experience the sun itself, but we can experience its rays and the qualities as held by those rays. Although the sun's rays are many, ultimately there is only one source: one sun.[2]

The most commonly worshipped deities are Vishnu, Shiva, Rama, Krishna, Ganesha, Kartikeya, Hanuman and the Goddesses Durga,

Lakshmi, and Saraswati. Three principle deities, representing the three fundamental powers of nature—creation, preservation, and destruction—play an integral role in running the cosmos: Brahma (not to be confused with Brahman) is the God of creation, Vishnu is regarded as the preserver of the universe, and Shiva is the God of destruction. Rama and Krishna are human forms of God at different times in history who appear to destroy evil, protect saints, sages, and devotees, and be role models for humanity by their lives and teachings. Each God or Goddess is associated with specific qualities; for example, Saraswati is the Goddess of arts, music, knowledge, and wisdom, and Lakshmi is associated with wealth, fortune, courage, and fertility.

The pluralistic nature of Hinduism further reinforces the notion of Hinduism as a way of life. As a result, there is greater acceptance of multiple faiths and ways of worship, and the beliefs that guide how one lives life is more important than how, where, or to whom worship occurs.

Hindus believe that existence is eternal and that each life is a cycle in the ongoing journey or quest toward *moksha*. *Moksha* or *mukti* (freedom) does not refer to liberation from sin, as in Christianity. Instead, it refers to release from the human condition and *karma* (good or bad) and into a condition where time and space cease to exist and all is seen as one.[3] The concepts of *karma* and *dharma* are central to how life unfolds. Karma is the universal law according to which every experience and action is the effect of a cause and is, in turn, a cause of an effect. The law of Karma essentially states that one's actions determine what fruits one gets. Life events are based on the integrity with which the person has lived current as well as previous lives.[4] Karma is everything that one has ever thought, spoken, done, or caused (intentionally or unintentionally) and is also that which one thinks, speaks, or does this very moment. Destiny, or *bhagya*, is different from karma, but is seen as a reflection of the fruit of karma. Thus, karma is not imposed by outside forces, either by God or by a punitive force, and it is not fate, as humans act with free will and therefore create their own destiny. Instead, it is accumulated through one's thoughts, words and actions, and throughout the various cycles of birth and rebirth.

Dharma is the path of righteousness: living life according to the moral universal principles described in the scriptures. These principles guide humans to live with integrity and progress on the spiritual path toward unity with Brahman.[5] A key principle involves refraining from attachment to the world as we see it. Worldly experiences are seen as temporary and illusionary (*maya*). The goal of detachment extends to materialistic things as well as relationships, given that all relationships and possessions are temporary; the objective, instead, is to turn toward Brahman. Living life without concern for the outcomes of the action is a way to foster detachment. *The Bhagavad Gita* (or *Gita*), a commonly quoted source of Vedic thought for Hindus, states in chapter 2, verse 47: "To action only you have right, not ever to its fruits. Let not fruits of actions be (your) motive (and let) not your attachment be to inaction."[6]

Hindu teachings provide guidance in all aspects of life, including health and illness, and there is no one Hindu scripture. The content of the *Gita* quoted above reflects the teachings of Lord Krishna with respect to the science of realization and the process by which human beings can establish their eternal relationship with God. From a practical perspective, the *Gita* presents wisdom needed for one to achieve self-realization. The *Vedas*, or *Books of Knowledge*, are considered to be the oldest texts, dating back to at least 1500 BCE. The term *Veda* does not refer to any one particular book; rather, the collective *Vedas* encompass the vast literature of the early phase of Hindu thought. The *Vedas* are not considered to be human compositions; they are regarded as supreme knowledge that was directly revealed by Brahman. Vedic teachings are found in several different compositions and compilations and serve as guides for people in all they seek. Recitation of relevant Vedic hymns is important at significant times in one's life, such as birth, marriage, death, or the start of a new venture.[7]

UNDERSTANDING OF PERSONHOOD AND HEALTH

In the Hindu view, personhood is composed of two distinct but cojoined entities: spirit (*atman*) and matter (*prakriti*). Even though spirit and matter come together in a person, the individual continues to possess a duality that consists of a real self (the pure spirit) and a false self, the composite of matter and spirit.[8] Internalized awareness of this is necessary to achieve enlightenment, at which point the soul is released from the cycle of birth and rebirth.

Relationship Between the Body and Soul (*Atman*)

To understand the relationship between Hinduism and health, one first has to understand how the religion views the person and his or her relationship with God. Generally, most religions in the western world refer to the person as a holistic being with a body, mind, and spirit that are intertwined and inseparable.[9] Alteration in any one element affects the other two and ultimately the whole person. Hinduism is similar in that the holistic view is important, but the relationship of various elements is understood differently, as described below. As well, there is a distinction between "spirit" and being spiritual; the term spirit may be translated as ghost or mental strength, but spiritualism is associated with the soul (*adhyatma*).

In Hinduism, the soul is the central entity. It is not the body that has a soul, but rather the soul has a body. The soul is the master of all activities, because the body can function only as long as there is soul within it.[10] The body is the environment of the soul and is mortal, whereas the soul is immortal or eternal. When the soul leaves, the body ceases to function and death occurs; however, death is not forever, as the eternal soul is part of Brahman, the absolute being. In this way, the world recognizes and understands the body, but people cannot truly know the soul as it exists beyond possible perception.

The other name for Brahman, *Paramatman*, provides a clear understanding of the soul's relevance to Hindus. The term is formed from *parama*, meaning "supreme" or "highest," and *atman*, which means individual spirit, soul, or self. In this respect, Hindus have a very personal relationship with God, the "supreme soul." After death, the objective is not to unite with family or any other person, as these physical relationships are temporary; instead, the objective is for the soul to completely reunite with the eternal *Paramatman*, without the need for further physical form. The soul is free of any illness or disease that the body may have had, but it carries with it the karma. This karma leads to the cycle of rebirth until eventually self-realization is attained, leading to *moksha*. With reference to the soul, the *Gita* states in chapter 2, verse 23: "Weapons cannot cut this (Self), fire cannot burn this, waters cannot wet and the wind cannot dry this."[11]

Another distinction in Hinduism is that the soul is not limited to humans, but exists in every living being, including plants and animals, and all are a reflection of the absolute being. One way of addressing God is *Sat-Chit-Anand*. *Sat* is existence (or truth), thus everything that exists (animate and inanimate) is part of God. *Chit* is consciousness, and thus *Sat-Chit* refers to existence plus consciousness, and all living beings are that level of God. *Anand* refers to bliss and is found within the existence of human beings; thus, *Sat-Chit-Anand* is existence-consciousness-bliss that can be experienced by human beings through self-realization.

Relationship Between Body and Mind

Hindus attach considerable importance to the relationship between the mind (mental activities) and the body (physical functions). Any disturbance in one affects the other and causes disease. Mental activities such as grief, fear, worry, anger, and sorrow are recognized as causative factors for physical illness, such as indigestion.[12] Therefore, for maintaining one's health, as well as for curing disease, it is required that both the mind and the body are kept in proper condition.

The mind plays a significant role in maintaining health by keeping itself and the senses under control. *Buddhi* is an important concept, and can be described as the combination of intelligence and understanding. It can also be thought of as the abstract notion of the brain; just as the brain is seen to have a central role in body functioning, all thoughts and actions come from *buddhi*. In this way, it is clear that there is a fundamental difference in how mind is understood in western thought and in Hinduism:

> This difference lies in the fact that western psychology identifies consciousness with mind, and being with thought, and thought with soul, or the Self; whereas Indian psychology distinguishes mind from consciousness. This distinction is due to the fact that western psychology recognizes only one plane of experience, and gives no consideration to what Hindus call the pure *cit*, the supreme unconditional consciousness, the Being, which they regard as the real Self, or the soul, different from the rationalizing mind and realized in the super-conscious, or transcendental state. Pure unconditional consciousness cannot be the property of the mind, they believe, for it is the source of the mind's apparent consciousness. Mind is said by the Hindu psychologist to be the "veiling power" of the pure consciousness, the Self, and it is associated with the Self only as a necessary condition of world experience.[13]

The distinction between mind and consciousness is important, since in western thought, mind is the route to achieving a peaceful and blissful state, and the unconscious or subconscious is a layer of the mind. For Hindus, however, the mind is important, but bliss and the un/subconscious are associated with soul and not the mind.

Health

In Hindu religion, health is described as the equilibrium of mind, body, senses, and soul with nature.[14] Given the intricate relationship between body, mind, and consciousness, it is not surprising that the concept of destiny is also salient to well-being. Destiny plays a key role in illness and disease. Destiny is what is meant to happen to one as a reflection of karma. Though it is, to some extent, outside one's control and unchangeable, one's response to present circumstance will influence what happens in the future, either in this or future lifetimes. Modern science identifies genetics as a salient factor in illness, but who or what determines one's genes? Hindu philosophy attributes this to karma. Thus it may be destiny to have particular experiences in life, including illness, but how one copes with, learns from, and responds to the illness will influence the future.

Good health is said to be at the root of virtuous acts (*dharma*), acquirement of wealth (*artha*), gratification of desire (*kama*), and liberation from the world (*moksha*).[15] *Gunas* is a term that denotes a set of qualities. The relative strength and combination of different *gunas* influences the nature of beings, including their actions, behaviors, and attachments to the objective world. In total, there are three *gunas*: The first *guna* is *tamas*, which is darkness, stupidity, and ignorance. The second *guna* is *rajas*, the stage when a person starts the active process of self-development, grows as a warrior, and then as a leader and organizer of other people. The third *guna* is *sattva*, which is purity, harmony, and bliss. The *gunas* are seen as the energies of the mind and are thus responsible for one's psychological constitution. In equilibrium, the three *gunas* preserve the mind (and thus indirectly the body), maintaining it in a healthy state. Any disturbance in this equilibrium can lead to illness.[16]

Ayurveda

A distinguishing feature of Hinduism is its fully fledged system of medicine. *Ayurveda*, or the science of healthy living, is a medical science that describes how to maintain one's health and vigor, and also how to deal with illness.[17] The term *Ayur* refers to life or lifespan, and *Veda* means knowledge. The knowledge of *Ayurveda* is said to be revealed by the creator, Brahma, and deals with subjects such as medicine, surgery, children's diseases, hygiene, and prevention of illness. This knowledge was written into *Samhitas* or compendia. There are two major *samhitas*: *Sushruta* (representing the surgical aspect of medicine) and *Charak* or *Caraka* (symbolizing the medical aspect). Estimates regarding the dates of origin of these texts range from 4th century BCE to 5th century CE.[18, 19] These writings are said to be "so clear, intelligent, and scientific . . . that they might fit into any modern textbook."[20] In addition to information about health and illness, *Carak Samhita* also outlines the "team concept of medical care"[21] by describing the fourfold nature of therapeutics as being comprised of physicians, patients, attendants (nurses), and drugs. This will be presented in greater detail later in the chapter.

Ayurveda's scientific approach stems from Hindu philosophy, according to which the universe is composed of five basic elements: earth (*prithvi*), water (*jala*), fire (*teja*), air (*vayu*), and ether or space (*akash*). These five substances also constitute the human body and correspond respectively to firm tissue, humor, bile, breath, and organic cavities. While earth and space are inert, the three other substances are active and mutually interactive. Wind, fire, and water exist in the body in the forms of breath, bile, and mucus. The actions of these body elements are also influenced by seasons, climatic changes, and hygienic conditions, as well as the person's particular constitution. Disequilibrium in any one of the elements invariably impacts on others and leads to various combinations of "troubles" or pathological conditions. This perspective is similar to Humorism, the ancient western theory regarding the makeup of the human body described by Greek and Roman physicians and philosophers. In this view, the human body is said to be filled with four humors—black bile, yellow bile, phlegm, and blood—that reflect the four elements—earth, fire, water, and air. Illness or disease was the result of excess or deficit in one of these humors.[22]

Ayurveda describes health as a multidimensional (physical, mental, social, and spiritual) positive state, not just as the absence of disease. There is an emphasis on prevention and health promotion; caring is privileged over curing; and quality of lifetime is more important than longevity. Each person is viewed as having a unique constitutional type and an unmatched set of life experiences; thus, health requires an individualized approach that consists of a total lifestyle and not just specific actions aimed at body, mind, or environment.[23]

In Ayurvedic thought, the body has two parts: physical (which includes biological/chemical processes) and the mind. The role of the mind is to activate, direct, and coordinate the sensory and motor organs, as well as to reason, deliberate, and discriminate. Body and mind make up the whole simultaneously, not sequentially, each being of equal value. Pathogenic factors of the body are attributed to *vayu*, *pitta*, and *kapha*, which are related to the elements of breath, bile, and mucus. Pathogenic factors of the mind are *rajas* and *tamas*, which are the first two *gunas*. All these pathogenic factors have their action in the body individually and in combination. Emotional states such as anger, fear, and anxiety can destabilize the physical domains, while pathogenic factors of the body can also produce mental disorders. In Ayurveda, there is no distinction between "physical" and "mental" illness; there is just illness. Consequently, pathogenic factors can be overcome in one of two ways. Therapies based on religious rights and physical propriety (medicines, proper diet, and proper daily routines) reconcile pathogenic factors of the body, and pathogenic factors of the mind require "spiritual and scriptural knowledge, patience, memory, and meditation."[24] However, given the integral relationship of the body and mind, one cannot effectively treat the body unless it is seen from the perspective of the spirit. Although it is acknowledged that addressing the psychic component may be elusive and time-consuming, dismissing it is considered bad medicine and unethical practice.[25]

The *Carak* also distinguishes between curable and incurable diseases and notes "no medicine is to be prescribed for incurable diseases."[26]

This guidance with respect to "'futile" treatment is for physicians, as it can be argued that there is no disease that cannot be cured with enlightened knowledge of sages who are well versed in the administration of elixirs and performance of spiritual acts.[27] Thus, even when treatment is futile, hope is maintained, and while death can be anticipated, it cannot be predicted with respect to specified time.

A comprehensive understanding of health in Ayurveda also includes a social dimension.[28] Control of sense organs and positive social relationships are part of good conduct, which is important for health and well-being. The fundamental belief is that humans are social animals who require positive social relationships to achieve physical and mental well-being. A person is expected to be happy and healthy on a personal level, but as the person is also a social being, the emphasis on personal health is extended to social health and involves concerns for the well-being of others in the community. Wrongful actions are seen as adding to stress and disharmony of the individual and the collective. Attributes of good conduct in Hindu philosophy range from good grooming and hygiene to engaging in good work that occupies the mind and reverence for the divine.[29]

In summary, medicine and morals are closely related in Hinduism. Health is complex, comprehensive, and a result of one's conduct in all spheres of life. Hindu philosophy encompasses an elaborate system of medicine, Ayurveda, which discusses health promotion, illness prevention, and also outlines elaborate curative treatments for specific conditions. As a science, Ayurveda's purpose is to ensure the health of body and mind; as a philosophy, its goals go beyond the preservation of health and curing of disease. Illness is viewed in holistic terms, with no distinction between physical and mental illness. Thus all treatment must also be holistic and inclusive of medicine, diet, daily rituals, spiritual and scriptural knowledge, prayer, and meditation. Health is both personal and social, and requires actions aimed at preserving personal as well as social morality.

Role of Person in Illness

Hindu philosophy gives significance to persons being active agents in their own lives. Health is defined as the state of equilibrium, and prevention of disease is achieved through diet, conduct, and regimens. Hygienic practices and other health measures are enforced through the regimens and religious observance.[30] However, although the person is expected to play a major role in maintaining health and well-being through thoughts and actions, a patient's role in recovery from illness or disease is less prominent. Of the four therapeutic factors (physician, medicament, attendant, and patient) described by the *Carak* as responsible for curing disease, patient actions are said to have the least important role. However, for optimal effectiveness, each factor needs to "have the requisite qualities."[31] The qualities of the patient are described as: "good memory, obedience, fearlessness, and uninhibited expression."[32] The use of the term "fearless" here is in reference to controlling mental stress, such as fear and anxiety, which would further aggravate the disease. In illness, the efforts of the patient are directed toward following instructions of the physician and in giving a correct history of the disease. Thus the role of a person in illness complements that of the physician, treatment, and attendant by adherence to therapeutic and *dharmic* regimens.

ENVIRONMENT

In Hindu philosophy, the environment is not separate from the person; all living things are part of the absolute being. The environment is also not limited to the physical environment that can be seen or felt, it extends to the unseen consciousness. Diet, climate, soil, season, time, and place are factors that need to be considered in relation to health, and the position of the individual in the universe is also important. Even in ancient times, Hindus had a highly developed knowledge of planets and the universe, and the relationship between the universe, its planets, and God is described in the *Vedas*. Thus, Hindus believe that a person's health may be influenced by many environmental factors, including astrological ones. Hindu astrology extends beyond the zodiac system found in western astrology and includes the *Nakshatra* system.[33]

A key concept associated with environment is that of purity. Hindus believe that it is important to keep mind, body, and environment pure and free of wrongdoing or toxins. Purity in thought is related to good intention. Purity in mind is important for trust. Purity of body is maintained through strict hygienic practices. For example, awakening before sunrise and cleaning feet and excretory organs frequently are practices that promote intelligence, purity, longevity, and auspiciousness.[34] Saliva and body discharges are considered to be impure and polluting (*tamsic*); in addition, menstruation is seen as very polluting and contributes to a negative attitude toward women. Purity also exists in different degrees, in that some objects are more pure (*suddha*) than others. For example, gold is considered to be more pure than copper. As well, some items (such as water from the Ganges river) are not only pure in themselves, but also have the ability to purify other objects that come in contact with them.[35]

A concept related to purity is that of auspiciousness (*subh*) and inauspiciousness (*asubha*). *Subha* is related to the time and manner in which events take place. There are days or times, based on the lunar calendar, that are considered to be either auspicious or inauspicious for critical events such as marriages or prayer rituals. Performing rituals (and treatments) at *subh* times is integral to the positive effects associated with the ritual. Purity/impurity and *subha/asubha* are part of one's daily life, thus the rituals of purification play an important role in maintaining dharma and well-being. For example, although childbirth is an auspicious (*subh*) event, it has many associated impurities, such as body fluid discharge, which renders both mother and baby impure. There are, however, several rituals and social ceremonies that are conducted to manage the impurities effectively. Overall, purity/impurity and *subh/asubh* can be described as two vital components of a Hindu person's life that are sufficiently complex and often require counsel of carefully trained persons such as priests.[36]

HEALER

Role of Physician

Ancient medical literature highlights four aspects of therapeutics: physician, medicament, attendant, and patient. Among these factors, physicians occupy the most prominent place by virtue of their knowledge, administrative position, and prescribing capacity. The desired qualities of physicians include: excellence in medical knowledge, extensive practical experience, dexterity, and purity.[37] Excellence in knowledge is achieved through learning from preceptors and studying scriptures. The virtue of purity is important, as it is associated with a spiritual force that the physician brings to healing. Although the actions of the physician are said to be all important, doctors do not have the right to be deterministic with respect to health outcomes or decision making; medical science cannot overshadow karma or the influence of forces of higher consciousness.

Medicament is something that exerts a therapeutic action when administered. The qualities of medicament to consider include abundance, suitability, multiple form, and potency. Medications should be potent, free from infection, and amenable to different forms to suit the nature of the patient and the illness. The physician is expected to acquire this knowledge and prescribe accordingly, after taking into consideration the physical and spiritual nature of the patient.

NURSING

There is no specific reference to "nurse" within the Hindu texts; however, the history of India is said to "reveal a more complete description of nursing principles and practices than that of any other ancient civilization."[38] The description of "attendant" in the *Carak* can be considered to be equivalent to nurse. The desired qualities of a medical attendant include knowledge of nursing, affection, and purity. Attendants were also expected to be "endowed with good conduct, cleanliness, character, devotion, dexterity, and sympathy and . . . (be) conversant with the art of nursing and good in administering therapies."[39] Other attributes of attendants include being:

> . . . endued with kindness, skilled in every kind of service that a patient may require, endued with general cleverness, competent to cook food and curries, clever in bathing or washing a patient, well conversant in rubbing or pressing the limbs, or raising the patient or assisting him in walking or moving about, well skilled in making or cleaning beds, competent to pound drugs, or ready, patient, and skilful in waiting upon one that is ailing, and never unwilling to do any act that they may be commanded (by the physician or patient) to do.[40]

Attendants were expected to be willing workers who did not speak ill of anybody and indefatigably followed instructions of the physician. In addition to attendants, hospitals also needed people who were well versed with music and the recitation of verses and stories.[41]

In ancient times, the attendants were generally male, or in rare cases, old women who belonged to subcastes of the Brahmin and priestly orders.[42, 43] Modern nursing was introduced in India in the 17th century by the Portuguese when they conquered Goa. For many years, nursing training was only given to European and Anglo-Indians. The first Indian female to have received nursing training was Bai Kashibhai Ganpat in 1891. In succeeding years, nursing schools were established all over the country; however, this was in the era of colonization and thus strongly influenced by Christian values. The Second World War led to an acute shortage of nurses in the country, and subsequently short intensive training programs were established for auxiliary nursing service where young women of "every caste and creed" were trained.[44]

It is important to acknowledge that nursing as a profession is not viewed very positively by contemporary Indian culture, particularly as it became a female-dominant profession. Nursing is viewed as having boundaries for physical, intimate tasks, and gender relationships that are different from those culturally acceptable for women, especially young women, in traditional Indian society. The lack of appreciation for contemporary nursing may also be associated with the notion that women, especially premenopausal women, are inherently regarded as less pure, which, in turn, may compromise the environment and the power of the spiritual force available for healing. The description of attendant as someone who carries out tasks that are "commanded by the physician or patient" suggests that nursing was largely viewed in a dependent role, with the nurse being regarded as a "handmaiden." This perpetuates the notion of a strong hierarchy, and privileges the physician role with significantly more respect and prestige.

Yet while the profession of nursing is only slowly gaining acceptance and stature within the modern community, the need for nursing services is clearly acknowledged and desired in the roots of Hinduism. Indeed, knowledge is clearly described as an essential quality of the attendant. Nurses were expected to possess knowledge and skill as well as virtue, and we can thus conclude that even in ancient times, the dependent role of nurses was augmented by the view of nurses as skilled knowledge workers. In addition, the *Carak* describes the four aspects of therapeutics in an integrated manner, with the reestablishment of equilibrium (health) depending on the strength of the total quadruple. Each of the four factors, including nursing, was therefore seen as a critical element in an integrated approach to health.

Although the need for nursing activities and nurses was recognized in the *Carak*, for most Hindus such functions are closely related to the concept of *seva*. *Seva* is translated as selfless service or work offered to God. In Indian culture, when one thinks of *seva*, particularly in the context of caring for the ill, one immediately thinks of family. The duty to do *seva* rests primarily with the son(s) and daughter(s)-in-law as it is their dharma. Such *seva* is akin to generating *punya* (good karma). Care giving thus becomes an obligation of the family, particularly for the males. From the traditional families' perspective, the nurse's role is to support the family and, as needed, direct them in particular aspects of care.[45] In today's society, however, the ability of family to do *seva* is becoming increasingly limited and reliance on outsiders is becoming increasingly needed and valued. This need further supports the recognition of nursing as a valued profession in contemporary society.

ETHICS

In Hinduism, there is no one source for moral authority. Hindu religious literature can be divided into two categories: *Shruti*: that which has been heard (revealed truth); and *Smriti*: that which has been remembered (remembered truth). The *Vedas* are considered to be the original scriptures of Hindu teachings (*Smriti*) and contain spiritual knowledge that encompasses all aspects of life. The highest authority is that of enlightened persons or incarnations of God (e.g., Rama and Krishna), as they are said to possess all knowledge, past, present, and future.

For the followers of the religion, the two most commonly used books to provide the day-to-day guidance are the *Ramayana* and *Gita*. Both books belong to the *Smriti* category as they are descriptions of historical epics. The *Ramayana* provides a description of Lord Rama's life, and in addition to showing the glory of God, it "provides a code of conduct, the role models for the family, and the philosophy for life here on earth and in the hereafter."[46] The *Bhagavad Gita* teaches the causation and the effects of karma and how to deal with its manifestations. It also teaches that human beings have free will and ability to make intelligent choices, which in turn may alter the manifestation of the karma.[47] The *Gita* is frequently regarded as the highest and most practical written expression of Hindu philosophy. For practical purposes, the conduct of Lord Rama and the teachings of Lord Krishna, both of whom took human form in times of need, serve as guides for conduct, decision making, and adherence to *dharmic* concepts for the average Hindu person.

In Hinduism, there is synergy between philosophical wisdom and ethical excellence, as the scriptures assert that moral and ethical excellence is a prerequisite to the pursuit of knowledge. Hindu ethics does not focus only on what is conducive or necessary for survival of a particular individual or species. Instead, it prescribes the disciplines for a spiritual life that should be observed both consciously and unconsciously.[48]

Hindu ethics is a systematic progression from the objective to subjective, and ultimately to super-ethical level.[49] Objective level ethics is described as social ethics and is guided by dharma. Each individual is said to pass through four stages of life: student, householder (family, procreation, obligations to kith and kin), forest-dweller (life of solitude and meditation, where demands of mind and senses yield to demands of the soul), and hermit (detachment to pursue the goal of self-realization). This scheme answers the moral question of how one should live. Thus morality, to some extent, is influenced by the stage of life and is relative.

In the first stage of objective ethics, "morality is represented by social codes demanding external conformity" and conscience is driven by fear of punishment for duties not done.[50] The subsequent stage of subjective ethics focuses on virtues as opposed to duties. Virtue is directed from within and arises from feelings of preference and self-respect; the "must do" orientation is transformed to "ought." Virtue has three parts: *Manasa* (mind), *Vacha* (speech), and *Karma* (action). Virtues of the mind are seen as kindness, detachment, piety; virtues of speech are evident through truthfulness, benevolence, and recitation of scriptures; and virtues of action include *seva*, social service, and good will toward others.[51] The third stage of ethics moves from social and personal, to transcendental. The transcendental has been characterized as the "post-ethical plane of being." At this level, ethics loses its substance as all empirical contradictions are transcended. It is important to note that this transcendence is not provided by an external source (as salvation is, e.g.); rather, the real self is already perfect but had been concealed by *maya* (illusion).

This duality of self is also evident in how truth is understood. Truth is of two kinds: scientific or empirical knowledge and transcendental or yogic knowledge. The former truth is perceived by the five ordinary senses or inferred from data they provide, and the latter is perceived by the subtle spiritual power of yoga.[52] Empirical knowledge is substantiated through inference and reasoning; transcendental knowledge comes with enlightenment.

Within Hinduism there is a call for promoting social welfare by helping society rid itself of selfishness, cruelty, greed, and other vices, thereby "creat[ing] an environment helpful to the pursuit of the highest good, which transcends society."[53] A person endowed with social consciousness is said to have a threefold debt to discharge. The first is a debt to God for all the natural amenities (sun, rain, wind, etc.), which is paid through worship and prayer. The second is the debt to teachers or saints from whom we inherit the spiritual culture, which is paid through the regular study of scriptures. Lastly, there is a debt to parents and ancestors from whom we receive our physical bodies, which is paid through procreation and ensuring the preservation of the lineage.[54] The notion of debt and duty to family takes on considerable importance in the day-to-day lives of Hindus. Despite having an ultimate spiritual goal of detachment, traditional Hindus have strong attachments and bonds to immediate and extended family in their current life. Strong families and family values are foundational to a strong society, which in turn is essential for good health.

ON BEING A HINDU AS PATIENT OR NURSE

Hinduism is largely a way of life with variations in rituals, traditions, and the particular deity of worship; thus, the influence of the religion on a patient or nurse can differ tremendously. It can also be independent of the degree of expressed religiosity of the individual. However, as the religion and way of life are so intertwined, even Hindus who may not be adherent to religious practices are likely to be inherently influenced to some extent by these core tenets. These individuals may thus display signs of influence without any concrete knowledge of the specific concepts mentioned in this chapter. The foundational concepts of karma and dharma will likely influence both patients and nurses in their responses and actions. In addition, Crawford identifies five principles as being of critical significance for most Hindus: purity, self-control, detachment, truth, and nonviolence (*ahimsa*).[55] These may further influence the day-to-day experiences and actions with respect to how one strives to meet their *dharmic* duties, particularly at times when health is compromised. For an individual in need of health care services, two key areas that are likely to show the influence of Hinduism are response to illness and decision making.

Response to Illness

A Hindu patient may view illness as karma and rely on the principles of dharma to respond to it. With this line of thinking, everything that happens is a result of karma. Illness is not random and questions such as "why me?" can be answered by "it is karma." Suffering can be seen as a way of releasing the debt for past negative karma as well as an opportunity to be tested and to learn from the difficult experience. Acceptance of pain can be viewed as progress toward the spiritual goal. The Hindu patient will acknowledge and may find comfort in the belief that while the body may be in pain, the soul is not harmed. In the *Gita*, Lord Krishna advises Arjuna to learn to endure fleeting things like pleasure and pain. The lesson is that when suffering and joy are equal, one has courage and is "fit for immortality."[56]

A potential challenge for patients with Hindu faith is experienced when karma is viewed as fatalism and passivity, or when the patients' belief in karma is interpreted by others as fatalism. The risk is that these patients will not get the support, education, and ongoing efforts to reduce the pain and suffering because they are seen as unmotivated. It is important that acceptance is not misunderstood as a desire for inaction. In fact, Hindu tradition guides one to avoid inaction and recognizes that while the consequences of past deeds must be accepted, actions taken today are important influences for the future. Patients can thus be encouraged to actively manage their condition, while accepting the outcome without the attribution of success or failure.[57,58] One's duty is always to do one's best and accept the outcomes, regardless of what they may be.

Challenges may also be encountered in discussions where quality of life is the salient principle for decision making regarding treatment. Given the belief that what is happening is Karma and that one's *dharma* is to accept it and live as best as one can, it may be difficult for a Hindu patient or nurse to see a poor quality of life as a valid argument for discontinuing treatment, such as long-term dialysis. Rather, such decisions are more likely to be influenced by the patient's age and stage of life.

The illness experience is also influenced by the understanding of the interrelationship between the body, mind, spirit, and even social conduct. The concept of holism is not just important in understanding the etiology of illness, but also in the response made to it. Desired interventions may be focused not only on biomedical therapies, but also on religious and spiritual rituals. Current health care discourse on religion and spirituality often differentiates between the two, with religion being described as a defined set of practices around a traditionally defined belief, and spirituality as a broad construct of lived experience with a focus on the *I*, the self, and one's relationship with the universe.[59] For Hindus, either as patients or nurses, the spiritual goal of consciousness is the essence of the religion. The quest for consciousness is associated with detachment and acceptance, where ultimately *I* ceases to exist as an individual and unites with Brahman.

The notion of spiritual distress may also be problematic for Hindu patients and/or nurses. The spirit or the soul does not have distress; these feelings are a result of pathogenic factors of the mind and the influence of the *gunas*. Thus, illness and distress are difficult to subdivide into mental, physical, and spiritual. The mind has a significant role in illness, not just because of its potential influence on the body, but also because *buddhi* is critical to the appropriate response. Thus, psychosocial and spiritual aspects of care are significant parts of the overall care experience and Hindus are also more likely to accept and desire a plurality of approaches to care. As noted in the *Carak*, pathogenic factors can be overcome by physical proprieties including medicine and diet, and religious rites, as well as meditation, prayer, and scriptural knowledge. Thus, the desire for a spiritual healer is likely to be seen as a natural part of care and not an "alternative" to medical care. Patients may also look to their doctors and nurses to integrate these spiritual aspects into prescribed treatments. Where physical and spiritual care is offered by different individuals or "specialists," integration of the two perspectives will be critical.

Hinduism also encourages self-healing, characterized by: testing the powers of one's mind constructively and positively; listening to the intelligence and wisdom of one's body; harnessing the creativity and positive energy of one's emotions; and finding one's place in the greater scheme of things.[60] Even though the *Carak* notes that the physician has the most prominent role in therapeutics, it is also clearly stated that the patient's actions must complement that of the physician. The patient is expected to have an active role in healing, and this role needs to be acknowledged and supported.

Decision Making

Hindu ethics is said to have a contextual structure, where the right or the dharmic thing to do is guided by the demands of the situation. Hindu ethics is not absolute and does not rely on authoritarianism or objective norms for conduct, nor is it relativist by privileging the individual and his or her preference and happiness. Instead, Hinduism gives importance to rational authority; reason is important but is augmented by revelation. Unlike western thought, where revelation is often though not exclusively seen as external, for a Hindu, revelation is an internal activity, similar to intuition and reflective of the holistic nature of the person. In the end, the individual is guided by both reason and teachings from the scriptures to determine what is of ultimate value in the particular situation.[61] Decisions may also be influenced by the extent to which a patient will still be able to carry out desired practices and rituals that are seen as being a critical part of one's dharmic life.

Hindu society and philosophy are characterized by the notion of *collectivism*, where decisions are based not on the individual good, but rather the good of the collective. Although this may seem like a paradox, as the ultimate objective is to achieve *moksha* as an individual, we must remember that the individual body is recognized as a "false self." The real self is one that is part of a larger consciousness. Thus, the decisions are guided not by what is right for the "false self" but by what will lead to revelation of the true self. Decisions are therefore based on what is "good" for others, family and society, and based on actions that fulfill one's duty toward others, including ancestors, teachers, and God. It is not surprising then that the stage of life may significantly influence the response to illness and treatment, such as pursuing more aggressive action when there are obligations to family, and a different response when the objective is a focus on detachment and self-realization.[62]

Notions of purity and auspiciousness can also influence decisions. For example: for a woman, dying before her husband is considered to be a more auspicious death and is preferred over becoming a widow. In addition, there are other attributes associated with what is considered "a good death." A good death is one that happens at home, and over which a person has control. Death is a social event and the collective expression of love and grief from the extended family allows the patient to participate in this ritual. Prolonging life artificially is seen to be of little value. However, it is important not to interpret this as leading to all refusals of resuscitation or mechanical support. Unless there is clear evidence of "fatal signs," extraordinary means are not prohibited on either moral or medical grounds.[63] Again, one has to view the situation holistically to determine the appropriate course of action.

An area of potential contention between western health care practices and Hindu beliefs is the area of "full disclosure" regarding a diagnosis and prognosis. Though western practitioners might feel obliged to offer complete information about prognosis including imminent death, Hindu beliefs would say that it is inappropriate to predict the timing of death. The impending death is not explicitly pronounced because words have power; "naming death may invite it too quickly."[64] All physicians can truly say is that there is nothing more they can offer with respect to treatment (as they know it). Western practitioners may see this as "withholding the truth" or offering false hope, but for Hindu patients, acceptance and hope can coexist. Even when the physician has nothing more to offer, interventions such as prayer and other religious rituals can still offer some hope. Death must neither be hastened nor resisted as an enemy of life;[65] instead, it is the last step in the journey of this birth and a step toward the ultimate destination of *moksha*. For these reasons, it is crucial that health care workers clearly ascertain the wishes of the patient before making any statements that can be interpreted as predictions.

The Hindu Nurse

Although Indian society does not see nursing as a high status profession, in our experience, Hindu nurses tend to view their role in very positive terms. Duty toward self and others is a salient feature of Hindu spirituality. In Christian faith, this may be a reflection of love. This love is unconditional despite the unattractiveness of the object/sinner; caring is to show God's love.[66] For Hindus, caring is serving God, who resides in each being. *Seva* is dharma. Nursing can be seen as an opportunity to provide the ultimate selfless *seva*, as there is little materialistic gain such as money or prestige.[67] The ability to provide such *seva* can be seen as a privilege, as it provides an opportunity for *punya* or doing righteous actions.

The ancient Hindu text *Caraka* describes the role of the nurse as subservient to the physician, but the fourfold nature of therapeutics clearly establishes this to be an interdependent and not a dependent role. The ancient view of nurses as attendants has evolved into nurses with professional knowledge and accountability that includes, but also extends beyond, doing what is commanded by the patient or the physicians. Nursing roles today comprise elements of both the attendant and the healer, and thus the desired attributes and expectations for Hindu nurses will likely be derived from the description of both attendant and physician.

A therapeutic relationship is at the heart of nursing, and for Hindu nurses, the relationship is not just with the individual but extends to a range of family members. Recognizing the value that may be placed on the family's role in care giving, the nurse is likely to encourage, and perhaps even impose, such a role for particular family members. Therefore, if the practice environment privileges individualism to the extent that family is excluded or defined very narrowly, Hindu nurses practicing in western society can be at risk of experiencing moral conflict. In addition, for Hindu nurses, the nurse–client relationship is likely to be characterized by a participative approach. Persons are regarded as both dependent and responsible and they are viewed as being "in equal need of beneficence and autonomy."[68] Concepts such as client empowerment, patient choice, and patient-centered care are consistent with Hindu thought and are likely to resonate with the Hindu nurse. The attendant functions also reflect actions that are characterized in the current nursing ethos as "being with" or "being present" to witness and share the illness experience, without a need for specific intervention. The interdependent nature of nursing and the team approach to care are concepts that are consistent with Hindu philosophy as outlined in the *Carak*. Authenticity and trustworthiness are crucial characteristics that patients may look for and nurses themselves will value greatly. For the Hindu nurse, compassion and kindness can be viewed as dharma. As well, the nurse may be more process-oriented than outcomes-oriented, as the outcomes are influenced not only by actions of the individuals involved, but also by karma.

The extent to which Hindu nurses are influenced by the traditional teachings is likely to influence how nurses view their role toward the patient, family, and even larger society. For example, acceptance is a foundational value in Hindu philosophy. Hindu nurses may therefore see it as their duty to help patients strive toward acceptance. This emphasis toward acceptance may, at times, be in contrast to patients who see disease and illness as something to be conquered. However, the contextual and situational nature of moral reasoning means that nurses may provide external guidance, but recognize that external opinions must be integrated into one's own, and ultimate decision making rests with the individual patient. For the Hindu nurse, body, mind, and spirit are intertwined in a way that they cannot be separated. The mind influences the body, but the physical conditions of one's environment also influence the mind. Spirituality is understood as much more than religion, yet the rituals associated with religion are also considered powerful.

Another area of potential influence is the Hindu nurses' understanding of knowledge development. There is general consensus in the nursing literature that there are several ways of knowing that can be classified as scientific and nonscientific, and both ways are equally important. This view is supported by western psychology in as far as there is recognition of the nonscientific approach to knowledge; however, the psychology literature privileges scientific knowledge and regards the nonscientific ways of knowing as celebrating the possibility of error.[69] For the Hindu nurse, both scientific and nonscientific ways of knowing are equally valid, but the nonscientific knowledge and reasoning extend beyond what has been characterized as professional craft knowledge to knowledge derived from one's consciousness and the soul.[70] Thus, the nurse is likely to hold intuitive and personal knowledge in high regard as it comes not just from the mind but from the soul.

On a broader social level, nurses influenced by Hindu thought are more likely to have a holistic understanding of health that includes a social dimension with a focus on prevention of illness and disease, promotion of health, and concern with the general well-being of persons in the community (social determinants of health). This understanding of rules of good conduct will likely extend to "an ethic of public health."[71] Promoting social welfare is an important element of Hindu ethics, thus creating a propensity for the Hindu nurse to be involved in public health and public policy initiatives.

Summary

In summary, even in illness, the central concepts of karma and dharma and holistic understanding of the person are paramount. These concepts can be expected to shape both the understanding of, as well as the response to, illness, including treatment decisions and who is involved in care. The illness experience is likely to be characterized by the co-existence of acceptance, hope, and a belief in possibilities beyond those offered by the mortal treatment team. Despite the odds or immediate outcomes, active commitment to one's duty is essential as the fruits of action extend beyond this life. This is applicable to both patients and nurses. Like all aspects of Hindu existence, illness experience is also characterized by holism where mental, physical, and spiritual health and illness cannot be separately distinguished. As a result, the desired treatment is likely to include support for the physical, mental, spiritual, and religious dimensions of one's being.

CONCLUSION

In conclusion, Hinduism has much to offer with respect to a holistic understanding of health, illness, and the human person. The relationship between religion, health, and health care is indistinguishable. Hinduism is more than a religion; it is a way of life, complete with its own indigenous system of medicine and a definition of health that extends beyond the body, mind, and spirit. For Hindus, it is not the body that has a soul, but rather the soul that has a body. While the body is mortal and subject to illness, the soul is eternal consciousness. The soul acquires karma through one's actions, thoughts, and deeds, and karma is responsible for the events of one's life, including illness.

Thus, it is clear that while Hindus accept what happens to them as karma, they also recognize that karma is not externally driven. Individual persons, through their own actions, take control of their destiny. Hindus are, therefore, advised to live their life according to dharma or righteous actions, which in turn will lead to self-realization and freedom from the cycle of birth and rebirth.

Hindu philosophy views health as something that is much more than the absence of disease. It is multidimensional and consists of physical, mental, social, and spiritual components that are interrelated to achieve a state of equilibrium with nature. Such a positive view of health requires an approach that is different from the disease-oriented view, where complaints are connected to pathology. For Hindus, how one lives life with respect to integrity and conduct are critical components of maintaining health and recovering from illness. Illness is also holistic in that there is no distinction between physical illness and mental illness. Recovery from all illness requires attention to the physical, mental, emotional, and spiritual domains in an integrated fashion.

Hinduism teaches one to be extremely patient-centered and focus on the illness experience. Every person is a unique being, not just in their constitution, but also in their life experience. Thus it is important to understand and address the total illness experience. Good medicine and care requires that the spiritual dimension of a person be addressed along with the physical, mental, and emotional aspects. It is clear that medicine has a moral structure and health care practitioners must also possess virtue along with knowledge and skills; thus, ethics, knowledge, and wisdom are intertwined.

Ancient Hindu texts describe with surprising clarity and detail the pathogenic factors of the mind and the body and how they can be addressed via the four elements of therapeutics: physician, medicament, nurse (attendant), and patient. Each of the four elements is critical and the patient is expected to play an active role in recovery. The role of nursing is to serve the patient well through knowledge of nursing, dexterity, affection, and purity and by promoting patients' and families' participation in care. Decisions related to health and healing are based on a collective orientation and influenced by many contextual factors, including the stage of life of the patient and perceptions of one's duty and righteous actions.

By drawing on the ancient texts and our own experiences, we have proposed some ideas on how Hindu religious beliefs might influence the understanding of health, illness, and care, for nurses as well as patients. We hope the discussion serves to explicate aspects of spirituality as the essence of humanity. Our intention is to provide insight and ideas for consideration, discussion, and further exploration. The degree to which any of the ideas presented would resonate in specific situations and with specific patients is difficult to anticipate, as the ways in which individuals adhere to and interpret the religious principles is subject to considerable variation.

NOTES

1. Kunhan, Raja C. *Survey of Sanskrit Literature.* Bombay: Bharti vidya Bhayan, 1962. 5.
2. Das, Shukayak N. "Why do Hindus Have so Many Gods?" *Hinduism* Web. 14 July 2010. http://hinduism.about.com/cs/basics/a/aa072103a.htm.
3. Dhavamony, M. *Hindu Spirituality.* Rome: Editrice Pontificia Università Gregoriana, 1999. 11.
4. Whitman, Sarah M. "Pain and Suffering as Viewed by the Hindu Religion." *The Journal of Pain* 8.8 (2007): 607–13.
5. Ibid., 607–13.
6. Srivastava, Bhartendu. *The Bhagavad Gita: Its Comprehension and Recitation.* Toronto: Pustak Bharti, 2010. 60.
7. Singh, B. *Hinduism and Western Thought.* New Delhi: Arnold Publishers, 1991. 29.
8. Lipner, J. "The Classical Hindu View on Abortion and the Moral Status of the Unborn." *Hindu Ethics.* Eds. H. G. Coward, J. J. Lipner, and K. K. Young. Albany, NY: State University of New York Press, 1989. 52.
9. Narayanasamy, Aru. "A Review of Spirituality as Applied to Nursing." *International Journal of Nursing Studies* 36 (1999): 117–125.
10. Rigved 1/164/38.
11. Srivastava 45.
12. Sharma, R. K. and Bhagwan Dash. *Agnivesas Caraka Samhita.* Vol. 1. Varanasi: Chowkhamba Sanskrit Series Office, 1976. xxxiii.
13. Prabhavananda, Swami. *The Spiritual Heritage of India.* 3rd ed. Hollywood: Vedanta Press, 1980. 201.
14. Pomerans, A. J. *Ancient and Medieval Science.* New York: Basic Books, 1963. 155.
15. Sharma and Dash 19.
16. Jayram, V. "The Triple Gunas, Sattva, Rajas, and Tamas." *Hindu Website,* 12 July 2010.
17. Murthy, N. A. and P. Pandey. *Ayurvedic Cure for Common Diseases.* New Delhi: Orient Paperbacks, 1997. 15.
18. Donahue, Patricia M. *Nursing: The Finest Art.* St Louis: CV Mosby, 1985. 58.
19. Dock, Lavinia L. *A Short History of Nursing.* New York: Putnam, 1920. 25.
20. Ibid., 62.
21. Donahue 61.
22. _____. "Humorism." Academic Dictionaries and Encyclopedias Website, 29 Sept. 2010.
23. Crawford, S. Cromwell. *Hindu Bioethics for the Twenty-first Century.* Albany, New York: State University of New York Press, 2003. 40–44.
24. Sharma and Dash 43.
25. Crawford 78.
26. Sharma and Dash 44.
27. Sharma and Dash 45.
28. Crawford 78.
29. Crawford 78.
30. Dock 27.
31. Sharma and Dash 183.
32. Sharma and Dash 9.

33. Das, Shukayak N. "Hindu Astrology I." A Hindu Primer 2007. 12 July 2010. http://www.sanskrit.org/www/Hindu%20Primer/hinduastrology1.html.
34. Crawford 68.
35. Coward 10.
36. Ibid., 11.
37. Sharma and Dash 187.
38. Donahue 62.
39. Sharma and Dash 187.
40. Donahue 62.
41. Sharma and Dash 290.
42. Dock 28.
43. Donahue 62.
44. Dock 306.
45. Joshi, Saraswati. Personal Interview. 25 July 2010.
46. Srivastava, Bhartendu. *Ramas Glory*. Toronto: Lugus Publications, 1998. xiii.
47. Hebbar, Neria Harish. "Ethics of Hinduism." *Hinduism* 2010. 12 July 2010. http://www.scribd.com/doc/45090568/Ethics-of-Hinduism.
48. Ramakrishna, Swami Nikhilananda. "An Essay on Hindu Ethics." *Understanding Hinduism.* New York: Vivekananda Center, 12 July 2010.
49. Crawford 13.
50. Crawford 19.
51. Crawford 20.
52. Sharma and Dash 227.
53. Ramakrishna.
54. Ramakrishna.
55. Crawford 22.
56. Whitman 607–13.
57. Whitman 607–13.
58. Crawford 106.
59. Narayanasamy 117–25.
60. Mysorekar, U. "Eye on Religion: Clinicians and Hinduism." *Southern Medical Journal* 99.4 (2006): 441.
61. Crawford 29.
62. Crawford 15.
63. Crawford 197.
64. Crawford 197.
65. Crawford 198.
66. Narayanasamy 117–25.
67. Sen, Purnima. Personal Interview. 10 June 2010.
68. Crawford 106.
69. Paley, John, Helen L. Cheyne, Len Dalgleish, Edward A. S. Duncan, Catherine A. "Nursing's Ways of Knowing and Dual Process Theories of Cognition." *Journal of Advanced Nursing* 60.6 (2007): 692–01.
70. Rycroft-Malone, Jo, Kate Seers, Angie Titchen, Gill Harvey, Alison Kitson, Brendan McCormack. "What Counts as Evidence in Evidence-Based Practice?" *Journal of Advanced Nursing* 47.1 (2004): 81–90.
71. Crawford 85.

10

Judaism and Nursing

Anita Noble and Chaya Greenberger

INTRODUCTION

Judaism is both a monotheistic religion and a culture. A religion is a "belief in a divine or superhuman power or powers to be obeyed and worshipped as the creator(s) and ruler(s) of the universe,"[1] whereas a culture refers to "nonphysical traits, such as values, beliefs, attitudes, and customs that are shared by a group of people and passed from one generation to the next."[2] The Jewish people are primarily the descendants of the biblical forefather Abraham and foremother Sara. Converts have, however, joined the fold throughout the centuries.

After enduring the 400 year crucible of Egyptian slavery (1400–1200 BCE), the Jewish people were forged into a nation and a religion by entering into a covenant with God and accepting the divinely ordained code on Mount Sinai. The latter, referred to as the Torah, includes the Ten Commandments as well as a written and oral code. The written code, originally composed of the five books of Moses, was canonically expanded to encompass the books of the Prophets and Writings to collectively form the written scriptures referred to as the *Tanach*.

The oral code comprised a basic oral teaching along with a compendium of exegetic techniques whose critical purpose was to enable the ongoing interpretation of the *Tanach*. Although initially handed down from one generation to the next by word of mouth, the code was eventually committed to writing. Over the centuries, as new situations evolved, the sages utilized these techniques to expand the code. The latter came to include a large intricate corpus of law, the *Halacha*, which is essentially an all-encompassing manual for daily behavior. In addition, the oral code included works of philosophy, ethics, parables, and folklore. These enrich the understanding of the *Halacha* and also provide general guidelines for leading a moral and fulfilling Jewish life. Some of its major opuses are the *Talmudic tractates*, specific codes of law, such as that of Maimonides (1135–1204 CE) and the *Shulchan Aruch* and the rich and varied *Responsa literature*, which is still accumulating. *Responsa* are crucial to the Jewish tradition, as they address head-on the new challenges facing each generation. Today, substantial parts of the *Responsa* address the ethical dilemmas posed by modern medical technology.

There are currently 13.2 million Jews worldwide, with the greatest concentrations in North America and Israel.[3] Europe, including the non-Former Soviet Union, and Latin America comprise the two additional major centers. Historically, the Jewish people have lived all over the globe. Varied ethnicities evolved, determining areas of origin. The two largest Jewish ethnic groups are *Ashkenazim*, formed of Jews of eastern or western European descent, and *Sephardim* (also known as *Edot Mizrach*), having origins in the Mediterranean countries, the Middle East, and northern Africa. A large concentration of Ethiopian Jews has immigrated to Israel over the last number of decades, and they constitute a distinct ethnic Jewish group. Customs and traditions vary with respect to ethnicity.

Cultural differences based on ethnicity run the gamut, from those of mundane matters such as culinary menus for festive occasions, to matters of the spirit, such as the makeup of the prayer book. The Jewish population also differs in the degree of their religious identity and the extent of adherence to religious, especially ritual, practice. In the United States, the main religious identity groups are categorized as Orthodox, Conservative, Reform, and Reconstructionist.[4,5] In general, the Orthodox are the most stringent adherents to the Jewish religion. The Conservative group is more liberal in interpreting the scriptures and oral teachings and less stringent in ritual observance, whereas Reform Judaism is the least stringent. Although its followers often celebrate Jewish holidays and religious rites associated with life changes, these practices often stem from cultural rather than religious values.

In Israel, the second largest Jewish population center, religious grouping is categorized as Ultra-Orthodox (*Haredi*), Religious, Traditional, and Secular. The Ultra-Orthodox applies "stringencies on the basic Jewish law to ensure adherence to the religious law and similarly [apply] such stringencies to dealing with the outside world to ensure protection from negative influences. Knowledge is primarily sought through religious study and religious life alone."[6] Israeli Jews who consider themselves Religious differ from the Ultra-Orthodox in relation to their "integration into the general society while maintaining their religious life and acquiring an education through non-religious and religious study."[7] Their "religious life" embraces full commitment to the *Halacha*, including its ritual aspects. The term Traditional refers to Israeli Jews who observe religious Jewish ritual practices out of respect for religious commands. Traditional practice differs from Religious practice in that traditional Israeli Jews do not place Jewish law in the forefront of everyday decision making.[8] Secular is attributed to Israeli Jews who disassociate themselves from "any connection between Jewish ritual and divine commandment. Secular Israelis can be sub divided into those that do not perform any Jewish ritual and those that perform Jewish ritual as a cultural rather than religious requirement."[9]

This chapter is not intended to serve as an authoritative guide to Jewish *Halacha*, although its underpinnings are rooted in classic Jewish sources. It is meant rather to assist health care professionals in understanding the mainstream Jewish conceptualization of health and illness that is to a greater or lesser extent embraced by most members of the Jewish faith. The decision-making process and behavior of both Jewish caregivers and care recipients are therefore reflected.

OUR OBLIGATIONS AS HUMAN BEINGS AND PROFESSIONALS FROM A JEWISH POINT OF VIEW

Human beings have innate compassion for fellow human beings by virtue of being created in God's image.[10] People are obligated to imitate God by bringing his compassion to fruition by their behavior. The *Talmud* in Tractate Shabbat (133:2)[11] states: "just as God clothes the naked, so must man, just as he consoles the mourners and visits the sick, so too must man." God created "one" Adam to teach two principles: the infinite value of every human being and the inherent equality of human beings.[12] Human compassion must be blind to such factors as color, culture, wealth, and health.

Commitment to compassion means acting, and if necessary, sacrificing to protect all facets of a fellow human's well-being. One must go out of one's way to help retrieve lost property, restore health, and forewarn a fellow human being of impending threats to physical and emotional safety. One is obligated to undergo discomfort, monetary expense, and if need be, a reasonable amount of danger, in order to aid those whose lives are threatened (Talmud Bavli, Tractate Babah Metziah, 30:2).[13]

Life and quality of life are paramount values that trump even autonomy. Maimonides taught that one has no right to say "I will endanger myself and it is no one else's business."[14] Maimonides further declares that to the extent that an individual is lacking in health and well-being (thereby diminishing quality of life), so will he or she be lacking in the ability to serve God in his or her lifetime.[15] We can extrapolate from Maimonides' teachings that individuals are obligated to intervene on behalf of others, assisting them in fulfilling obligations to themselves. Destitute, alone and/or physically or emotionally handicapped people may perceive life as futile. Social solidarity as a religious obligation dictates that it is the entire community's business to do everything in its power to ensure that individuals receive the emotional and physical support necessary to empower individuals to choose health and life.

Leaving the sick alone is ungodly.[16] The religious duty to visit the sick, even in non-life-threatening situations, applies even to those individuals who are exempt from other obligations toward fellow beings.[17] The duty is comprehensive, including assessing and tending to mundane and aesthetic needs, providing emotional and spiritual support, and praying.[18,19] These echo the nursing process. Nurses, however, are obligated to "visit" the sick on a level commensurate with their knowledge and experience. Their profession is a divine calling, reflected in the commandment "Thou shalt surely heal."[20] Alleviating pain and suffering is central to healing. This is reflected in the Hebrew root for healing—*rafo*—which also has means "to ease."[21]

In Tractate Nedarim (40:1), the *Talmud* tells of Rabbi Akiva who was the sole visitor of a gravely ill individual. After carefully assessing and meticulously caring for his needs, the individual regained health and proclaimed with gratitude: Rabbi, you have given me life! Akiva, experiencing an epiphany, gathered round his disciples and preached that refraining from visiting the sick is tantamount to bloodshed.

The Art of Empathy

Rashi (1040–1105 CE), the great medieval commentator, relates that the meaning of the name "Puah," one of the two biblical Israelite midwives mentioned by name in the Bible (Exodus 1.15), is a cry imitating that of women in childbirth.[22] Midwives would habitually mimic the sounds made by the birthing women, displaying empathy in a way that could be experienced by the care recipient on the most fundamental level.

The *tanaic* work of Avot De Rabbi Natan[23] gives insight into how difficult empathy can be by relating a story about a visit that the righteous but most otherworldly, Shimon Bar Yochai paid to a sick individual. Finding him in the midst of cursing God for his plight, Bar Yochai preached: rather than curse, you should pray for mercy. The offended individual responded: if only God would smite you with my illness. Bar Yochai admitted his failure in fulfilling the commandment of visiting the sick. The "caring occasion" and the "teachable moment," which could have been utilized to help the patient find meaning in his suffering, were missed. The deeply spiritual Bar Yochai was incapable of appreciating the fundamental mundane needs of his fellow human being. True empathizers shoulder part of the illness burden, thus lightening the load.[24] Although all are obligated to pray for the sick, righteous visitors are expected literally to "become ill" along with their fellow human beings.[25] This intimates that supreme empathy is a sacrificial act that is concomitant with sublime moral stature.

Empathy comes most naturally in situations where sick individuals and their visitors share similar world views culturally, spiritually, developmentally, or by virtue of strong family ties or a very deep friendship.[26] Yet empathizing can be a great challenge, even for individuals possessing close ties with the sick. The biblical book of Samuel (I Samuel 1.1–2.10) relates the story of Hannah, a barren woman, very beloved of her husband, who attempted to console her with the words: "Do not cry, I am better for you than ten sons."[27] Although well meant, these words were lacking in empathy. Reading between the lines of the biblical verses, the *midrash* puts these words in Hannah's mouth: "Dear God, everything that you created in women, you created for a purpose. Eyes to see, ears to hear, a nose to smell, hands to labor, legs to walk, and breasts to nurse the young. Please grant me a child so that I may put these breasts to use."[28] Her husband missed the point; a husband is not a substitute for a child.

NURSES AS PROFESSIONAL EMPATHIZERS

Despite the fact that nurses will naturally differ in many ways from their care recipients, the ability to empathize is central to their profession. Nurses need to develop super-sensitivity to their own "blind spots," so that they impinge as minimally as possible on the ability to empathize. The Jewish tradition relates to empathy very much like Watson, who champions transpersonal caring, transcending one's own world in order to enter the world of the other.[29] The carer is self-sacrificial, giving up his or her own world view, at least temporarily, so as to enter the world of the "other." The carer is, however, also rewarded by growing as a human being.

The quality of care nurses provide for the sick is thus partially determined by their ability to accept the legitimacy of the entire gamut of human responses to misfortune. Individuals approach suffering in different ways. Biblical examples are of some who do not question and suffer silently (like Abraham); others pray that the suffering be ended (like King Hezekiah); some actually ask God for continued suffering in order to be cleansed of sin (like King David); while still others rebel openly and self-righteously (like Job). Yet all are called children of God.[30] Job's friends who ostensibly came to console him were counterproductive, for they would not accept the possibility that there was no direct and proportionate correlation between Job's deeds and the tragedies that befell him.

WHY DO BAD THINGS HAPPEN?

Individuals confronted with serious illness naturally ask this question, either consciously or subconsciously. They may choose to share their thoughts with their nurse. The written scriptures delineate a simplistic causal relationship between righteousness and health and prosperity. After the Israelites were freed from Egyptian bondage, God promises them: "If you will heed my commandments, I will spare you all the diseases with which I have smitten Egypt, for I am your healer" (Exodus 15:26); "If you serve God, he will bless you with ample sustenance and eradicate disease from among you" (Exodus 15:26). Conversely, straying from God's teaching will lead to catastrophic consequences, including deadly infectious diseases (Exodus 23:25). Metaphysical causation of misfortune is summed up in Deuteronomy: "I [God] bring death and give life, I smite with illness and I heal, none can escape my hand" (32:39).

The *Talmud* in Tractate Berachot (5:1–2), however, paints a much more complex picture of why bad things happen and outlines the appropriate human response. An individual struck with misfortune is initially to reflect upon his or her behavior, in case there is a need to right a wrong. For those individuals who have achieved a high level of spirituality, even lack of devotion in prayer and study can be a sufficient cause for misfortune. However, if after having sincerely considered the issue, they conclude that they are not deserving of punishment, they may assume their own righteousness and regard their misfortune as a labor of love, intended to cleanse them and bring them closer to God. Judaism acknowledges that "bad things can happen to good people."

A *Modus Vivendi*: Finding Meaning in Suffering and Learning From the Sick

An individual struck with illness is to be treated as a noble person.[31] Visitors, lay people, and professionals are to sit before them as a student sits before an expert.[32] Why is this so? Healthy individuals naturally lull themselves into a false sense of immortality. The experience of a serious illness, however, presents itself as a rude awakening; it is a lonely rendezvous with one's own mortality. Coming face-to-face with this fact of life brings one, almost naturally, to take stock of how one has lived one's life; it is a cleansing experience. For example, it may bring one to ask: has my time been devoted to truly meaningful things? Are there wrongs that have to be righted in terms of human relationships?

A tragic event such as an illness can thus serve as an impetus to transcend oneself, give altruistically to others, and vicariously experience their joy and accomplishments. Sick people are challenged purposefully to turn a negative situation into a meaningful and positive experience. If accomplished, this is a noble act. Rabbi Joseph D. Solovechik (1903–1993 CE), a giant among modern Jewish scholars and existential philosophers, stresses repeatedly that the reason why tragedies befall people is often unclear. He likens it to looking at a magnificent tapestry upside down.[33] Although Jewish philosophy espouses ultimate divine justice, how that justice is meted out, how much of it sooner, later, in this world, or in the world to come is beyond the scope of human knowledge. It is certain, however, that suffering as experience must not be wasted. It can be used to relearn the value of time and relationships, reprioritize goals, and learn submission to the divine will. Judaism perceives a person to be a dialectic being; he or she finds greatness in conquering the world, but can also find greatness in being conquered, that is, accepting suffering and loss, yet coping nobly. A nurse's presence at the bedside supports individuals through this process. This is not to imply that illness is a welcome guest. Rather it is noble to make constructive use of whatever suffering cannot be alleviated after all options have been exhausted.

The *Talmud* (Tractate Berachot 5:2) (22) relates a dialogue between Rabbi Yochanan and his colleague, Rabbi Chiah, who was suffering a serious illness. Chiah bluntly stated that he would gladly forgo the rewards for his suffering and instead be free of it now. Rabbi Yochanan stretched out his hand and Chiah was immediately relieved. The story suggest that suffering can potentially take such a heavy toll on a person that even a righteous sage would be willing to forgo its reward for relief.

Additional insight can be gleaned from the answer the *Talmud* gives to why Rabbi Chiah, a righteous sage in his own right, was dependent on Rabbi Yochanan for relief. Someone who is imprisoned, states the *Talmud*, is incapable of being freed from prison. Suffering can be so totally debilitating as to render people incapable of facilitating their own healing process, both on a physical and metaphysical plane. Nurses can be potent facilitators for such individuals. In many instances, therefore, individuals resort to prayer, which is indeed a central vehicle both for expressing one's feelings as well as beseeching God for the return of good health.

HARNESSING NATURE AND "CONQUERING GOD" FOR HEALING

Although God is the ultimate creator, he willingly invites human beings—indeed commands them—to be his partners in creation by improving nature. Although this may seem paradoxical on a theological level, God purposefully limits his omnipotence in order to make room for people to reign over earth.[34] By manipulating the forces of nature to improve quality of life, people do God's will and essentially realize their godly image as creators. Hence, curing illness and caring for those who suffer, using technologies that "fool mother nature," does not constitute rebellion against God according to the Jewish tradition, but on the contrary, celebrates God's desire, so to speak, to be conquered by humans.[35]

If illness is a result of people's imperfect deeds or the need for catharsis, bypassing the metaphysical realm by using natural means of cure might be perceived as useless at best and immoral at worst. This, however, is not the case. Judaism recognizes the simultaneous existence of two planes of causality, the physical and the metaphysical, equivalent to two avenues of treatment. Good deeds and prayer are indeed the order of the day whenever catastrophe strikes, but one is obligated at the same time, and with no less rigor, to utilize all that the art and science of healing have to offer in terms of care and cure.[36]

The *midrash* relates a discussion between two great sages of the *Mishnah* and an anonymous ailing individual who accompanied them on a journey.[37] He asks the sages, "how can I heal myself?" They proceed to recommend a certain medicinal potion. The anonymous man challenges them with the question: "who smote the man with illness?" They answer, "God of course." "If so," said he, "you are asking God to interfere with God's will." The sages inquire with regard to his livelihood, to which he responds that he was a farmer. "How do you allow yourself to interfere with God's world by working the land so that it may bear fruit?" they ask. The impatient man responds "how else can I survive?" "So is the case," say the sages, "with respect to one's health. Natural avenues of healing are legitimate and a necessary part of life no less than toiling the land." An individual or a community that disregards this are deemed negligent both morally and religiously.

It is not surprising that the study of medicine was very highly regarded by Jewish scholars. The legendary Talmudist Shmuel, the great codifier Maimonides, and the classic biblical commentators Nachmanides (1194–1270

CE) and Avraham Ibn Ezra (1092–1167 CE) were physicians, to name a few. Throughout the ages, Jewish tradition has avidly advocated fighting natural causes of illness by practicing good hygiene, maintaining a healthy life style, and using science in the service of humankind. Jewish sages championed the discovery of the smallpox vaccination, hailing its discoverer a saint.[38] The modern and post modern era have seen an explosion of life-saving and life-enhancing discoveries, many of which have been championed by Jewish *halachic* authorities. They work in collaboration with scientists and health practitioners to ensure ethically and *halachically* appropriate use of technology.

Judaism is nevertheless sensitive to the negative potential lurking in the recesses of manipulating nature. The Bible (Genesis 2:15) tells that the Garden of Eden was given to Adam for him *"L'ovdah u'lishomra,"* literally, to "work" in the garden and care for it. He was given the right, indeed the duty, to utilize the garden's potential creatively for his own benefit, but with great care. With respect to this verse, the *midrash* relates that "When God put man in the Garden of Eden, he took him on a so-called guided tour of the garden and said: See how beautiful and praiseworthy are my works; and all that I have created, I have created it for your sake.[39] Take heed not to destroy or damage my world, for if you do, there will be no one to repair it or restore it after you." Thus Adam, and with him all humanity, received ultimate free choice and also ultimate responsibility. Beyond its ecological implications, the *midrash* has relevance to the preservation of a just and moral social order.

This can be illustrated with the use of organ transplant technology, which can be a double-edged sword. Donating an organ to save a life, both during one's lifetime and postmortem, is perceived by many contemporary Jewish scholars as a potentially appropriate and even noble act.[40] There are, however, possible pitfalls. Scrupulous care must be taken to harvest for transplant only after definitive death has occurred so as to preserve the sanctity of life.[41] Autonomous decisions by individuals not to donate must also be respected. Other concerns relate specifically to transplants from live donors, but to elaborate on them would be beyond the scope of this chapter. Suffice it to point out one central issue is the extent to which one may or should risk one's life for donation. Minimal risk is not viewed as an impediment and is seen by many scholars as the fulfillment of several religious commandments, including "Do not stand by idly while your brother's blood is being spilt" (Leviticus 19:16). Individuals are, however, commanded to give priority to their own life; hence exposure to substantial or grave danger is not permissible, even in order to save another human being.[42]

The *Talmud* (Tractate Babah Metziah 62:1) tells a heart-rending story of two friends who were traveling in an uninhabited land with only one canteen of water. The canteen belonged to one of the two; if he alone would drink, he would survive until reaching civilization. If, however, they would share the water, neither would survive. Ben Petorah thought that the owner of the water should demonstrate solidarity with his companion and share his water. Rabbi Akiva (50–135 CE), whose opinion prevailed, ruled that the "owner" is obligated (or according to an alternate interpretation, permitted) to drink all the water in order to assure his own life. The noble camaraderie echoed in Ben Petorah's opinion is well-taken. Nevertheless, as Rabbi Akiva stands, individuals are not *halachically* obligated (perhaps not even permitted) to risk their lives by donating an organ. Certainly, they should not be pressured to do so by health professionals under such circumstances.

However, if individuals choose to endanger themselves for family members, especially parents for children and vice versa, this seems so basic to human nature that it is difficult not to perceive it as a moral and indeed noble act. Rabbi Chaim David Halevi insightfully pointes out that sacrificing oneself for a child is tantamount to sacrificing for oneself and hence does not pose any *halachic* problem.[43] Jewish literature abounds with stories of individuals who endangered themselves for the sake of others in a variety of special circumstances, such as for great leaders in times of national crisis. These are indeed recognized by *halachic* authorities as exceptional circumstances in which risking one's life for a greater cause is championed.[44] In Israel, advanced practice nurses serve as organ transplant coordinators. They must possess expertise both in scientific and ethico-*halachic* aspects of transplantation, as well as the religious and cultural vantage points of donors and their families. This knowledge is essential for facilitating technologically successful transplants, while maintaining pluralistic sensitivity and high moral standards.

The *Responsa* literature contains abundant principles and specific guidelines regarding the ethically appropriate use of health sciences. These include but are hardly limited to artificial life support mechanisms, fertility technologies, and genetic engineering.

USE OF PRAYER AND AMULETS FOR THE MAINTENANCE, PRESERVATION, AND RESTORATION OF HEALTH

Prayer

Prayer plays an important role for many Jews in all aspects of life. Even Jews who do not consider themselves religious are apt to turn to prayer in times of illness or other turmoil.[45] God is traditionally believed to be the source of health and illness and all that pertains to the maintenance, preservation, and restoration of health is ultimately in God's hands.[46] Jewish prayer contains many verses asking God to maintain or restore health in oneself, that of a family member or a nonrelated individual. The *Tanach* contains many instances where prayer for a sick person promoted their healing. Biblical examples are Moses who prayed for his sister's Miriam recovery from her affliction with leprosy (Numbers 12:13), the Shunamite woman's son recovered due to Elisha's prayer (II Kings 4:33), and King Hezekiah's prayers gained him 15 additional years of life after he prayed to God to be healed (II Chronicles 32:34).

Halachic Jewish prayer occurs three times daily and contains prayers for health. The *Amedah*, considered the core of daily prayer, is a compilation of 18 prayers, including a specific prayer asking God to restore health and allows for specific names to be inserted.[47] Other prayers pertaining to health and illness are said at specific times or in specific places (e.g., the grave of a righteous person, when praying for the sick). Prayers or the recitation of Psalms, which serve the same purpose, may be offered by patients themselves, relatives, friends, or those who are unfamiliar with the patient. Additionally, many people offer personal prayers for the restoration of health.

Kavanah is a critical aspect of Jewish prayer and refers to the concentration, devotion, intention, and conviction that one uses in praying to God.[48] It is common during a hospitalization for traditionally observant patients and their families to be seen with a prayer book or Book of Psalms in their hand so that they can turn to fervent prayer. Many prayers laud the work of the physician but acknowledge that God is the ultimate physician who has the power to heal even those illnesses that are deemed incurable.[49]

In times of need, many Jews pray at holy sites such as the Western Wall (the remnant of the Jewish Temple, also known as the Wailing Wall) and gravesites of a righteous biblical personality named in the Bible.[50] These burial sites are located in Israel and include the Cave of the Patriarchs, where patriarchs Abraham, Isaac, and Jacob and their wives, the matriarchs Sarah and Rebecca, are buried. The matriarch Rachel is buried in Bethlehem and pilgrimages are common for the purpose of prayer. Additionally, pilgrimages are made to gravesites of Jewish scholars, such as the *Tannaim* and *Amoraim* (10–220 CE) whose teachings are recorded in the oral law, and many rabbinic figures of early and recent dates.[51] The purpose of praying at the grave of a great sage is not to pray to that individual, as prayer is always directed to God, but to have these righteous personalities act as spiritual intermediaries or to have their merit intercede on their behalf.[52] Blessings given by a living rabbi, whether in the presence or absence of a sick person, are held in high regard, as this represents a living intercedent with God. Additionally, dedication to religious study, righteous deeds, and other spiritual acts, such as giving charity and helping others, performed with *kavanah*, is an attempt to gain additional merit with God and overturn any evil decree.

The Jewish mysticism of *Kabbala* is also a source for customs to help cure the sick by spiritually changing the "evil decree."[53] For example, according to *Kabbala*, a person's name is considered to have spiritual importance, as the name's meaning has a connection to the person's character. Jewish baby boys traditionally receive their name on the 8th day after birth when they are ritually circumcised, and infant girls are named in the synagogue during the first week after birth. In times of illness, the name may be altered or changed entirely in order to give the person a spiritual renewal and with that a hope he or she is considered a "new person" who is no longer under the evil decree.

Jewish religion obligates patients to seek care from health care professionals; although the centuries old texts use the term "physicians," in later times this has also referred to other health care professionals. For that reason, health care professionals are duty bound to become proficient in their profession and are mandated to heal the sick.[54] The "Daily Prayer of a Physician" acknowledges God as the creator and ultimate healer and beseeches God to grant the physician wisdom, confidence, gentleness, and support in the great task of caring for God's created beings.[55,56] The prayer is attributed to Maimonides, a 12th century Jewish physician and philosopher. This is also the prayer that is recited at many medical school graduations.

Differences in cultural values, such as those pertaining to prayer, may exist between the nurse and patient. As intra-cultural variation is larger than inter-cultural variation,[57] these cultural clashes may occur even when the nurse is a member of the same cultural group. For that reason, nurses who share the same culture might experience dissonance between their own and the patient's prayer customs and values. Just as nurses care for the physical and mental needs of patients, so too, the nurse must provide for the spiritual needs of the patient.[58] Obtaining a cultural history, on every patient, not only those from a different culture than the nurse, will assist in understanding the specific cultural needs of each patient. On a practical level, for patients who pray at certain times of the day, organizing care with this in mind should be facilitated. If a patient partakes in ritual prayer, planning the nursing care with consideration of the prayer times will prevent disturbance of the prayer session. If the patient wants to attend a prayer service, if possible, make this feasible. Formal Jewish prayer ritual includes specific customs such as ritually washing hands with a cup prior to prayer and praying in the direction towards Jerusalem. Nurses who have cultural knowledge about these rituals, as well as others, can contribute significantly to an atmosphere that promotes spiritual and cultural comfort for the patient.

Amulets

Jewish writings include many anecdotes concerning the use of amulets in order to maintain, preserve, or restore health. Amulets are "sacred objects, such as charms, worn on a string or chain around the neck or wrist to protect the wearer from the evil eye. Amulets may also be written documents on parchment scrolls."[59] The practice has been in use for centuries and was considered a component of medical care. There are Jews who refrain from this practice, as there are rabbinic authorities doubting its effectiveness; however, the *Talmud* (Tractate Shabbat 61:2) lends it legitimacy.

For those who believe in them, *segulot* (supernatural cures or folk remedies) are engaged in with much *kavanah*. Some consider such acts as changing or altering one's Jewish name, giving charity, and performing good deeds as *segulot*. On a supernatural level, *segulot* also include such actions as placing a holy book near or under the pillow of the patient, wearing a red thread around one's wrist or ankle, wearing or pinning to one's clothing a medallion with an amulet to ward off the evil eye, and obtaining from a rabbi a bottle of "holy water" or "holy oil" that is rubbed onto the patient's skin.[60] These actions are believed to promote healing on a spiritual level. Health care professionals need to assess their patients for the importance they put on spiritual actions, such as prayer and amulet use, and incorporate these practices into the total health care management.[61,62]

SUMMATIVE REMARKS

This chapter focuses on selected topics in which Judaism interfaces with nursing practice. These were chosen from a wide range of options. Caring and curing is a primal religious duty for all, especially professionals. The underpinning for this obligation is that both the caregiver and the care recipient are made in God's image. Caregivers are commanded to imitate God by demonstrating kindness and compassion to others. "Presencing" and displaying empathy are mandated to the degree possible; they are challenging but rewarding actions that join caregivers with the sick as they question and ultimately find meaning in their difficult situation. Caregivers are commanded to explore all avenues for improving quality of life and longevity, including modern technology, taking heed to examine the ethical ramifications.

It is remarkable that although these are religiously rooted principles, many have become deeply engrained in the Jewish collective culture and are espoused by Jewish individuals who do not perceive themselves as religiously observant. An elegant reflection of this phenomenon was enacted by the "secular" Israeli legislation. On 28 Sivan 5758 (June 22, 1998), the Knesset, the governing body of Israel, passed its unique version of the "Good Samaritan Law." Its name is somewhat unwieldy: The "Do not stand idly by the blood of your neighbor law" (*Lo Ta'amod 'al Dam Re'ekha Law*). Yet these words were deliberately chosen as they are the words of the biblical law in Leviticus (19:16). The Act stipulates that if one witnesses a sudden life-threatening situation befalling any individual, one is law-bound to do everything possible in order to extend direct or indirect assistance as needed, barring risking one's own life. Individuals are obligated both to exert themselves physically as well as to incur financial expense as necessary, for which one is by law reimbursed, either by the benefactor or the government. Although other countries have Good Samaritan laws, the Israeli version is inspired by the biblical edict and is the only one that stipulates that the act of omission—failing to do what is necessary and possible to save life—is not only immoral, but illegal and punishable by a fine.

Familiarity with the Jewish *halachic* approach to health and well-being and the prevalent cultural customs and practices is important for nurses and others providing health for Jewish care recipients. When ministering care to all patients, however, a thorough cultural assessment is of primary importance rather than relying on outward appearances or other superficial indicators. As with all cultures, intra-cultural variation is greater than inter-cultural variation. This chapter addresses a nonexhaustive but representative core of Jewish principles, commandments, and practices. Its importance lies in serving as a vehicle for nurses of various faiths and cultures to enrich their understanding of issues related to nursing as a whole through the Jewish prism.

NOTES

1. Spector, Rachel E. *Cultural Diversity in Health and Illness*. 7th ed. Upper Saddle River: Pearson Prentice Hall, 2009. 352.
2. Ibid., 348.
3. Tal, Rami. The Jewish People Policy Planning Institute: Annual Assessment 2008. Jerusalem. The Jewish People Policy Planning Institute. Web. 20 June 2010. http://www.jpppi.org.il/JPPPI/Templates/ShowPage.asp?DBID=1&LNGID=1&TMID=150&FID=341.
4. Selekman, Janice. "People of Jewish Heritage." *Transcultural Health Care: A Culturally Competent Approach*. Eds. Larry D. Purnell and Betty J. Paulanka. Philadelphia, PA: F.A. Davis, 2003.
5. Shuzman, Ellen. "Perinatal Health Issues of Jewish Women." *Transcultural Aspects of Perinatal Health Care: A Resource Guide*. Ed. Mary Ann Shah. Tampa, FL: National Perinatal Association, 2004.
6. Zarembski, Laura. The Religious-Secular Divide in the Eyes of Israel's Leaders and Opinion Makers. Jerusalem: The Floersheimer Institute for Policy Studies, 2002, 11. Web.
7. Ibid.
8. Ibid., 13. Web.
9. Ibid., 11. Web.
10. Talmud Bavli, Tractate Shabbat 133.2.
11. Ram Brothers, and the Widow Ram. *Talmud Bavli: Vilna*. Jerusalem: Tel-man, 1981.
12. Talmud Bavli, Tractate Babah Metziah 30:2.
13. Talmud Bavli, Tractate Sanhedrin 73:1; Tractate Babbah Kamah 81:2.
14. Maimonides, Moses. *Mishneh Torah hu Ha-Yad ha-Chazakah le-haNesher ha-Gadol Rabbenu Moshe bar Maimon*. Jerusalem: Eshkol, 1968. Hichot Rozeach U'Shemira al Hanefesh 11:5.
15. Maimonides, Hilchot Deot 4:1.

16. Chacham, Amos. *Sefer Tehilim, Daat Mikrah.* 7th ed. Jerusalem: Mosad Harav Kook, 1990. Psalm 41(4).

17. Talmud, Tractate Nedarim 39.

18. Ram Brothers, and the Widow Ram. *Shulchan Aruch: Vilna.* Jerusalem: Tel-man, 1981. Yoreh Deah 335, 338.

19. Asher Ben Yaakov. "Arbaah Turim." Eds. A. Samet, D. Bitton (eds). Jerusalem: Machon Yerushalayim, 1990. Yoreh Deah 335, 338.

20. Samet, Aharon, and Bitton, Daniel. *Mikraot Gedolot Hamaor, Chamisha Chumshai Torah.* Jerusalem: Hamaor, 1990. Exodus 20:19.

21. Babylon Free Online Dictionary. Web. 3 June 2010. http//:www.babylon.com/definition/ease/Hebrew.

22. Talmud, Tractate Sotah 11:2, Rashi commentary.

23. Schecter, Shomo Zalman. *Avot D'Rabi Natan,* 41. 2002. http://www.daat.ac.il/DAAT/mahshevt/avot/shaar-2.htm. Web.

24. Talmud, Tractate Babba Meziah 30:2.

25. Talmud, Tractate Berachot 12:2.

26. Global Jewish Data Base. *Commentary on the Torah, Siftei Cohen Genesis 48:2.* 14th version. Jerusalem: Taklitor Torani, 2009. CD-ROM.

27. Kil, Yehuda. *Daat Mikrah, Book of Samuel.* Tel Aviv: Mosad Harav Kook, 1990. 11:9.

28. Talmud, Tractate Berachot 31:2.

29. Watson, Jean. The 10 Carative Factors. 1985. Web. 30 May 2010. http://www.angelfire.com/bc3/nursinginquiry/carative.htm.

30. Masechet Semachot. 8 (Evel Rabati). Web. 22 May 2010. http://www.hebrewbooks.org/pdfpager.aspx?req=37970&pgnum=655.

31. Ashkenazi, Bezalel. Sefer Shitah Mekubezet. Web. June 2010. http://www.hebrewbooks.org.14057.

32. Kook, Avraham Yitzchak. *Ein Ayah,* 32. Yafo: Machon Herziah, 1999.

33. Soloveichik, Joseph Dov. *Divrei Hagut V'Haarach: Kol Dodi Dofek.* 9–19. Jerusalem: Beit Zion Hadar, 1982: 65–70.

34. Kaplan, Lawrence. "Motifim Kabbalaiim B'Haguto shel Harav Soloveichik." *Emunah B'Zmanim Mishtanim:al Mishnato ahel Harav Yosef Dov Soloveichik.* Ed. A. Sagi. Jerusalem: Maor Valach, 1996. 75–94.

35. Soloveichik. 65–70.

36. Waldenberg, Eliezer Yehuda. *Responsa Tsits Eliezer, Ramat Rachel, Part 5:20.* 16th version. Bar-Ilan. University Responsa Project. Ramat Gan: Bar-Ilan Publishers, 2008. CD-ROM.

37. Buber, Shmuel. *Midrash Shmuel.* 4:7. Vilna: Ram, 1925. Web. 20 June 2010. http://www.ebrewbooks.org. 33213.

38. Eisenberg, Daniel. The Ethics of Smallpox Immunization. 2009. Web. 23 May 2010. http//:www.aish.com/ci/sam/48943486.html.

39. Vagshal, C. "Midrash Rabbah." *Kohelet.* Ed. C. Vagshal. Vol. 6. 7:28. Jerusalem: Vagshal Publishers, 2001.

40. Yosef, Ovadia. *Yechaveh Daat (Responsa).* Jerusalem: Chazon Ovadia, Porat Yoseph, Machon Yerushalayim, 1973, 84:3.

41. Zweibel, Chaim Dovid. A Matter of Life and Death: Organ Transplants and the New RCA. "Health Care Proxy". Web. 1 July 2010. http://www.hods.org/pdf/A%20Matter%20of%20Life%20and%20Death.pdf.

42. Eisenberg, David. Does Jewish Law Permit Donating A Kidney? Web. 31 May 2010. http//:www.aish.com/ci/sam/48954401.html.

43. Halevi, Chaim David. Asai Lechal Rav. 1989. Web. 20 May 2010. http://www. hebrewbooks.org/home.aspx. *44Bar-Ilan Judaic Library*. Responsa Mishpat Cohen 14. 18th version. Bar Ilan University Responsa Project. Ramat Gan: Bar-Ilan Publishers, 2010. CD-ROM.
44. Spector. 2009.
46. Rosner, Fred. "Complementary Therapies and Traditional Judaism." *Mount Sinai Journal of Medicine*. 66:2 (March 1999): 102–05.
47. Hanefesh Community, National Assembly Jewish Students. The Shema Prayer & the Amidah Prayer. Web. 7 July 2010. http://www.hanefesh.com/edu/amidah.htm.
48. Zehavy, Tzvee, Kavvanah (concentration) for prayer in the Mishnah and Talmud: New Perspective in Ancient Judaism. 1987. Web. 20 June 2010. http://www.tzvee. com/Home/kavvanah.
49. Sulzbach Siddur. *Prayer for a Pregnant Woman. Compiled in Aneni: Special Prayers for Special Occasions*. Nanuet, New York: Feldheim Publishers, 2003.
50. Noble, Anita, Lawrence Noble, Rachel E. Spector, Rachel Yaffa Zisk-Rony, Anna C. Woloski-Wruble. *Traditional Customs Used by Jewish Women to Facilitate the Childbirth Continuum*. Book of Abstracts as presented at The First Global Conference of Doctoral Midwifery Research Society, Northern Ireland, 2010.
51. Bacher, Wilhelm, Jacob Zallel Lauterbauch, Joseph Jacobs, Louis Ginzberg. *Tannaim and Amoraim*. Jewish Encyclopedia. Web. 13 June 2010. http://www. jewishencyclopedia.com/view_friendly.jsp?artid=59&letter=T (2002).
52. Noble, Anita, Lawrence Noble, Rachel E. Spector, Rachel Yaffa Zisk-Rony, and Anna C. Woloski-Wruble. *Traditional Customs Used By Jewish Women to Facilitate the Childbirth Continuum*. Book of abstracts, The First Global Conference of Doctoral Midwifery Research Society, Northern Ireland, September, 2010.
53. Friedman, Azriel Hirsch. My New Jewish Name, Aish Hatorah. Web. 17 June 2010. https://www.aish.com/print/?contentID=48943666&section=sp/so 2010.
54. Rosner, Fred. "Complementary Therapies and Traditional Judaism." *Mount Sinai Journal of Medicine* 66: 102–05. Web. 3 November 2009. http://www.mymson sitehealth.net/msjournal/66/04_Rosner.pdf 1999.
55. Friedenwald, Harry. "Oath and Prayer of Maimonides." *Bulletin of the Johns Hopkins Hospital* 28 (1917): 260–61. Delhousie University Libraries. Web. 17 June 2010. http://www.library.dal.ca/kellogg/Bioethics/codes/maimonides.htm.
56. MedicineNet.com. Definition of Maimonides prayer. MedicineNet.com (1998). Web. 20 June 2010. http://www.medterms.com/script/main/art.asp?articlekey=4247.
57. Campinha-Bacote, J. (2007). *The Process of Cultural Competence in the Delivery of Healthcare Services: The Journey Continues*. Cincinnati, OH: Transcultural C.A.R.E. Associates.
58. Spector. 2009. 82–83.
59. Spector. 2009. 82–83.
60. Barr, Joseph, Matitiah Berkovitch, Hagi Matras, Eran Kocer, Revital Greenberg, Gideon Eshel. "Talismans and Amulets in the Pediatric Intensive Care Unit: Legendary Powers in Contemporary Medicine." *Israel Medical Association Journal* 2:4 (April 2000): 278–81.
61. Spector. 2009.
62. Noble, Anita, et al. 2010.

11

Christianity and Nursing

Janice Clarke

INTRODUCTION

The essence of Christianity is to live in relationship with God and each other, and from this flow the principles that have made the Christian community ripe for the development of nursing. They are principles such as love for your neighbor, hospitality to the stranger, compassion, and a holistic view of the person in which the body cannot be divorced from the spirit. Western nursing has grown out of the Christian church and so Christianity and nursing have historically had strong associations. This chapter aims to show how these core principles have influenced the development of health care, as well as informing Christian health ethics. It will also show how Christian principles have the potential to inform nursing theory and practice for all nurses, enabling them to practice their art to the highest level. Nursing has always taken its knowledge from a variety of sources and theological models have their own contribution to make in nursing. However, for Christian nurses, these principles will not only be an informing factor, but also an obligation.

The chapter falls into six main parts:

1. The core beliefs of Christianity and the authority for those beliefs. This section focuses on those beliefs that are most likely to affect health care practices.
2. The individual and the community: hospitality to the stranger.
3. Health and medicine in the Christian tradition.

4. Christian health care ethics.
5. Nurses in the Christian tradition.
6. Christian patients.

Christianity is an ancient global religion. Consequently, a wide range of practice and belief exists among Christians and even within groups belonging to the same denomination or subgroup of belief. This is not a negative factor but rather reflects the variety of human experience and character. Different denominations tend to place emphasis on different aspects of belief. The sources used here have deliberately been taken from a variety of denominations.

CORE BELIEFS AND AUTHORITY IN CHRISTIANITY

Christianity may be unique in its central belief that God lived on earth as a man and a Jew. This man was Jesus Christ; Christ means, anointed by God. The names Jesus, Christ, and Jesus Christ are used interchangeably by Christians. Christians believe that they know God principally through the fact that he was born on earth as a human being. God is known not only because a person somewhere was told about him, or because he invisibly acted through any event; God's purpose and nature is known primarily because God lived as a human here on earth.[1] The eye witness accounts about his life and death contained in the scriptures of the New Testament are, however, not the only basis for Christian beliefs. Accounts or "revelations" have been reflected on and written about by theologians and other Christians for 2000 years. Such writings, together with the lives of saints and martyrs, the rituals and prayers used in services of worship, and many other sources have formed a living repository of knowledge that are collectively known as the Tradition. This knowledge, which has been subjected to inspired and devoted interpretation, together with study, prayer, and sacramental practice is imbued, Christians might say, with the Holy Spirit. Tradition is the result of participation, relationship and fellowship with Christ, in the community of the *Church* (italicized words are explained in the glossary at the end of the book). It is the continuation of the scriptures, making the scriptures "understandable and meaningful"[2] and bringing the revelation in the scriptures into the present day, facing present day situations. Therefore, the *New Testament* and *Old Testament* with the Tradition form the main historical source of Christian belief.

Tertullian (160–220 CE), an early theologian, said that scripture was easy to understand correctly if it was read as a whole, but that read in parts, it was possible to make it mean anything you wished, thus correct interpretation, with reference to the Tradition, was crucial.[3]

The first clue about the importance of the concept of relationship to Christian spirituality comes from the fact that Christ called God his Father and related to him as his son. After Christ was crucified, the Bible teaches that the Holy Spirit descended to his disciples. Here is the second clue about relationship, because here is born the idea of the Trinity of Father, Son, and Holy Spirit. Not three Gods, but one. The Christian God is a communion of "persons," "divine and human, in loving relation."[4] It is this idea of equal, reciprocal, and mutual relationship which, as Downey, a Catholic theologian, referred to above, says forms a template for relationships between people and is the basis of Christian ethics.[5] This understanding of a community of persons is not only an example for Christians to follow, but in a mystical sense, is also seen as a pattern stamped on humanity that should be fulfilled in our lives in order to be fully human. "I need you in order to be myself."[6]

Similarly, the person is also understood as being a composite or "community" of three parts: body, soul, and spirit, each part being in relation or communion with the other two. In Eastern Orthodox Christian theology, each "person" of the Holy Trinity is said to relate to the two others by a process of *perichoresis,* meaning the soul and spirit always transmigrating into the body, and the body into the soul and spirit. This notion of being constantly permeated by spirit, as well as the belief that humans are made in the image of God (Genesis 1:27), gives rise to the belief that human beings are equally spiritual and material. People therefore live in a paradox that they are constantly striving to resolve. They are higher than the angels because they possess a body and so contain potential that not even the angels can aspire to.[7] As *imago mundi* (an image of the world) reflecting the two different aspects of the created universe, Maximus (580–662 CE) said that each person was a microcosm of the whole universe, a laboratory "in which everything is concentrated." The person's unique ability to move between the two levels of matter and spirit, linking the two levels "as a natural bond," defines their vocation as mediator between heaven and earth.[8]

Christian theology tells of how at some point humans chose to rebel against God's will, an event depicted in the Garden of Eden when Adam and Eve ate from the tree of knowledge of good and evil from which God forbade them to eat. Therefore humans came to reflect the cosmos in a disordered way. However, through the practice of love, Christians believe that they can renew their relationship with each other and restore their relationship with God. This Christian love is called *agape:* the unconditional act of will that is indifferent to the value of the thing it loves, whereas *eros* is the love dependent on attraction and yearning.[9] Thus, Christians are commanded to love even their enemies.

The Christian life is not only about looking inward but also about looking outward toward other people. It is about community rather than individuality and the only purpose in perfecting the inner spiritual life is to learn how to love others more and better. Christianity is a religion of encounter: with God, with other human beings, and encountering our own selves. Christian living is dominated by learning about how to live closer to God and more in alignment with what are perceived to be God's wishes for us.

The relationship portrayed in the Trinity and told about in the *Gospels* gives a template and guide for how people should act. The scriptures and the Tradition teach that God loves humanity and wants only the best for people, tolerates their faults, seeks their spiritual growth, is forgiving and just, and gives us freedom, therefore we know that this is how we should relate to others.

THE INDIVIDUAL AND COMMUNITY: HOSPITALITY TO THE STRANGER

Hospitality is a natural part of Christian practice because it describes how people should act in encounters with the stranger: with welcome, protection, help, and comfort. To Christians, Christ's image is in each person perceived as a stranger. When Christ described how people will be judged in the future he said, "For I was hungry and you gave me food; I was thirsty and you gave me drink; I was a stranger and you made me welcome, naked and you clothed me, sick and you visited me in prison and you came to see me. . . . In so far as you did this to one of the least of these brothers of mine, you did it to me." (Matthew 25, 34–40)[10]

What is known as the "great" or "first" commandment, that is, "to love God and also to love your neighbor as yourself" led to Christ being asked "who is my neighbor?" (Luke 10:29), to which he told the story of a Jew who had been set upon and beaten by thieves. A priest came across him, as well as a man from his own country who both ignored him. Then a Samaritan saw him, treated his wounds and took him to an inn where he cared for him overnight, then gave the innkeeper instructions to continue his care for payment on his return (Luke 10, 30–35). The Samaritans and the Jews reviled each other and were in constant dispute over how they interpreted religious laws, yet it was a Samaritan who cared for the Jew, showing how a neighbor could be any stranger.

In an increasingly diverse society, the concept of hospitality to strangers comes into sharp focus bringing a powerful message about the need for love and inclusiveness. It speaks of how those who are outside our immediate circle should be treated. Sutherland uses the theology of the stranger to explore how people relate to different types of people on the margins of society, be they ill, poor, or foreign. He suggests that what these "outsiders" have in common is that their appearance "is disconcerting and confusing to others; they cause consternation and discomfort."[11] They challenge our settled ideas and ordered lives. They force us to think about our own mortality and how easily our own contentment could be upset.

HEALTH AND MEDICINE IN THE CHRISTIAN TRADITION

The Protestant theologian Karl Barth (1886–1968) argues that human beings should strive toward health as the way to exercise being fully individual, fully satisfying their needs, and fully using their reason and the way to be fully human.[12] Christians see it as their vocation to be fully what God has made them, that is, fully human, seeing it as an obligation to seek good health.

Thus, medicine has a long history in Christianity, beginning with the healing miracles in the New Testament setting the example of the importance of healing disease. The first known hospital in the Christian world, the Basileias, was established by Basil the Great, Bishop of Caesarea in Cappadocia in 372.[13] Basil begged the authorities for permission to provide a place for strangers and "people who need attendance in consequence of infirmity . . . nurses, medical attendants and a means of conveying them."[14] Such hospitals were built as parts of monasteries because Basil believed that caring for the sick and suffering was part of the *monk's* calling, putting the message of love into practice. Early Christians were encouraged to care for the sick and their enthusiasm for doing so has often been called reckless. For instance, Eusebius writing during 263 CE records how Christians acted during a plague in Caesarea. "Everything is tears and everyone is mourning, and wailings resound daily through the city because of the multitude of the dead and dying . . . our brethren were unsparing in their exceeding love and brotherly kindness. They . . . visited the sick fearlessly, and ministered to them continually, serving them in Christ."[15]

Bishops were well-known for organizing health services and relief in times of pestilence. Smith and Cheetham give the example of how Placilla, the Christian wife of Emperor Theodosius (347–395 CE), cared for the sick not by delegating the task to others lower than herself, but by working with her own hands in the hospital. She "handled the pots" of those confined to bed, preparing food, feeding and washing the sick; doing work which was "generally done by domestics."[16] The Emperor Julian (332–363 CE) was scathing, saying of Christians that they "give themselves to this kind of humanity . . . starting from what they call love" in order to create converts.[17] Nevertheless, it is clear from these accounts and many others that by the 4th century, Christians had become known for their care of the sick both as individuals and in institutions, as well as their tendency toward "hands on" care and their willingness to sacrifice their own safety and dignity to help others, and not only their family and friends or soldiers, but also strangers. What was also revolutionary about early Christians and what put them in opposition to the surrounding culture was the belief that everyone was of equal status and equally deserving of care when in Greco-Roman society status was based on citizenship, family, and virtue.

The first nurses came from religious orders, such as the charity of St. Vincent de Paul in the 17th century. In the 1830s, a Lutheran pastor in Kaiswerwerth in Germany established an order of deaconesses (female church officials able to carry out some of the functions of clergy, such as helping at baptisms) to nurse the sick and it was when Florence Nightingale saw this that she went on to create her secular version of this model. As supernatural explanations for disease gave way to scientific reason, Christian doctors embraced the new order so that there are now few differences in medical practice between secular and Christian doctors.

The origin for much Christian health care and ethics lies in the stories of Christ's healing ministry in the *Synoptic Gospels*. Gill (2006) has analyzed the repeated themes of these stories to see what they have to say that is distinctly Christian about behaving ethically toward sick and disabled people.[18] His qualitative analysis reveals that incidents of healing were often accompanied by displays of emotion by Christ himself, together with touching, despite notions of uncleanness, and acting with faith, compassion, care, and humility. There is also an element of being willing to act outside the law, to do something different from the expected, to be prepared to shock and to take a risk. Christ's actions seem to demonstrate commitment to the person you feel compassionate about and a willingness to risk your own reputation or freedom to help them. For example, Christ healed a woman in the synagogue on a Saturday (the Jewish Sabbath), an act that was outside the Jewish law. He did this not in some discrete place, but in full view of the officials (Luke 13:10–17), causing shock and consternation that he was willing to counter fearlessly.

Gill used the word compassion to describe how Christ not only expressed sympathy at the predicament of the people he met, but he was willing to take action to allay it. Christ often showed anger during these incidents, forming a common combination of sympathy, action, and anger. For instance, in Mark's account of the healing of the leper (Mark 1:40–45), the characteristics of care, compassion, touch, anger, and the willingness to touch someone who is considered ritually unclean, come together. A number of things could render a person ritually unclean, such as menstruation, sexual activity, or death. To touch someone who was ritually unclean in ancient times would have been seen as shocking. For instance, ritual bathing was required before visiting the temple. The theologian Hooker[20] suggests that the anger is indignation at the cause of disease. To Jews at this time, lepers were outside the rest of society and anyone who touched them took on, not only the possibility of disease, but according to Mosaic law (the law that came from God through Moses), also their unclean state. Yet, Jesus voluntarily touched the man. Gill makes the point that given the persistent belief in some nations that disease is associated with uncleanness of spirit, it is not surprising that most health care in those nations is delivered through Christian agencies. The common demands for faith on behalf of those being healed or their family and friends, Gill argues, should be interpreted as confidence or trust rather than faith, meaning religious belief.

Gill's analysis shows that the core of these stories is compassion, a slightly mistrusted concept in modern health care where it has somehow come to be associated with disempowerment and dependence. Gill argues that even Christian health ethics has failed to give compassion the importance it deserves and suggests that "principled scruples" and empathy have often been placed before it.[21] Whereas empathy means that we can identify with the feelings of the sufferer, compassion can be a spur to action to alleviate the suffering. Davies analyzes the theology of compassion and suggests that "In compassion we see another's distress (cognition), we feel moved by it (affectively) and we actively seek to remedy it (volition)."[22] Mercy is sometimes used in the Bible to mean compassion, but it should be seen as compassion shown to someone over whom you have power.

In the stories of healing in the Synoptic Gospels, Christ is seen being moved to anger at the suffering before him, then seeking to find a solution. These notions of compassion, care, touch, righteous anger, the willingness to deal with the "unclean" and the need to inspire trust, all have something to teach nurses; however, arguably it is compassion that lies at the core of Christian ethics.

CHRISTIAN HEALTH CARE ETHICS

One of the problems for Christians in finding solutions to ethical problems that do not contradict their religious beliefs, is in harmonizing the relief of suffering with the upholding of principles. In a belief system where all life is valued, infused with God's spirit and in the image of God, the question of how to reduce suffering when it seems the only way is to end life, have always perplexed Christians. To Gill, holding to principles must give way sometimes to compassion, which is a more risky ethical stance underpinned by the notion that rules and principles were created to smooth the path of humankind on the earth. When they become obstacles to compassionate care, they may need to be discarded. This calls for discernment and judgment with love; clearly a difficult path. As Christ says in the Gospel according to Mark, "The Sabbath was made for man, not man for the

Sabbath." (2:27) This might mean that treatments should be discontinued when they cease to bring benefit and the burden of misery they impose is overwhelming.[23]

Borg puts the dilemma in a historical context. He argues that in the dominant paradigm of the Jewish *Torah* (the first five books of the Old Testament), holiness gave way to the "compassion code." This new paradigm was ushered in by the "new covenant," meaning a new relationship with God mediated by Jesus Christ. Jesus contrasts holiness with compassion in the Synoptic Gospels saying "I desire mercy (compassion) not sacrifice," (Mathew 9:13).[24] Healing on the Sabbath was allowed because it was exercising compassion even though it was against the religious law. Borg reminds us that Christ taught that we were children and should do as children do, imitating their father, making a compassionate God their role model. "The fitting response of those who lived under the compassion of God was compassion"[25] as demonstrated in the *parable* of the wicked servants who were criticized by Jesus because instead of releasing their debtors from their debt as their master had done to them, they forced their own debtors to pay up on pain of punishment (Matthew 18:23–35). Whereas Leviticus 9:2 states "Be holy as God is holy," Luke says "Be compassionate as God is compassionate." (6:36)

Another characteristic of the new covenant is inclusiveness. The compassion demonstrated in the *Torah* is usually compassion for your own social group, starting with your family and ending with your tribe. Whereas the compassion of the New Testament is to be offered to everyone with whom you come into contact and anyone can be seen as your neighbor, if they are in need.[26] As Matthew (5:45) has, "God causes his sun to rise on bad men as well as good, and his rain to fall on honest and dishonest men alike." Thus, Christian ethics is inclusive and dominated by compassion rather than slavishly following principles.

This viewpoint is reflected in the principles proposed by the Anglican bishops of the Lambeth Conference, the decision-making body of the Church of England, in 1998, which suggested some principles that should guide ethical decision making:

1. Life is God-given and therefore has intrinsic sanctity, significance, and worth.
2. Human beings are in relationship with the created order and that relationship is characterized by such words as respect, enjoyment, and responsibility.
3. Human beings, while flawed by sin, nevertheless have the capacity to make free and responsible moral choices.
4. Human meaning and purpose is found in our relationship with God, in the exercise of freedom, critical self-knowledge, and in our relationship with one another and the wider community.

5. This life is not the sum total of human existence; we find our ultimate fulfillment in eternity with God through Christ.[27]

Such principles describe compassionate decision making where moral freedom is respected, the wider community acknowledged, and the responsibility to each other and the sanctity of life endorsed. The bishops proposed that the first, second, and fourth principles made all forms of euthanasia wrong. Yet in some circumstances, it was acceptable for treatment to be refused or stopped by patients because the fifth principle reminds us that Christians do not "need to cling to life at all costs."[28]

THE NURSE IN THE CHRISTIAN TRADITION

Nursing has struggled to describe a truly holistic and integrative model of the human person, and the modern imperative to include spirituality has produced a flurry of updating that has not yet produced models that sufficiently account for how people's spirit articulates with their body and their mind.[29] Nursing is essentially about caring for embodied selves. Therefore, any model of nursing must be capable of encompassing and explaining the body not only as a mechanical and chemical system but as an embodied self which, for Christians anyway, contains spirit. Recent interpretations of nursing have tended to emphasize psychological and spiritual states in separation from the body.[30] However, in the Christian model of the person, body, soul, and spirit are inextricably interrelated. Christians believe that God came to earth in human form, and so sanctified the human person, including the body.[31] Because of the way that soul, spirit, and body constantly pour into each other, to care for the body means to touch both the soul and the spirit of the person: in caring for the physical body we care for the whole person. Therefore, a Christian theology of care is arguably innately holistic. The body is not just a housing for the soul; the body is the very condition of human existence. The body does not keep the person "earthbound," because Christians believe that one can become close to God in this life, with a body. Luther saw the whole person as being spiritual, including the body,[32] and Nouwen, a modern day writer about spirituality, thought that Christianity takes the body more seriously than other religions and wrote "the way one lives in the body, the way one relates to, cares for, exercises, and uses one's own and other people's bodies, is of crucial importance for one's spiritual life." The body is seen as a glorified place, a temple, a means of sanctification. Loving care of the body is a spiritual act.[33] Therefore, Christian nurses are not repulsed by the physical body and do not consider it innately unclean; care of the body is an important activity and not to be denigrated or delegated to the least qualified or those of the least status.

Thus physical care is careful, attentive, and unflinching touch of the body, rather than a mechanical, instrumental, distracted touch that attempts to keep a person at arm's length. The philosopher Levin proposed that through this kind of touch we can learn to know a person better and come into better relationship with a person. He suggests that when bodies are handled appropriately, the true nature of another person is allowed to emerge. He says, ". . . careful touch, which is open to feeling what it touches and uses, gets in touch with a thing's essential nature more deeply and closely than the hand which willfully grasps . . . or than the hand which is indifferent to the beauty of the thing in the wholeness of its truth."[34]

However, realizing this link between the body and the person—a truly embodied self—is only possible within a paradigm that is capable of valuing the body. Groenhout, Hotz, and Joldersma have analyzed interactions between patients and nurses using the framework of the Protestant tradition, and suggest that how nurses use the right level and type of touch affects their relationship with patients and governs the level of dependency between the two parties. This "dance" between two partners can contain elements of self-sacrifice and mutuality that make these embodied encounters spiritual. Physical care performed in this spirit can become a *sacramental* act.[35]

The parallel aspect of the nurses' work, besides working with the body, is in relationship. Nurses constantly encounter "the other," the stranger, and their work is devoted to bringing each "other" into relationship. Nurses have to engender trust quickly and inspire their patients to have faith in their helpers on whom they may depend. Campbell suggests that for all practitioners who work in this way, their task is almost religious whether they believe or not, because they hope for an end to suffering, however illusive. He calls the love, or agape, that gives birth to this hope "moderated love" and suggests that all good professionals will need this.[36]

Nurses straddle the "normal" or "outside" world of their home and family, and the world of disease, disorder, and taboo every working day. Nurses bring this outside world to patients and become their bridge to the outside. This is not only the physically outside world, but the world of normality, sanity, and certainty from which patients may feel estranged. Maximus, the 6th century theologian, said that the human being was the natural mediator between all the levels of the cosmos by holding the two poles of the material and the spiritual, transcending both by uniting them and aiming always toward unity and God. Because of the unique work that nurses do, they could be called a quintessential mediator, reminding people, by loving care of their body, that they are valued. Christian care of the whole person is not only aimed at healing the body, but through careful caring, to contribute toward healing of the whole person enabling them to move along their own path toward God. The principles of hospitality and holistic and compassionate care for strangers, who reflect the image of Christ, and the inclusivity that these principles encompass, bring each person in from the margins, direct the encounters of Christian nursing and provide an ethical backdrop to the nurse–patient relationship.

Care within this paradigm cannot stop at the bedside. The Old Testament, as well as the New, contains many exhortations to speak up for those whose voice is not heard or who are poor or strangers.[37] Nurses working within this model will seek to eradicate the poverty and injustice that cause illness and disability and that may involve them in political and social action. This care transcends sentimentality. The righteous indignation of Christ, when he saw injustice, urges Christian nurses, using Christ as an example, to be prepared to face criticism to advocate on behalf of patients and to be prepared to fight for a better society. Similarly, at home after work, or in church, Christian nurses may pray for patients, bringing the world of their patients into their own world as though deriding the division.

Nursing seen in this light could truly be called a vocation. This is a spiritual calling that not only affects the person being cared for, but which could also affect nurses, helping them on their own path to God by giving the opportunities to practice what Christians might call the virtues of compassion, self-sacrifice, tolerance, and love.

THE CHRISTIAN PATIENT

Christians aim to place themselves in God's hands and may see times of illness and anxiety as tests of their faith or as opportunities to come closer to God. Therefore, they are likely to try to be stoical and accepting about illness. However, in a paradoxical world, such trials may also cause loss of faith for some people as they face the reality of believing that God's purpose is to provide what each person needs, and not to give each person what they want. Christians, as with any believer, who have not thought about their faith for a long time may rediscover it at times of crisis. Nurses serve these patients by prompting them to remember what had given them strength in the past and providing the circumstances for patients to reconnect with those things and, if they wish, practice their faith. As with all religions, devotional and scriptural reading, music, and nature can all help people to immerse themselves in their faith, or to rediscover it.

Of suffering, Weil says, "The extreme greatness of Christianity lies in the fact that it does not seek a supernatural remedy for suffering but a supernatural use for it."[38] While Christianity teaches that Christians should unashamedly pray to be relieved of suffering, they might at the same time pray that God's will be done and that they will have the strength to accept it. Christians might feel that suffering is part of life, but that like all aspects of life, it must be capable somehow of being put to the service of God. Christians may try to find meaning in suffering by seeing it as an opportunity to draw closer to God and deepen their faith by increasing their dependence on God. Roman Catholics in particular may see suffering as redemptive and as punishment for their own or others' sins. Therefore, although suffering should not to be sought or idealized, it can be seen by Christians to be an opportunity to learn more about themselves, to deepen their relationship with others, to empathize with others who are also suffering, to appreciate their own dependence on God, and to enable them to appreciate the preciousness of life. Consequently, for Christians, suffering could be tinged with hope, because there is always hope of a better reality to come.

If nurses are to be respectful of patients' religious views, they must be able to accept those views, not necessarily believe them, but accept that their patients' beliefs are a response to the sacred, and not just a response to social and psychological conditioning. Religious belief means living within a particular world view; it is not just a means of expression or a lifestyle choice. Just as nurses have had to learn to accept the modern definition of pain—that it is what the patients says it is and exists when the patient says it does—so nurses have to accept that religion is about responding to the sacred, as the patient sees the sacred, and is not a psychological or social need or prop.[39] To people who live within the perspective of Christianity, the symbols of their religion are not just illustrative of a divine reality, nor are they only symbols of or for that reality, but they are pointers to an actual reality, which in some ways may be more real to them than daily life. To Christians, the sacraments, such as *Holy Communion* (also called *Eucharist* or the *Lord's Supper*), are not just illustrative or symbolic of a truth, but they actually manifest a truth. As Florovsky writes, "The Eucharistic Sacrament is neither a mere remembrance nor a 'repetition' of the Last Supper. It is rather its 'manifestation' or extension. Worshippers are, as it were, taken back to the Upper Room and made participants of the same sacred Supper."[40]

Because of this, Christian rituals should be treated with seriousness and solemnity because to Christians, these are not just a comfort but are actually supernatural events that put them in touch with God. Therefore, it may be very important to receive Holy Communion, and especially at times of illness and crisis, because it is seen to have a healing function. In Eastern Orthodoxy, the last words the priest utters before giving Holy Communion are "for the healing of our souls and bodies." Christians may experience a feeling of completeness and fulfillment after receiving Holy Communion, and following the service they should be given privacy for a while to contemplate what has taken place and to return slowly to the material world from the spiritual world.

The true meaning of sin is not to do with being bad, but it literally means "to miss the mark." It is a paradoxical aspect of being human that as soon as we begin to interact with other people, we are constantly "falling short" of where we want to be. As St. Paul said "I cannot understand my own behavior. I fail to carry out the things I want to do and I find myself doing the very things I hate" (Romans 7:15–16). Christians have the chance to deal with this paradox and the guilt it may engender by seeking confession to a priest and being given absolution (forgiveness) or by seeking Holy Communion or other forms of blessing, and anointing with oil, so that they can face the world anew. Especially when Christians are faced with the reality of their own mortality and their need for God, they may suddenly feel the need for confession, anointing, and forgiveness as part of a healing process that sees the whole person as in need of healing, not only the body. In the Roman Catholic and the Orthodox Churches, and in recent decades in Protestant Churches, a priest or pastor may be summoned to pray with a person and give a blessing by placing a hand on their head and making the sign of the cross; this may be accompanied by the anointing with oil on the forehead and hands. In the Roman Catholic Church, this is particularly requested by patients to prepare for death, but may also be requested in times of illness where it is called the sacrament of the sick. This is a subtle form of healing, where healing is seen as an acceptance of the burden life has placed on them and a willingness to place themselves in God's hands and learn what this illness has to teach. Healing may mean receiving the courage to work with and through the illness and the fortitude to deal with whatever pain may be involved. In this way, it could be argued that if healing means to feel better, then it is possible to be healed by these means, although materially the disease may be the same. Likewise, prayer is a healing way to communicate desires and needs and therefore the privacy to pray is important, as well as the freedom from embarrassment. People may need to be invited to voice their religious needs in a world that is increasingly secular and where they may not wish to stand out. During illness and anxiety, prayer may become much more important and can be a great source of help in managing physical and spiritual pain.

CONCLUSION

Christian theology is innately holistic and relational. It offers ways of understanding the person and society that can enhance any nurses' understanding of their role. Christianity holds deeply integrative views of the person that honor the body, the site of most nursing care. In addition, Christian models of relationship are inclusive and compassionate toward strangers. Indeed,

Christian ethics holds that acting compassionately is more important than rigidly following principles. For non-Christian nurses, Christian theology offers pragmatic and comprehensible reasons to care and meaningful models of relationship. For Christian nurses who consciously works within the paradigm, their beliefs will motivate and enrich their daily work and they will strive to offer the best care, unconditionally, because that way they are every day fulfilling God's purpose in their lives.

NOTES

1. Ward, Keith. *Religion and Revelation*. Oxford: Oxford University Press, 1994.
2. Meyendorff, J. *Living Tradition*. New York: St. Vladimir's Seminary Press, 1978. 16.
3. McGrath, Alistair, E. *Christian Theology: An Introduction*. Oxford UK: Blackwell, 2001. 15.
4. Downey, Michael, *Understanding Christian Spirituality*. New Jersey: Paulist Press, 1997. 39.
5. McGrath 326. Op. cit. McGrath also gives an overview of a number of classical and modern ideas on The Doctrine of the Trinity. 318–344.
6. Ware, Kallistos. "The Trinity: Heart of our Life." *Reclaiming the Great Tradition: Evangelical, Catholics and Orthodox in Dialogue.* Ed. James S. Cutsinger. Illinois: Intervarsity Press, 1997. 141. 125–146.
7. Ware, Kallistos. "The Transfiguration of the Body." *Sacrament and Image*. Ed. Allchin, A. M. London: The Fellowship of St. Sergius and St. Alban, 1967. 25. 17–33.
8. Maximus the Confessor. *Difficulty 41,1305A* in Louth, Andrew. *Maximus the Confessor*, London: Routledge, 1996. 157.
9. Nygren, Anders. *Agape and Eros, (Parts 1 and 2).* London: SPCK. 1953. ix.
10. All biblical quotations are from *The Jerusalem Bible, Popular Edition*. London: Darton, Longman & Todd, 1974.
11. Sutherland, Arthur, M. *I Was a Stranger: A Christian Theology of Hospitality.* Abingdon US: Abingdon Press, 2006. 13.
12. Barth, Karl. *Church Dogmatics*. Edinburgh: T & T Clark, 1961. 3/4. 357.
13. Amundsen, Darrel W., and Gary B. Ferngren. "The Early Christian Tradition." *Caring and Curing: Health and Medicine in the Western Religious Traditions.* Eds. Ron L. Numbers and Darrel W. Amundsen. Baltimore: The Johns Hopkins University Press, 1998. 49. 40–64.
14. Basil the Great's Epistle 94, quoted in William Smith and Samuel Cheetham. *A Dictionary of Christian Antiquities.* Vol 1, London: John Murray, 1875. 786. Web. 12 Sept. 2011. <http://www.archive.org/details/christianantiqui01smituoft>
15. Eusebius. Chapter 7. "Ecclesiastical History," *Nicene and Post Nicene Fathers Series II Vol 1.* Ethereal Classics. Web. 12 Sept. 2011. <http://www.ccel.org/ccel/schaff/npnf201.iii.xii.xxiii.html> Book 7, Chapter 7, p. 307. NPNF2-01. Eusebius Pamphilius: Church History, Life of Constantine, Oration in Praise of Constantine | Christian Classics Ethereal Library.
16. Smith and Cheetham 786.
17. Fragment from Emperor Julian, quoted in Smith and Cheetham. 786.

18. Gill, Robin. *Health Care and Christian Ethics*. Cambridge, UK: Cambridge University Press, 2006. 62–93.

19. Gill.

20. Hooker, Morna, D. *The Gospel According to St. Mark*. London: Continuum, 1991. 80.

21. Gill 94.

22. Davies, Oliver. *A Theology of Compassion*. London: SCM Press, 2001. 17–18.

23. Gill 116.

24. Borg, Marcus. *Conflict, Holiness, and Politics in the Teachings of Jesus*. Harrisburg, US: Trinity Press International, 1998. See: 135–151 for a biblical exegesis of the move from holiness, as the main content of religious life, to compassion.

25. Borg 138.

26. Borg 140.

27. Anglican Consultative Council. *The Official Report of the Lambeth Conference July 18-August 9, 1998, Lambeth Palace, Canterbury, England*. Morehouse: London. 1999.

28. Gill 110.

29. Graham, Ian. V. "The Relationship of Nursing Theory to Practice and Research within the British Context: Identifying A way Forward." *Nursing Science Quarterly*, 16. 94. (2003): 346–350. Oldnall, Andrew. S. "On the Absence of Spirituality in Nursing Theories and Models." *Journal of Advanced Nursing* 21. (1995): 417–418.

30. Allen Shelly, Judith, and Arlene B. Miller, *Called to Care: A Christian Theology of Nursing*, Illinois: Intervarsity Press. 1999. 17.

31. For a detailed explanation of the spirituality of the body see pages 90–110 in Ware, Kallistos. "'My Helper and My Enemy': The Body in Greek Christianity." *Religion and the Body*. Ed. S. Coakley. Cambridge: Cambridge University Press. 1997. 90–111.

32. Tripp, David. "The Image of the Body in the Protestant Reformation." *Religion and the Body*. Ed. S. Coakley. Cambridge University Press: Cambridge, 1997. 131–155.

33. Nouwen, Henri, J. M. *The Road to Daybreak: A Spiritual Journey, Memorial Edition*. London: Darton, Longman & Todd, 1997. 202.

34. Levin, David, M. *The Body's Recollection of Being: Phenomenological Psychology and the Deconstruction of Nihilism*. London: Routledge and Kegan Paul, 1985. 128.

35. Groenhout, Ruth, Kendra Hotz, and Clarence Joldersma. "Embodiment, Nursing Practice, and Religious Faith: A Perspective from One Tradition." *Journal of Religion and Health* 44.2 (2005): 147–160. 152.

36. Campbell, Alistair.V. *Moderated Love*, London: SPCK, 1984. 14.

37. For example, see Isaiah 1 v17. "Search for justice, help the oppressed, be just to the orphan, plead for the widow."

38. Weil, Simone. *Gravity and Grace*. London: Routledge, 2002. 81.

39. Clarke, Janice. "Religion and Reductionism: A Discussion Paper about Negativity, Reductionism and Differentiation in Nursing Texts." *International Journal of Nursing Studies* 43. (2006): 775–785.

40. Florovsky, Georges. "The Worshipping Church" in *The Festal Menaion*, Mother Mary and Archimandrite Kallistos Ware. Pennsylvania: St. Tikhon's Seminary Press, 1969. 21–38. 29.

12

Islam and Nursing

Muntaha K. Gharaibeh and Rowaida Al Maaitah

SETTING THE SCENE

The Philosophical Views of Islam

Islam means the submission or surrender of one's will to the only one and true *Allah* (God) worthy of worship, and anyone who does so is termed a "Muslim."[1] The two main sources for Islamic law, *Shari'a*, are the *Qur'an* and *Sunnah*. *Shari'a* is a complete detailed code of conduct, based on the rules and regulations that were revealed to the Prophet Muhammad. The *Qur'an* is the sacred book of Islam and the highest and most authentic authority in Islam. It is the word of Allah revealed to the Prophet Muhammad, via the angel Gabriel, written in Arabic, and is the essential guide for all aspects of a Muslim's life. The *Sunnah* is a collection of deeds, words, and traditions of the Prophet Muhammad and his followers, checked for their authenticity and passed down over time.[2,3]

Jurists and scholars in Islam agree that the aim of Islamic Shari'a is to safeguard the five sublime objectives of life, namely: faith, body, offspring, property, and mind. The scholars of Islam express these five objectives in terms of the five essentials, by which they mean what is fundamental and without which life may not be possible. When any of these fundamentals is undermined, life will be compromised and may become chaotic and humanity will suffer. The loss incurred will be either short-term in this life or long-term in the hereafter.[4]

For Muslims, Islam is not only a religion but a complete way of life with values that advocate peace, mercy, and forgiveness. For Islam, a Muslim can be defined as a person who accepts the Islamic way of life and complies with the will of Allah without question. All Muslims have to fulfill five essential religious duties that include declaring that there is no other God but Allah, and that the Prophet Mohammed is his messenger; praying five times a day: at dawn, midday, late afternoon, after sunset, and late evening; fasting during the month of Ramadan, (with some flexibility or exemptions for sick and elderly people, pregnant women if they cannot tolerate it, and young children); giving money to charity (*Zakat*) amounting to 2.5% of an individual's annual income and savings; and going on a pilgrimage to Mecca (*Hajj*), at least once in a lifetime if one can afford it.[5] Based on the *Qur'an*, *Hadith* (sayings), and *Qiyass* (analogy), Islamic jurists classify human actions into one of five categories on a spectrum: obligatory (*Wajib*), recommended (*Mustahab*), permitted (*Masmoush*), disapproved but not forbidden (*Makrouh*), and absolutely forbidden (*Haram*).[6]

Although the *Qur'an* is not a book about medicine or health sciences, it contains information that leads to guidelines in health and diseases. The traditions of the Prophet Muhammad in matters of health and personal hygiene are also a guide for his followers; a vital component of human life is being healthy, which enables us to undergo our daily life while carrying out our responsibility and duties in the community. According to the *Qur'an*:[7]

> God has bestowed on humans his blessings, both hidden and apparent. Of these blessings the greatest is that of health, which the prophet regarded as one of the two graces, the importance of which was not appreciated by many people. Divine law in matters of blessings does not change: because God will never change the grace which he hath bestowed on a people until they change what is in their own souls. (8:53)

This verse stresses that God has enjoined humankind to worship and thank him in accordance with the precepts enshrined in his *Shari'a*. This message targets the individual and the community of Muslims to promote their spiritual and material aspects and to achieve their well-being in this world and the hereafter.

Some common and essential Islamic terms need to be clarified for health care providers who do not know Arabic and who do not have an Islamic background.[8]

> *Hadith*: Saying(s) or action(s) ascribed to the Prophet Mohammad or act(s) approved by the Prophet.
> *Fatwa*: Formal religious rulings that are produced by Muslim Scholars.

Fiqh: Islamic jurisprudence, that is, knowledge of practical Islamic rulings deduced from detailed statements and religious texts. Literally, it is the understanding and acquisition of knowledge.

Schools of Fiqh: The schools of Islamic thought or jurisprudence. The four most important were founded by Malik, Abu Hanifa, Al-Shafie, and Ibn Hanbal.

Haram: Prohibited, banned, illegal, and impermissible, from a religious standpoint, generally applied to actions or things considered sinful to Muslims.

NURSING PARADIGM CONCEPTS: ISLAMIC VIEWS

Health

Islam considers health as one of the greatest blessings that has been given to human beings by God after faith itself. The prophet says: "There are two blessings which many people do not appreciate: health and leisure." [9] He also says: "No blessing other than faith is better than well-being." [10]

One of the most important texts from which the *Fiqh* of health may be deduced is the verse in the Qur'an: "And he enforced the balance. That you exceed not the bounds: but observe the balance strictly: and fall not short thereof." (55:7–9)

This comprehensive verse emphasizes the balance that God established in the universe, with its different forces and influences, including humankind; it draws our attention to God's balance that applies to everything, making it clear that any disturbance of the balance, whether by increase or decrease, may lead to terrible consequences. God says: "Mankind! Your transgression will rebound on your own selves." (10:23)

Ali Ibn Abbas (died approx. 994 CE), a Persian physician and psychologist, in his book, *Kamil As-Sina'ah*, concludes that health means that the body is in a state of equilibrium. The state of equilibrium was further explained by Ibn Sina (known in the west as Avicenna) in 1093 CE as dynamic: The state of equilibrium that a human being enjoys has a certain range with an upper and a lower limit, meaning that it is like a balance that moves between two extreme limits. [11]

In order to maintain the state of equilibrium, protect it against imbalance, and restore it to its proper position, a human being must have a "health potential." This is referred to in the *Hadith* by the Prophet as saying: "And store up enough health to draw on during your illness." [12] "Health potential" in Islam takes different forms: proper nutrition, good immunity, physical fitness, as well as mental and personal security and stability, which enable a person to deal and cope well with the stressors; therefore the concept of health in Islam is not restricted to curative aspects, but implies aspects of restoration, preservation, and maintenance of health.[13]

Health Restoration, Preservation, and Maintenance in Islam

The importance of the concept of health restoration is evident in a number of *Hadiths* that have come down to us from the Prophet Muhammad, prescribing certain medicines for certain diseases. The Prophet emphasized the importance of seeking medical care. In an authentic (trusted) *Hadith* he says: "God has not created a disease without creating a cure for it"[14] raising the hopes of patients and making it clear that all diseases may be cured.[15]

The Prophet also placed the whole issue of the treatment of diseases in its proper context, as he made it clear that supplication (a humble prayerful request), medication, and methods of prevention are also parts of God's will. It is evident that Islam leaves no room for fatalism, even though it may be mistaken for reliance on God. The Prophet also opposed so-called "faith-healing" but approved medical practice that relies on study and experimentation, seeking to relate causes to effects.[16]

The preservation of health as a blessing can only be achieved through taking good care of one's health and taking every measure to maintain and enhance it. Based on this principle, Muslims are required to comply with physician recommendations regarding the preservation of good health. Both the *Qur'an* and *Sunnah* include teachings that clarify important health issues for Muslims, ranging from health maintenance to caring for each organ of the body.

The body, offspring, and mind cannot be completely safeguarded without maintaining good health, viewed as a top priority by the Prophet, and to maintain good health requires the provision of developmental needs such as good food, drink, clothing, shelter, marriage, transport, security, education, and income. He instructs Muslims to pray to God for forgiveness and sound well-being, "No blessing other than faith is better than well-being."[17] The Prophet says: "Wealth is appropriate to a God-fearing person, but good health is better for the God-fearing than wealth."[18] He further says: "He of you who finds himself enjoying good health, is secure in his community and has daily sustenance, as if he had the whole world at his fingertips."[19]

Therefore, it is no wonder that the *Qur'an* and the traditions of the Prophet include many statements to protect and promote health to preserve the properly balanced position in which persons are created. If we study these statements carefully and apply them properly, as we are required to do, we will find at our disposal a large volume on the *Fiqh* of health. This is based on the fact that the *Shari'a* is embodied in clear statements, whereas the *Fiqh* is the result of careful study of such statements and implementing them.

Health Accountability

Good health is something for which we are accountable to God. The Prophet says: "The first thing every servant of God will have to account for on the Day of Judgment is that he will be asked by God: Have I not given you a healthy constitution and have I not quenched your thirst with cold water?"[20] The Prophet also says: "No one will be allowed to move from his position on the Day of Judgment until he has been asked how he spent his life: how he used his knowledge: how he learnt and spent his money: and in what pursuits he used his health."[21] It is part of the duty of all Muslims, therefore, to safeguard this blessing and not to allow any chance to overcome it through ill usage, otherwise they will be severely punished according to God's immutable laws. The Qur'an states: "Anyone who tampers with God's grace after it has been bestowed on him will find God to be stern in punishment" (2:211) and "God would not alter any grace he has bestowed on a folk unless they alter what they themselves have." (8:53)

Holistic Health

It is well known that Islam attempts to solve problems within their proper context and not in isolation. This Islamic approach to social problems integrates health within the concept of social development. For example, the health of the community cannot be improved unless there is a marked improvement in income, education, nutrition, housing, clothing, as well as the improvement in the supply and distribution of clean water, sanitation, proper disposal of rubbish, and other important human needs. This Islamic approach to health care is based on the essential features of Islamic society, discussed later.

THE INDIVIDUAL, HUMAN RIGHTS, AND SECURITY

Islam considers the individual within the context of human rights and human security. The Islamic *Shari'a* aims at obtaining benefits for individuals and societies while protecting them from harm. For this reason the rules of *Shari'a* explain the rights of human beings, whether as a fetus, child, young or old person, and male or female. Islam emphasizes that the existence of any right implies the existence of a duty; hence it is the duty of individuals, societies, and states to protect these rights from harm caused by others. A verse in the Qur'an says: "who quickens a human being, it shall be as if he has quickened all mankind." (5:32) This "quickening" in Islam is not only physical; it is also mental and social. All members of a Muslim society (including non-Muslims) are considered brothers in Islam and in humanity, and this brotherhood implies many duties. A brother, to use the words of the Prophet, "cares for his brother and protects him" and "he does not fail or forsake him."[22] In Islam, the individual is entitled to respect as a human being, irrespective of race or religion.

In its essence, and by virtue of its rules and regulations, Islam provides the individual, especially children and elderly people, with a protective environment. A highly authentic *Hadith* by the Prophet indicates that: "Your body has a (human) right."[23] This means that human rights were recognized by Islam 14 centuries before the international Universal Declaration of Human Rights. On the care and protection of children, the Prophet says: "Allah will (on the Day of Reckoning) question each person in a position of responsibility about what he or she was responsible for in this life."[24] Likewise, Islam values the care of aged people. According to the second Caliph, Omar Ibn Al-Khattab (589–644 CE) "it is unfair to exploit the youth of a human being and then to forsake him when he becomes old."[25]

Although Islam clearly distinguishes between the individual as a separate entity and as a member of the community, these two realities are nevertheless deeply interrelated. This explains why community actions have a spiritual value for the individual, and vice versa. Two traditions of the Prophet seem to be quite relevant in this respect: (a) "The faithful in their mutual love and compassion are like the body; if one member complains of an ailment all other members will rally in response,"[26] and (b) "The faithful to one another are like the blocks in a whole building; they fortify one another."[27] God describes the Faithful in the Qur'an saying: "They give priority over themselves even though they are needy." (9:59)

The preservation of any individual's life should embrace the utmost regard to his and her dignity, feelings, tenderness, and the privacy of sentiments and body parts. Patients are therefore entitled to full attention, care, and a feeling of security while with their physician. The physician's privilege of being exempt from some general rules is only coupled with more responsibility and duty, which they should carry out in conscientiousness and excellence in obeying God, and worship God as if they see him.

Environment

God warns against corruption of the earth and pollution of the environment in several places in the *Qur'an*. This is also evident in God's directives, such as: "Eat and drink of the sustenance God has provided and do not corrupt the earth with evil" (2:60) and "Do not corrupt the earth." (7:85) Other Islamic directives on keeping the environment healthy concern water sources and roads. There is a complementary order to keep the environment clean and pollution free, as reflected in the Prophet's *Hadith*: "the removal of harmful objects from the road counts as an act of benefaction."[28]

Truth, Knowledge, and Research

Islam urges people to learn, making learning an obligation for all Muslims (men and women) while emphasizing truth and knowledge. The Prophet says: "Seeking knowledge is obligatory for every Muslim, male or female."[29] He also says: "Whosoever has three daughters or three sisters, whom he teaches and brings up until Allah provides them with the means of independence, will definitely be rewarded with an admission to heaven."[30]

Truth is defined as what benefits humankind in this present life and in the life to come. God says: "what has been sent down to you by your Lord is the truth" (13:1) and "those who are endowed with knowledge believe that has been revealed to you by your Lord is the truth." (34:6) Knowledge is part of the knowledge of God "who taught man what man never knew" (96:5), which reveals God's signs in his creation: "And in yourselves do you not see?" (51:21)

The Qur'an also states that: "It is only those who have knowledge among his slaves who fear Allah. Verily, Allah is all-mighty, oft-forgiving," (35:28) and "my Lord, increase me in knowledge." (20:114) We also find rich evidence of the same idea in the tradition of the Prophet. He says: "When the son of Adam dies, his work ceases, except for three: [leaving behind] continuous charity; [leaving behind] knowledge that is of benefit [to humankind], or [leaving behind] a righteous child who would make invocation on his behalf."[31] Therefore, knowledge of health is part of the knowledge of God "who taught man what man never knew" (96:5) and the study of medicine entails the revealing of God's signs in his creation.

The Qur'an recommends the prayer: "O my Lord, advance me in the knowledge" (20:114) and the Prophet Muhammad decrees that: "the pursuit of knowledge is a mandate on every Muslim man and woman."[32] There is no censorship on scientific research in Islam, be it academic, to reveal the signs of God in his creation, or applied, aiming at the solution of a particular problem. Islam is a religion that is open to scientific progress: God encourages people to find solutions to their problems, and God will help them.

Community and Society

The views on community in Islam are founded on the pillars of solidarity, cooperation, self-sufficiency, and perfection or ihsan. Solidarity is based on the view that a society comes into existence when every individual becomes a person, without losing the identity of individuals within the community. Solidarity establishes a bond of unity among members of the society as emphasized in the Qur'an: "He it is who has made you strong with his help, and rallied the believers round you, making their hearts united. Had you spent all the riches on earth you could not have so united their hearts, but God has united them together. He is indeed almighty and wise." (8:63)

The Prophet highlights the meaning of the concept of "society of believers" by saying: "In their mutual love, compassion and sympathy for one another, believers are like one body: when one part of it suffers a complaint, all other parts join in, sharing in the sleeplessness and fever."[33] The second Caliph, Omar Ibn Al-Khattab decreed that if a man living in a locality died of hunger, being unable to sustain himself, then the community should pay ransom money (*fidiah*), as if they had killed him. This explains the social responsibility of individuals and societies to protect their members, especially the disadvantaged.

Cooperation is based on the concept of the "brotherhood of believers," as written in the Qur'an: "Believers are indeed brothers." (49:10) This is clearly explained by the Prophet who says: "None of you attains to the status of faith until he wishes for his brother whatever good he wishes for himself."[34] Islam does not allow any of its followers to take a passive or indifferent attitude toward social responsibility.

Self-sufficiency requires that the Muslim community should be in a state of progress and development, and to give practical effect to the description first expressed in the Bible and related in the Qur'an. The Muslim community is described "as the seed which puts forth its shoot and strengthens it, so that it rises stout and firm upon its stalk, delighting the farmers." (48:29) This means that every member of the Muslim community is like a shoot or a branch of a tree, not representing a burden to it, but on the contrary, fulfilling its duty of strengthening it. The underlying principle in all this is that Islamic society places a duty on every individual to support the community and its members until it has reached the stage of self-sufficiency. A Muslim, as the Prophet says, is one who "works with his own hands to benefit himself and to give others in benefaction."[35]

Islam provides safeguards for keeping Islamic society healthy through charity and setting things to right, as stated in the Qur'an: "no good comes, as a rule, out of secret confabulations save for those who are devoted to enjoining *sadaqa*, or *maa'rouf*, or setting matters to rights between people." (4:114) *Sadaqa* means "charity" as stated by the Prophet: "Every individual must give with every rising sun *sadaqa* for his own soul."[36] *Sadaqa*, right behavior, is a strong indication of individual commitment and belonging to the society. The Prophet further stresses *perfection* or *ihsan* as the fourth concept for safeguarding Islamic society when saying "God has decreed that whatever human beings do should be done with *perfection*."[37]

Family and Marriage

The family in Islam is viewed as the building block of society. Marriage is the foundation of Islamic society that provides stability and security. The *Shari'a*, as in the Qur'an and the traditions of the Prophet, enjoins a man who seeks to set up a family to focus his attention primarily on looking for a woman who is virtuous and of sound conduct. The Prophet stresses that choosing a wife who is of virtuous conduct and high morality is a great accomplishment for men as he says: "Acquire the woman who is religiously observant and you will succeed."[38] As for the woman's choices for a husband, the Prophet says: "When you are approached for marriage by a man whose religiosity and manners are acceptable to you, then do accept his proposal and marry him."[39] This reflects the equity between women and men in relation to women's rights in choosing their spouse.

ISLAMIC ETHICAL PRINCIPLES

Value systems drawn from religious, philosophical, ideological, and other cultural systems are the main sources of health ethics also in Islam, with the main professional health ethical principles being respect, justice, and beneficence.[40]

Respect for human dignity means that a human being should be treated as a person or individual who has rights to claim and duties to perform; this entails independent decision making and continuous protection of such independence, as well as taking full responsibility and accountability for all one's actions. Individuals have the right of independent decision making, which is clearly spelled out in the following verses of the Qur'an: "Do whatever you may wish" (41: 40); "You are not the one to impose on them" (88:22); and "You are not the one to compel them" (50:45). The right to take full responsibility and accountability is stated in the following verses: "Each individual is accountable for his deeds" (52:21) and "Every soul is responsible for its deeds." (74:38)

These important Islamic principles fit within the main principles of dealing with patients; they imply recognition of the patient's fundamental right as a person or individual, entitled to rights and committed to duties. Persons have the right to know the details related to their health problems, receive proper treatment, safeguard their confidentiality with respect to their medical condition and treatment protocols, and to obtain adequate care.

The principles of justice and beneficence are also among those strongly stressed by Islam. They are mentioned together in the Qur'an:

"God commands justice and beneficence" (16:90) and are highly regarded in contemporary medical ethics. Justice means equity in meeting patients' needs and in delivering quality care. This is reflected in maintaining, as much as possible, equality in the distribution of health care resources and the provision of preventive and curative opportunities without discrimination for sex, race, belief, political affiliation, social, or other considerations.

Beneficence involves the fulfillment of one's duty toward one's brothers and sisters in humanity, particularly those who are weak or helpless, as indicated in the following verse:"And why should you fight for God's sake in the cause of the deprived men, women and children?" (4:75) This verse presents beneficence as a noble Islamic value that is closely related to the duty of nurses and health care providers who should acquaint their patients with their rights and enhance their health and well-being. In addition, beneficence also entails perfection, as far as possible, both in performance and in kindness, as stated by the Prophet: "God has decreed perfection on everything."[41]

However, the prohibition of causing harm is stated in the following two verses in the Qur'an: "My Lord has forbidden all atrocities, whether overt or disguised, and harm (*ithm*)" and "abandon all harm (*ithm*), whether committed openly or in secret." (6:120) The Prophet also warns against self-harm or harming others, as stated in the *Hadith*: "there shall be no infliction of harm on oneself or others"[42] and "Cursed be everyone who causes harm to a believer or scammed [cheated] him."[43]

The principles of respect, justice, and beneficence and other related values are the main pillars of biomedical ethics in Islam. Currently, religious scholars in Islam are considering emerging global health issues and their relevance to and application in Islam.[44]

Islamic Stance on Selected Ethical Issues

The flexibility of Islamic law is not accidental: it is an essential part of the *Qur'an*, where it reveals that Islam is for all people at all times. Consequently, its jurisprudence must be capable of responding to widely diverse needs and problems. Islam was revealed gradually. This fact illustrates the divine recognition of the human difficulty in adjusting to sudden change. Hence, flexibility and evolution are inherent characteristics of this religion. Based on this, Islamic juridical tradition seeks to address and accommodate the demands of justice and public good for every ethical dilemma. Thus legal doctrines and rules, in addition to analogical reasoning based on theoretical cases, enable a Muslim jurist to resolve ethical dilemmas about issues concerning, for example, life and death and reproductive issues. The *fatwa* can explore and reveal the insights of a jurist who has been able to analyze and connect cases to an appropriate situation of linguistic and rational principles and rules that are able to provide keys to a more valid conclusion for a case under consideration.[45]

This section presents the Islamic views on some of the debated issues such as life and death and reproductive health issues, including abortion, contraceptives, reproductive assisted technology, and female circumcision. These issues are discussed within the philosophical foundation and principles of Islam with less emphasis on the technical aspects of their nature.

Life and Death

Morality in Islam is expressed in the intentions of the person who is performing the action, therefore morality is determined by intentions, and actions are considered moral if intentions are good and genuine. Muslims believe in life after death and that they will be judged by their actions on the Day of Judgment. They also believe that life in heaven is everlasting and is the main reward for their good deeds; this explains the intimate connection between morality and the fact that God is the creator and law-giver, whose precepts humans should abide by.[46]

Life and death are in Allah's hands, and human beings should not "play God." Life and death are considered as the two main guiding principles in Islam, supported by the following verses from the Qur'an: "Blessed be he in whose hands is the Dominion, and he has Power over all things. He who created death and life that he may test which of you are best in deed, and he is Exalted in Might, Oft-Forgiving" (67:1–2) and "No soul can die except by Allah's permission." (3:185) God is the creator of humankind who gives and ends life as indicated in these verses: "Does not man see that it is we who created him from sperm? Yet behold! He stands as an open adversary! And he makes comparisons for us, and forgets his own creation. He says who can give life to (dry) bones and decomposed ones? Say, 'he will give them life who created them for the first time, for he is versed in every kind of creation.'" (36:77–79) Hence, human life is regarded as precious and sacred in Islam and taking a life is considered a major sin, including intrauterine life of the embryo and fetus, which should not be willfully taken unless indicated by Islamic jurisprudence that should not be compromised by the medical profession. The Qur'an says: "Whoever kills a human soul for other than slaughter or corruption on earth, it shall be as if he killed all mankind." (5:32)

Muslims believe that in life sickness and suffering are God's ways to test their faith; they are seen as a form of purification or recompense for wrong deeds and a time to make peace with Allah. The Islamic stance on the issue of life and death is clear to health care providers and it guides their practice. For example, Muslims believe and realize that:

- Spiritual and physical needs should be accommodated in the care of terminally ill people who should be treated with sympathy, care, and compassion.
- "Mercy killing" in Islam is prohibited and is not considered one of the legitimate indications for killing (because life is in God's hands).
- Islam allows resuscitation; a space should be left for the will of Allah, which should be allowed to prevail in case the person does not wish to be resuscitated.
- Muslims believe that individuals with brain-stem death should not be kept alive artificially.[47]

Abortion, Assisted Reproductive Technologies, and Female Circumcision

It is important here to clarify the two main principles that provide a framework for much of the discussion and rulings on reproductive issues in Islam: first is the preservation of posterity and second is the ensoulment and the sacred nature of human life. A detailed examination of these foundational principles provides a comprehensive background for delving into an examination of specific reproductive issues.[48] The preservation of one's lineage through marriage, family formation, and procreation is of the utmost importance in Islam. The Qur'an states: "Wealth and progeny are the allurements of this world." (18:46) The importance of progeny within the context of Islam is twofold: first, it is critical to understand the effect of some modern reproductive technologies on blood relationships, and second, an emphasis on lineage helps one to understand the root of the need for many reproductive technologies based on the significant hardship of infertility.[49]

Abortion is not permitted in Islam because human life is highly valued, even in cases of rape or incest, as Muslims believe that the child has the right to live. The Qur'an does not explicitly refer to abortion but offers guidance on related matters. In some cases, abortion is allowed when the pregnancy threatens the mother's life. In that case, Islam recommends abortion before the fetus is 120 days old, leaving only two options: to let either the mother or the fetus survive, but not both. Scholars argue that such a case can only be determined by a specialist who is a trusted and committed Muslim doctor.[50] This is supported by the Qur'an: "Kill not your children on a plea of want. We will provide sustenance for you and for them. Come not near shameful deeds whether open or secret. Take not life which God has made sacred except by way of justice and law. Thus he commands you that you may learn wisdom." (6:151)

Contraception

Contraception and family planning are allowed and there has not been a direct explicit opposition to contraception in the Qur'an. Muslim couples are encouraged to have children, who are referred to as their "wealth." Muslims believe that every baby comes with his or her own provision. Muslims are influenced by the Prophet Mohammed's call to "get married and multiply," and believe that procreation is one of the most important objectives of marriage.[51]

Within Islamic legal interpretation, the use of some forms of birth control is allowed. Birth control is not forbidden, but some interpretation considers tubal ligation and other nonreversible techniques as unlawful.[52,53] Although the use of reversible contraception is not forbidden in Islam, it is regarded as undesirable, and its use must have medical reasons and must not cause harm to the user.[54] The consent of the marital partner is essential for the use of any contraceptive method, including withdrawal, because the husband's or wife's one-sided decision may jeopardize the rights and interests of the other partner, including the right to full sexual enjoyment.[55]

Even though ensoulment is at 120 days of conception, many Muslim authorities prohibit the use of postcoital methods of contraception, such as the intrauterine device because these could result in the abortion of a fertilized egg. For Muslim scholars, the rhythm method and *coitus interruptus* are acceptable forms of contraception provided they are performed with the consent of the wife.[56] The coil and emergency contraception (the morning-after pill) are considered unsuitable, as they effect abortion. Instead, barrier methods are advocated, as they do not interfere with the body's natural function.

Assisted Reproductive Technology

One of the debated reproductive issues that arises and creates a gap between religion and science is assisted reproductive technology (ART), which relies on the use of technology to assist infertile couples to conceive a much longed-for child.[57] ART is essential if it involves the preservation of procreation and treatment of infertility in one partner of the married couple.

Although Islam views infertility as a "serious disease" and "a threat for families," adoption is not acceptable as a solution to the problem of infertility; therefore fertility treatment is acceptable, allowed and encouraged, and attempts at curing infertility are not only permissible but even believed to be a duty.[58] Based on this, the prevention and treatment of infertility is encouraged and becomes a medical priority because it will ensure an uninterrupted process of procreation. Islam encourages the affected man or woman to seek medical treatment.[59]

The guiding principles of ART in Islam involve using it with a married couple only; it must be conducted within the context of a valid marriage, performed by a competent medical team in order to reduce the chances of failure, and to decrease risks of multiple pregnancies. Freezing of the remaining fertilized ova is permissible as long as they are only used in subsequent cycles for the same couple, and the couple is still married.[60–62] The Qur'an states: "Then has he established relationships of lineage and marriage.... " (13:38) The use of donor sperm, eggs, or embryos will result in the biological father or mother being different from the "married couple." According to Islamic law, this is similar to adultery in confusion of the lineage.

ARTs have created religious bioethical problems and dilemmas and Islam has presented a middle of the road solution, moderating between the two extreme views. Allah says: "Thus we have appointed you a middle nation, that you may be witness against mankind, and that the messenger may be witness against you." (2:143) The advances, availability, and the wide status of ART may create conflict between different options, not only for clients and their families but also for health care providers. Therefore, Muslim couples' decision regarding ART options is influenced by many factors, including the socioeconomic context, knowledge of the moral, ethical and legal status of ART, and sex preference of the baby. To facilitate ethical decisions, a thorough assessment of these factors is needed. Counseling services that integrate Islamic principles on ART are essential to eliminate ambiguities and ensure credibility of health care providers, as well their practices. The need of individual *fatwa*, rather than general counseling statements, which integrates the individual needs and beliefs, may seem to be more effective. This approach necessitates the development of specific protocols, guidelines, and counseling materials that are designed by Muslim scholars and qualified health care providers. These materials need to be aligned with Islamic principles and based on the philosophical views of Islam on life and death, and the belief that procreation is the objective of marriage, to facilitate the couples' informed choices within their diverse contexts, especially if they live in non-Muslim countries where the official legal stance on reproduction varies. Therefore, health care providers need to observe the principles of respect for human dignity, security of human genetics, and inviolability of the person whenever a new reproductive technology is being introduced.

Female Circumcision or Female Genital Mutilation

Circumcision in Islam is obligatory for males and there is no single verse in the Qur'an that relates explicitly or implicitly to female circumcision. Female circumcision or female genital mutilation (or cutting) is a forceful procedure that involves removal of a part of a girl's genitalia at an early stage in life and is one of the most harmful practices for a female child. The position taken by a great number of scholars in the absence of any *Hadith* that may be authentically attributed to the Prophet is that female circumcision is neither required, obligated, nor a *sunnah* in the sense of Islamic tradition. Despite this fact, it is practiced in some Muslim countries such as Egypt and Sudan where misconceptions and false beliefs prevail that female circumcision removes redundant organs. Female circumcision causes medical complications, including pain, hemorrhage, urine retention, dryness of the vagina, pain during intercourse, difficulty delivering children, and vaginal and anal fistulas. Female circumcision violates women's rights in an Islamic perspective. Because marriage is considered a sacred relationship in Islam, women have every right to psychological, moral, and emotional considerations, and their right to be sexually fulfilled must be respected on an equal footing with the right of the man.[63,64]

THE MEDICAL AND NURSING PROFESSIONS IN ISLAM

The *Islamic Code of Medical Ethics* was developed by WHO as a guiding tool to maintain all health care professionals' behavior within the boundaries of Islamic teachings. It is also considered as a code of conduct for medical and nursing students in their professional life to acquaint them with what to do and what to avoid when facing pressures, temptations, or uncertainties.

This *Islamic Code of Medical Ethics* defines *therapeusis*, or the medical profession, as a noble profession, honored by God, who made it the miracle of Jesus, son of Mary. Al-Ghazali (1058–1111 CE) considered the profession of medicine as *fardh kifaya*, meaning a duty incumbent upon on society that some citizens carry out on behalf of all. As medicine is about preserving health and well-being of individuals, this means that the profession of medicine in Islam is a religious necessity for society. It is a unique profession and should never yield to social pressures motivated by enmity or personal, political, or military feuds.[65]

The medical profession has the right and owes the duty of effective participation in the formulation and issuing of religious verdicts concerning the lawfulness or otherwise of unprecedented outcomes of current and future advances in biological sciences. These verdicts should be reached between Muslim specialists together with Muslim specialists in jurisprudence and biosciences. One-sided opinions have always resulted in a lack of comprehension of the technical or legal aspects of those verdicts. The guiding rule in unprecedented matters falling under no text or law is the Islamic dictum: "Wherever welfare is found, there exists the statute of God."[66] Therefore, physicians must have a broad knowledge of jurisprudence, worship, and essentials of *fiqh*. This knowledge will enable them to counsel patients seeking guidance about health issues with a bearing on Islamic rituals of worship such as views pertaining to pregnancy and prayer, fasting, pilgrimage, family planning, and so forth.

Hence, medical practice becomes an act of worship and charity in addition to being a lifelong career. The medical profession operates along the single track of God's mercy, never hostile and never punitive, never taking justice but mercy as its goal, in whatever situations and circumstances.[67] It follows that the roles and responsibilities of physicians in Islam are well delineated: they are seen as catalysts through whom God, the Creator, works to preserve life and health. Physicians are merely instruments of God in alleviating people's suffering, therefore they should be grateful and forever seeking God's help, with an attitude of modesty, free from arrogance and pride and never falling into boasting or hinting at self-glorification through speech, writing, or direct or subtle advertisement.[68] In addition, their responsibilities are focused on their commitment to update their knowledge and strive to keep abreast of scientific progress and innovation. They must also know that the pursuit of knowledge has a double indication in Islam: apart from the applied therapeutic aspect, this pursuit of knowledge is in itself worship. The following verses from the Qur'an highlight this: "My Lord, advance me in knowledge" (20–114) and "Among his worshippers the learned fear him most" (35:28) and "God will raise up the ranks of those of you who believed and those who have been given knowledge." (58:11)

Medical education, despite being a specialty, is a tiny part in a whole mesh of knowledge founded on belief in God; God's oneness and absolute ability, and that he alone is the creator and giver of life, knowledge, death, this world and the hereafter. Yet, medical education has to be protected and purified from every positive activity toward atheism or infidelity.[69]

Windows of Opportunity for Muslim Nurses

It is clear that physicians efficiently used the underpinning philosophical views of Islam to shape the medical profession and further advance it to a theoretical framework for their practice. They are strongly involved in the juristic Islamic system by being educated about the sources of conflict and ethical dilemmas arising from advances in biosciences, participate in formulating appropriate *Fatwa*, and integrate these within the ethical components of the medical education and practice systems.

Unlike the medical profession, Muslim nurses did not utilize the existing knowledge and frameworks of health in Islam to develop the nursing profession. The failure of Muslim nurses to shape the practice, education, and the regulatory system within the Islamic views can be attributed to many factors, among them the fact that Muslim nurses were women who were struggling for social status, professional identity, and societal approval and recognition. Muslim nurses have been using western practice, education, and ethical models rather than integrating the holistic views of Islam.

Muslim nurses did not examine, utilize, and conceptualize the Islamic traditions on the views of care and caring practices; caring in Islam is the manifestation of love for God and the Prophet Muhammad. The caring concept is reflected in various traditions and means more than the act of empathy. It is viewed within the concept of a society of brothers and sisters, based on solidarity, cooperation, self-sufficiency, and perfection or *ihsan*. These views reflect that caring requires nurses to be responsible for, sensitive to, and concerned with people in need, especially the weak, the suffering, and those outcast from society.[70] In addition to what physicians do in relation to preserving health and the well-being of individuals and communities, nurses have an extended role in caring for human responses and provide a unique service to society that meets the requirements of *fardh kifaya*. Muslim nurses need to educate themselves within the views and traditions of caring in Islam and the Islamic juristic system, and create partnerships with Muslim scholars to participate effectively in the formulation of and issuing of religious verdicts concerning the health of populations and pay their duties to the Muslim society.

Although the *fiqh* of Islam does not explicitly define nursing and nurses within the perspective of Islam, there are many lessons that can be learned from the Prophet traditions in acknowledging women's role in times of peace and of battles. *Therapeusis* was practiced by the "Lady-Healers" who joined the Prophet's army in battle, caring for the casualties and dressing their wounds. Rufaidah Bint Sa'ad was among those "Lady-Healers" who lived at the time of the Prophet Muhammad and was the first professional nurse and founder of the nursing profession in Islam. Her practice was influenced by her father, who was a physician, from whom she learnt the care while working as his assistant. She then trained a group of women companions as nurses and established her own field hospital tent, caring for the injured referred by the Prophet Mohammad and became very famous during the main Islamic battles. The Prophet assigned a share of the booty to Rufaidah and the other nurses, and Rufaidah's share was equivalent to that of a soldier who had actually fought in battle. This was the first unique recognition of women in Islam reflecting gender equity while working side by side with men that could have been a golden opportunity for Muslim nurses to develop the nursing profession.

Rufaidah's history illustrates all the attributes expected of a good nurse: she was kind and empathic, a capable leader and organizer, mobilizing resources and involving others to produce good work. She had clinical skills that she shared with other nurses whom she trained and worked with. She extended the nursing scope of practice beyond caring for sick people to caring for people in the community to solve the social problems that affected their health and well-being. In that sense, one could say she was a public health nurse and a social worker. She is an inspiration for the nursing profession in the Muslim world for her distinguished role in war and peace. During peace time, she set up her tent outside the Prophet's mosque in Medina where she cared for the sick and was involved in social work at the community level. With her kind personality, she cared for the poor, orphans, and handicapped people. Islamic history acknowledges her role in mentoring other nurses in Islam.[71]

THE WAY FORWARD

It is evident that Islam has placed great value on ethics as a core concept in medical practice. Islam laid the foundation of the meaning of health and ethics within the five religious duties that form the theoretical principles and references for health care organizations, health care providers, patients, and Muslim communities. Islam is considered a flexible progressive religion in responding to new biomedical challenges and provides a framework of values and ethics derived from religion. Ethical practice is the responsibility of all nurses, and developing a framework of nursing ethics within an Islamic perspective can play an important role in understanding the meaning and practical applications of ethics for nurses caring for Muslim patients all over the world.

Within the context of Islamic ethical principles, it is important that registered nurses recognize and understand that their ethical decision-making is not done in isolation, and occurs within a context of Islamic care that can bring a unique perspective to the decisions that need to be made with Muslim individuals and their families. Muslim nurses need to realize that there is no way to strengthen their profession and improve care without integrating the Islamic ethical principles in their own practice. Failure to develop and implement theoretical frameworks to guide decision making and ethical practice impair any initiative to ensure morally responsible nursing practice. This requires that nurses be informed and examine emerging religious values to revise or develop an Islamic nursing regulatory system, including laws, bylaws, codes of ethics, and standards of care to be aware of, and being responsive to ethical dilemmas that are part of their daily life. Nursing is part of the health care system and nurses have a religious moral duty to participate in issues of health policy and to contribute to religious verdicts regarding health, illness, health care, policy, and ethics.

Teaching ethics must become an essential requirement in clinical practice. Nurses must actively take part in clarifying ethical dilemmas and become scholars in utilizing Islamic essentials and ethical guiding principles to shape their practice and expand the field of *fiqh* of health to serve their profession. This will empower them in leading their societies to a healthier future in working side by side with other health care providers. Nurses have a critical role in generating evidence through research, in order to refine and strengthen ethical guiding principles to be responsive to the Islamic social context of health care that is continuously dominated by science and technology, similar to that of western societies, with a preference for factual and testable data and lesser attention to religious influences and human relationships. This requires stronger cooperation among all nurses from different countries and different religions to build synergies through an integrated approach in identifying the concepts of health, ethics, and nursing from various religious perspectives. This is a new paradigm shift that requires commitment and leadership of nurses to move to a higher level of investment in nursing. Scholar nurses are at the heart of these efforts and need to take this opportunity to contribute to the ethics of care as an integral part of education, socialization, and the practice of professional nursing.

NOTES

1. Majali, M. *Islamic Culture and Thought. The Conversation of the Holy Qur'an Society.* University of Jordan, Amman Jordan, 2006.
2. Foley, R. "Muslim Women's Challenges to Islamic Law the Case of Malaysia." *International Feminist Journal of Politics* 6.1 (2004): 53–84.
3. World Health Organization. *The Right Path to Health: Health Education through Religion. An Islamic Perspective.* Alexandria, Egypt: Eastern Mediterranean Regional Office, 1997.
4. Foley, R. "Muslim Women's Challenges to Islamic Law the Case of Malaysia." *International Feminist Journal of Politics* 6.1 (2004): 53–84.
5. Oxford Islamic Studies online. "Pillars of Islam." Web. May 5. 2010. http://islamicpath .org/pillars-of-islam/
6. Sachedina, Zulie. "Islam, Procreation and the Law. " *International Family Planning Perspectives* 16.3 (1990): 107–11.
7. The Holy Qur'an, English translation of the meanings and Commentary, published by Al Madinah Al Munawarah. Saudi Arabia: King Fahd Holy Qur'an Printing Complex, 1984.
8. World Health Organization. *The Right Path to Health: Health Education through Religion. An Islamic Perspective.* Alexandria, Egypt: Eastern Mediterranean Regional Office. 1997.
9. Narr. Al-Tirmidth, Altermizi, Book 39, on Zuha (Piety), Chapter 1, Number 2311.
10. Narr. Ibn 'Abbas, Volume 8, Book 76, Number 421.
11. Ullmann, Manfred. *Islamic Medicine.* Edinburgh: Edinburgh University Press, 1978. Rpt. (1997): 55–85.
12. Narr. Al Bukhari, Imam Nawawi's Chapter 1, Hadith number 40.

13. World Health Organization. *The Right Path to Health: Health Education through Religion. An Islamic Perspective.* Alexandria, Egypt: Eastern Mediterranean Regional Office. 1997.

14. Narr. Al- Burkhari Volume 7, Book 71, Number 582.

15. World Health Organization. *The Right Path to Health: Health Education through Religion. An Islamic Perspective.* Alexandria, Egypt: Eastern Mediterranean Regional Office. 1997.

16. Ibid.

17. Narr. Ibn 'Abbas, Volume 8, Book 76, Number 421.

18. Narr. Ibn Majah, Al Hakim and Ahmad Following Mouaz Ibn Abdullah Ibn Khubaib.

19. Narr. Ibn Majah, following Abdallah Ibn Al Ansari following his father.

20. Narr. Tirmidhi, Book 50, Chapter 88, Number 3369.

21. Narr. Al Tirmidhi, Book 40, Chapter 1, Number 2425.

22. Narr. Al Tirmidhi, Book 30, Chapter 18, Number 1934.

23. Narr. Al Tirmidhi, Book 39, Chapter 65, Number 2421.

24. Narr. Al Tirmidhi, Chapter 4, Number 208.

25. UNICEF & Al Azhar University. *Children in Islam: Their Care, Upbringing and Protection.* ISBN (Egypt) 11119. New York: United Nations Children's Fund, 2009.

26. Narr. Al Bukhari, Book 73, Volume 8, Number 5665.

27. Narr. Bukhari Volume 3, Book 43, Number 626.

28. Narr. Termidhi. Book 30, Chapter 36, Number 1963.

29. Narr. Ibn Majah, Chapter 1/81, Number 224.

30. Narr. Al-Tirmidhi. Book 30, Chapter 13, Number 1919.

31. Narr. Al-Tirmidhi. Book 15, Chapter 36, Number 1381.

32. Narr. Tabarani. 4/245, Number 4096.

33. Narr. Al Bukhari. Book 73, Volume 8, Number 5665.

34. Narr. Al Bukhari. Book 2, Volume 1, Number 13.

35. Agreed Upon by al Bukhari and Muslim as reported by Abu Mousa al ash'ari.

36. Narr. Ahmad following Abu Zarr.

37. Narr. in Muslim, Abou Dawood, Al Termizi, Al Nassa'i, Ibn Maja and Al Darimi, by Shaddad Ibn Aous.

38. Narr. Tirmidhi. Book 11, Chapter 4, Number 1088.

39. Narr. Al Tirmidhi. Book 11, Chapter 3, Number 1086.

40. World Health Organization. "Ethics of Medicine and Health." *Eastern Mediterranean Regional Office* Series 4. 1998.

41. Narr. Ahmad following Abu Zarr.

42. Narr. Daragutni, following Saeed Al Khudri.

43. Narr. Al Tirmidhi. Book 30, Chapter 27, Number 1948.

44. World Health Organization. Ethics of Medicine and Health. Series 4. *Technical paper presented at the Forty-Second, Session of the Eastern Mediterranean Regional Office.* Alexandria, Egypt. 1998.

45. Sachedina, A. "End-of-Life: The Islamic View." Lancet 366.9487 (2005): 774–79.

46. Kamali, M. H. *The Sanctity of Life in Islam: The Dignity of Man; The Islamic Perspective.* Malaysia and the Islamic Foundation, UK: lmiah Publishers, 1999.

47. World Health Organization. "Ethics of Medicine and Health." *Eastern Mediterranean Regional Office* Series 4. 1998.

48. Haseltine, S. "Islamic Ethics and Reproductive Technologies." *Ivy Journal of Ethics* 7.1 (2007): 27.

49. Ibid.

50. Madkur, M. S. *Al-Janin wa al-Ahkam al-Muta'allikah bihi fi al-fiqh al-Islami.* Cairo: Dar al-Nahdhah al-Arabiyah, 1969. 301–302.
51. Kridli, S. A., and S. E. Newton. "Jordanian Married Muslim Women's Intentions to Use Oral Contraceptives." *International Nursing Review* 52. (2005): 109–114.
52. Mughees, Abdul. "Better Caring for Muslim Patients." *World of Irish Nursing & Midwifery* 14.7 (2006): 24–25.
53. Alamah, H. W. "Bridging Generic and Professional Care Practices for Muslim Patients Through use of Leininger's Culture Care Model." *Contemporary Nurse* 28.1–2 (2008): 83–97.
54. Mughees, Abdul. "Better Caring for Muslim Patients." *World of Irish Nursing & Midwifery* 14.7 (2006): 24–25.
55. Mehryar, A. H, S. A. Nia, and S. Kazemipour. "Reproductive Health in Iran: Pragmatic Achievements, Unmet Needs, and Ethical Challenges in a Theocratic System." *Studies in Family Planning* 38.4 (2007): 352–361.
56. Mughees, Abdul. "Better Caring for Muslim Patients." *World of Irish Nursing & Midwifery* 14.7 (2006): 24–25.
57. Haji-Ahmad, Norhayati. "Assisted Reproduction–Islamic Views on the Science of Procreation." *Eubios Journal of Asian and International Bioethics* 13 (2003): 59–60.
58. Samani, R., M. Ashrafi, L. Alizadeh, and M. Mozafari. "Posthumous Assisted Reproduction from an Islamic Perspective." *International Journal of Fertility and Sterility* 2.2 (2008): 96–100.
59. Inhorn, Marcia C. "Making Muslim Babies: IVF and Gamete Donation in Sunni Versus Shi'a Islam." *Culture, Medicine and Psychiatry* 30 (2006): 427–450.
60. Schenker, Joseph G. "Religious Views Regarding Treatment of Infertility by Assisted Reproductive Technologies." *Journal of Assisted Reproduction and Genetics* 9.1 (1992): 3–9.
61. Haseltine, Sarah. "Islamic Ethics and Reproductive Technologies." *Ivy Journal of Ethics* (2007): 27.
62. World Health Organization. *Female Genital Mutilation. A Joint WHO/UNICEF/UNFPA Statement.* Geneva. 1997.
63. Ibid.
64. Kasule, Omar Hasan. *Empowerment and Health: An Agenda for Nurses in the 21st Century.* Paper presented at the 3rd International Nursing Conference. Brunei Dar as Salam. 1998.
65. Jan, R. "Rufaida, Al-Asalmiy, The First Muslim Nurse." *Journal of Nursing Scholarship* 28.3 (1996): 267–268.
66. Ibid.
67. Kasule, Omar Hasan. *Empowerment and Health: An Agenda for Nurses in the 21st Century.* Paper presented at the 3rd International Nursing Conference. Brunei Dar as Salam. 1998
68. Jan, R. "Rufaida, Al-Asalmiy, The First Muslim Nurse." *Journal of Nursing Scholarship* 28.3 (1996): 267–268.
69. World Health Organization. *The Right Path to Health: Health Education through Religion. An Islamic Perspective.* Alexandria, Egypt: Eastern Mediterranean Regional Office. 1997.
70. Jan, R. "Rufaida, Al-Asalmiy, The First Muslim Nurse." *Journal of Nursing Scholarship* 28.3 (1996): 267–268.
71. Ibid.

13

Sikhism and Nursing

Savitri W. Singh-Carlson and Harjit Kaur

"Seva with Akal Purkh's Grace"

The purpose of this chapter is to present the foundations of the Sikh tradition that inform health practices and issues of ethical concern, with the aim of providing guidance to health care professionals who care for Sikh patients, or who themselves are Sikh. The ethical constructs of justice and selflessness are strong for the Sikh, and are rooted in the code of conduct that orchestrates the life of the Sikh follower, whether in India or in one of the diasporic Sikh communities found around the world.[1] The chapter begins with an overview of the Sikh religion, including the sociopolitical context in which the religion originated 500 years ago, and the location of Sikh communities around the world today. After outlining key tenets of the faith as developed by the 10 Gurus, the chapter proceeds to provide the link between these foundations and present Sikh practices that relate to health care and nursing ethics. Findings from a Canadian study conducted with South Asian women's perceptions of respect within a clinical setting will be used to illustrate how women from this population experienced respect when in relationships with health professionals.[2]

OVERVIEW OF SIKHISM

Currently, there are 20 million Sikhs in the world, most of who live in the Punjab region of India. The Sikh diaspora has spread over England, Australia, United States of America, and Canada, with the majority of migration taking place over the period of 1940–1980s.[3]

Gurus and the Historical Development of Sikhism

Guru Nanak Dev Ji founded the Sikh religion in the 15th century with the belief in *Ek Ong Kar* (one creator) who is *Nirankar* (without form). A succession of 10 Gurus, each named by the former Guru himself, established the core tenets of the Sikh faith. Collectively, the 10 Sikh Gurus acknowledged themselves as human beings with the capacity and wisdom to share the universal teachings of the one creator. They gave the Sikhs spiritual, social, economic, and political guidance during the period of 239 years from the 1st to the 10th Guru. Table 13.1 provides an overview of the Gurus and their individual contributions in the creation of the Sikh religion. In the Sikh tradition, the title *Guru* is extended beyond the Hindu understanding of a wise, authoritative, and knowledgeable person who guides others. In Sikhism, a Guru includes understanding or knowledge imparted through any medium.

The Moral Teachings of Sikhism

Further understanding of the Sikh religion is offered by the symbolism embedded in the *Khanda*. This Sikh emblem speaks to how a Sikh will conduct his or her life within the realms of moral and ethical responsibilities to the self, family, community, and humanity at large (see Table 13.2).

This symbol represents Sikhism as a religion based on the integrative individual identity of the constructs of *miri* and *piri* that correlate to the "warrior and saint" philosophy of the religion.[4] The moral authority of the warrior includes acts of social justice and being a competent protector, and the saint as the compassionate healer. The warrior and the saint connectedness bring the togetherness as a whole person who is a learner, a seeker, and is striving to achieve balance or harmony.

Sikh virtues and ethics are taught by *Sri Guru Granth Sahib Ji* (SGGSJ), the holy book of Sikhs. To quote the holy teachings:

Virtues are Priceless and are not for sale for any price at any store.

O Nanak, their weight is full and perfect.[5]

Five moral virtues form the ethics of the Sikhs namely kindness/compassion (*daya*); righteousness and morality (*dharma*); courage (*himat*); self-confidence, organization (*mokham*); and nobility and grace (*sahib*). These virtues have a historical significance from the Amrit ceremony of 1699 by Guru Gobind Singh Ji when the five beloved (*panj pyare*) names of the first five initiates to the *khalsa* corresponded to these virtues.[6] Building on these virtues, the *khalsa* code of conduct (*Rehat Maryada*) is held as core

TABLE 13.1 Sikh Gurus and Their Contributions

Sikh Gurus	Contributions
1. Guru Nanak Dev Ji (1469–1539)	• First Guru whose principal message was for Supreme universality of One God and equality of all humans.
2. Guru Angad Ji (1539–1552)	• Advocated selfless service, piety, and universality. • Introduced Gurmukhi (written) and Punjabi (spoken language) of Sikhs.
3. Guru Amar Das Ji (1552–1574)	• Promoted *krit* (earning an honest living), *dasvandh* (sharing 1/10 of earning's for community cause) and *vandkaychakna* (the virtue of sharing). • Emphasized participation in *sangat* (congregation) to recite *kirtan* and Gurbani from Sri Guru Granth Sahib Ji (SGGSJ) and partake in *langar* (community kitchen) (sitting and eating together). • Advocated equality of women by denouncing the practice of *sati* (widow burning on her husband's pyre) and use of veils while promoting monogamy and remarrying of widows.
4. Guru Ram Das Ji (1574–1581)	• Active in *seva* (voluntary service). • Established the township of Amritsar and began construction of *Harmindar Sahib* (Golden Temple).
5. Guru Arjan Dev Ji (1581–1606)	• Completed compilation of the SGGSJ. • Sacrificed his life for the independence of community against false accusations, which was the beginning of martyrdom and sacrifice within Sikhism.
6. Guru Hargobind Ji (1606–1644)	• Conceptualized the identity of a warrior–saint (*miripiri*). • Introduced martial arts (G*atka*). *Gatka* guides the discipline to defend self and others in upkeeping human rights and the freedom to practice religion. • Formalized warrior–saint identity by building *Akal Takhat* (the seat for social/political decisions) facing the Golden Temple, which is the center of spirituality.
7. Guru Har Rai Ji (1644–1661)	• Promoted healing and peace.
8. Guru Harkrishan Ji (1661–1664)	• Became the youngest Guru at age 5.
9. Guru Teg Bahadur Sahib Ji (1665–1675)	• Sacrificed his life to prevent the forced conversion of Hindus to Muslims by the Mughal ruler, Aurangzeb. • Reinforced commitment to religious tolerance and peaceful living.
10. Guru Gobind Singh Ji (1675–1708)	• Bestowed Sikhs with present code of conduct and the ceremony of *Amrit* (baptism), where a Sikh becomes a *Khalsa* (baptized Sikh) and commits to *Rehat Maryada* (discipline of a *Khalsa*). • Formalized the last name of *Singh* for all males and *Kaur* for all females.
11. Sri Guru Granth Sahib Ji (1708–eternity)	• In 1708, SGGSJ, the *Shabad* (Word) was bestowed the Guruship. Is revered as the Supreme Spiritual Guru of the Sikhs. • Holy scripture embodying teachings of the Gurus.

TABLE 13.2   The Khanda

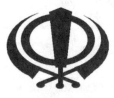

The *Khanda* is the Sikh emblem comprising a solid inner circle (*Chakra*), two interlocked swords (*Kirpans*) on each side, and one double-edged sword (*Khanda*) in the middle.

- The inner circle *(Chakra)* signifies infinity and reminds all Sikhs of the creator, *Ek Ong Kar* (one God) and to embrace all creation compassionately. It encompasses the values of oneness, unity, justice, humanity, and morality. The two *Kirpans* (outer swords) around the Chakra represent the two swords of *miri* (warrior) and *piri* (saint), signifying the spiritual/political sovereignty thereby imparting a conceptual balance between the *miri* (left) and *piri* (right).
- The two-edged inner sword, the *Khanda*, symbolizes the disintegration of ego and elimination of inequalities. The right edge of the *Khanda* symbolizes freedom and authority governed by moral and spiritual values. The left edge of the *Khanda* symbolizes divine justice, which chastises and punishes evil oppressors.

to the faith: not cutting one's *kesh* (hair); refraining from meat, alcohol, and other stimulants; remaining celibate until married and maintaining a monogamous relationship with one's spouse; respecting all other women as mothers, daughters, or sisters according to their age; and committing to *naam simran* (daily meditation and prayers).[7] *Seva* (volunteering for humanity) and *simran* (meditation) guide the service to community and the importance to seek connection to *Guruji* and the Universal God. The five inner moral virtues that a Sikh is to refrain from are lust, jealousy, greed, attachment, and anger. Quoting from the SGGSJ:

> It is through reflection that awareness; mind and intellect are created and formed.

> The seeker develops discrimination and differentiation of evil from noble.[8]

The warrior–saint teachings are reflected in the *bana* and *bani*, which are central to the moral teachings of Sikhism. The *bani* symbolizes the baptized Sikh's inner self that signifies the ethical values and virtues that a Sikh person embraces.[9] The *bani* involves the recitation of *kirtan*, which is the singing of *shabads* or sacred hymns in a complex musical structure.[10] Guru Nanak Dev Ji, the first Guru introduced the daily practice of the recitation of a collection of five *banis* (prayers) in the ambrosial hours after taking a bath, *rehraas sahib* (evening prayer) at dusk (before dinner), and *kirtans Sohila* (night prayer) before bed. *Bana* symbolizes the baptized Sikh's outer dress code that signifies the moral and ethical code of conduct, which a baptized Sikh abides by and is referred to as *the five Ks*:

- *Kesh* (uncut hair, usually tied and wrapped in the Sikh Turban, *dastar.* A symbol of saintly qualities).
- *Kanga* (wooden comb, usually worn under the *dastar.* A symbol of cleanliness).
- *Kachhera* (characteristic shorts, usually white in color. A symbol of chastity/sexual morality).
- *Kara* (iron bracelet, which is a symbol of eternity, strength, and restraint. A reminder of the Sikh's bond with the Guru).
- *Kirpan* (curved sword, from 1 to 3 feet in length. A symbol of justice and protection).

DIVERSITY WITHIN THE SIKH COMMUNITY

As with other religious communities, especially those with histories of migration, a range of diversity exists within Sikh communities. Sikhs today have migrated from various parts of the world, bringing with them the cultural and traditional practices of their previous homeland. With migration, they may adapt cultural nuances of the new social environment while retaining the foundational code of conduct and principles of Sikh religion. Stereotypical notions of all Sikhs observing the same traditional and cultural practices need to be understood from the individual perspective.

Along with migration, another variation within the Sikh community pertains to baptism. Sikhs are baptized in the *Gurudwara* (temple) at any age, with similar rituals as the first baptism of the *khalsa* that was performed by Guru Gobind Singh Ji in 1699. Sikhs who take the *Amrit* (baptism) commitment aspire to the highest level of self-discipline and dedication to SGGSJ. Being baptized also involves following a strict dietary, dress, and social *khalsa* code of conduct of Sikhism. Adherence to the *bana,* the outer dress code, and *bani,* the recitation of SGGSJ, strengthens one's inner morals and ethics. A compilation of daily prayers are found in the *Gutka* (small book of holy prayers), which Sikh patients may carry with them. Because the practice of the daily prayers is a part of the code of conduct and the *Gutka* is a holy book, the Sikh patient will want to prepare for these prayers with cleanliness and to place the *Gutka* in a clean space. In this practice, nurses will need to respect the *Gutka* by providing a clean place for it and handling it with clean hands.

However, not all Sikhs are baptized. The last names of Singh and Kaur, originally indicating baptism, are now used by many non-baptized Sikhs as well. It is therefore important to confirm with the patient if he or she is baptized since the nurse will have to care for the patient accordingly to facilitate religious observance. A Sikh could abide by all the five visible outer dress code Ks and not be a baptized Sikh. In fact, almost all Sikhs wear the *Kara* (steel or iron bangle). It is important to respect the religious observations of all Sikh patients; however, it is even more critical for a nurse to ask the patient or his/her family about their religious requirements. There is much diversity among the sub-groups of this population, and therefore nurses must go beyond dress and outer appearance to avoid making assumptions.

SIKH PHILOSOPHY (ETHICS) IN THE RELATIONAL CONTEXT OF HEALTH CARE SERVICES AND NURSING PRACTICE

In view of the Sikh ethics outlined above, the topics that we have chosen to focus on—selfless service, karma cycle and fate, treatment decision making, and respect in the contexts of the profession of nursing and gender more generally—are germane to the social relational context of health care services and nursing practice in any setting, whether clinical or community nursing practice.

Selfless Service

The principle of selfless service (*seva*) is voluntary, intertwined with community unity, and is a large part of the underlying philosophical principle for Sikhs; it is the moral and social ethical duty of being a Sikh. The concept of *seva* is also the underlying motivation for the Sikh individual to choose the nursing profession. Serving humanity, and thus a fellow human in need of health care, speaks to the mindset of the nurse.

This concept of service to the community, inclusivity, and equality for all is the *Gurudwara*, the door of peace, door of livelihood, door of learning, and the door of grace, which are always open to the community, regardless of denomination, race, caste, sex, or religion for food, rest, and shelter at any time. The sense of the *Gurudwara* as the anchor to the individual and community is actualized when the hospitalized patient's family have prayers conducted at the *Gurudwara* along with other community members.

Gurudwara is not only the place of worship, as other religious places of worship, but is also the place of social, economic, political, and community gatherings for the individual and their families and encapsulates the philosophy of humanitarianism and selflessness of Sikhism. It is the temporal place where the warrior and the saint identity come together to integrate the warrior and saint principles of faith by acquiring spiritual knowledge and wisdom and to provide care for the sick, elderly, and handicapped. The *Gurudwara* is also a place for discussing problems facing the Sikh community. Infringement of the Sikh code of discipline may be considered and suitable *seva* decided upon by the *panjpyare* (five baptized leaders, either male or female).[11]

Sense of Community—Concepts of Seva and Dasvandh

Communitarianism is valued over individualism in the Sikh tradition.[12] This value has implications for moral agency in contrast to the individualistic ethical and humanistic responsibility that presides in Western cultures. For nurses, this may mean that they have to advocate for families at visiting hours, in the palliative ward or the intensive care unit, because the patient may receive condolences from the community at large.

The philosophy of universality is practiced in the Sikh community to provide service (*seva*) and monetary contributions (*dasvandh*) in local and global communities. These principles form the basis for daily prayers and earnings—where a 10th of one's 24-hour day and earnings shared with the community. To illustrate the enactment of these principles, we draw on recent examples from Canada.

Support for the Individual Community Member

The case of Mr. Libar Singh, a Sikh from Punjab, India, who was a visitor to Canada in 2007–2008, exemplifies the Sikh sense of community and justice.[13] Singh was paralyzed when he suffered a stroke during his stay in Canada. Because he would ultimately receive better medical attention in Canada, he sought refuge at the *Gurudwara* where he was cared for by the Sikh community. His supporters were concerned about visits by Canadian Border Services Agents to the Sikh temple where he sought sanctuary. The community at large became involved in supporting his cause. In 2008, 11 cities across Canada participated in actions, delegations, and events in solidarity with Mr. Laibar Singh, demanding that the Canadian Border Services Agency (CBSA) and Minister Stockwell Day respect Mr. Laibar Singh's sanctuary, and that Mr. Laibar Singh be granted permanent residency. Across Canada, protesters showed their solidarity, inspiring mobilizations, led by the South Asian community.

Support for the Larger Community

The Sikh community residing in Surrey, British Columbia, Canada has together donated their time and money to fund the expansion of the Surrey hospital, which will serve one of the largest Sikh communities in Canada. "For three years in a row, the South Asian community has shown its generosity through the radio-thon fundraiser for Surrey Memorial Hospital," said

Red FM owner Kulwinder Sanghera, who is also a board member at Surrey Memorial Hospital Foundation. "This was a very moving experience to witness the number of people who came together to give generously. What a powerful show of generosity," says Foundation President/CEO Jane Adams. "We saw children donating piggy banks, businesses joining forces to give, and families contributing what they can."[14]

Supporting the Communities Globally: British Columbia Sikh Community Donates $1.5M for Haiti

Also exemplifying the moral concepts of *seva* and *dasvandh*, here expressed in global humanitarianism, the Sikh community, the *Gurudwara*, and three South Asian radio stations in the Metro Vancouver area raised $1.5 million in donations and pledges for victims of the Haitian earthquake.[15] In these ways, the teachings of Sikhism regarding universality and communitarianism provide clear guidance for service for the individual as well as for local and global communities.

Karma Cycle and Fate

The notion of karma and rebirth is important for the Sikh patient, with ramifications for nursing ethics. This is visible in the fundamental idea that each person is repeatedly reborn so that his or her soul may be ultimately purified and eventually join the divine cosmic consciousness.[16] In fact, the belief that what a person does in each life influences the circumstances and predispositions experienced in future life; therefore, action, thought, or behavior whether good or evil, leave a trace in the unconsciousness that is carried forward into future lives[17] and translates into the practice of ethical principles and actions that a Sikh strives for in life. As we read in the SGGSJ, "Those who understand the Lord's Court, never suffer separation from him. The True Guru has imparted this understanding. They practice truth, self-restraint and good deeds; their comings and goings are ended."[18]

Sikh women diagnosed with breast cancer in a study conducted in Canada accepted suffering related to the psychosocial impact of breast cancer as a part of life, as part of the karmic cycle and of fate.[19] Most Sikh women in this study believed that suffering and pain are things that every human being goes through. One woman explained:

> We all want God to look after us and keep us healthy, it is our fate, but we have to do our part. God listens to us as we go through this life and we are re-born after this life depending on how we have been in this life. We are all part of the same God

Whatever was in my karma, if after giving pain god gives us happiness, even then whatever happens, happens, what would I get by shouting it out to everyone and crying about it, it is our suffering.[20]

Religion and fatalism went hand in hand for some of the women, both older and younger, because of the high value they placed on doctors' advice and their strong belief in God.[21] Such beliefs seemed to form a contextual part of these women's previous health care experiences. Both for participants who were English speaking, and for those who were non-English speaking it seemed important that, although they believed that God and their own fate might play a part in their cancer conditions, their belief in God alone would not get them through the cancer condition.

Women related their personal belief in fatalism and God to the importance they placed on their relationships with health professionals. Some women felt nurtured by health professionals who were attentive and listened to their stories unconditionally while caring for them during their clinical visits.[22] On the other hand, some of the women's previous health care experiences in Canada included receiving unclear explanations about their illnesses, and perceptions of being "brushed off" by some physicians.[23] They stated their physicians did not always take the time to provide them with information needed to explain their symptoms, but rather referred them to yet another specialist. Women suggested that some health care providers stereotype South Asian women, assuming most do not speak English and know little about their health care. Previous unpleasant health care experiences with a few health care providers left some women untrusting and uncertain about accessing health care in the future.

Suffering may be considered a part of health and illness and of the karmic cycle of birth, death, and rebirth.[24] This will also reflect on the concept of death and dying. A Sikh understands that it is the physical body that perishes and the spirit or soul is undying. This concept is elaborated during the *Amrit* ceremony where the body, mind, and soul are offered to the Guru. This practice of the philosophy encourages the nurse to be present for the family at the time of imminent death of a patient and to provide space for the Sikh family to perform *kirtansohila* (prayer for bed time), *ardas* (formal prayer), and hymns for a peaceful journey of the soul.

Treatment Decision Making

The concepts of communitarism and karmic cycle come together to influence treatment decisions for the Sikh patient and family, especially in light of the extended family. It is common practice for the Sikh family to provide family members with social support and financial security. The concept of extended family as community extends to the honor given to the elderly and extended family connectedness provides help and support to elders of the family. When the patient is intimately integrated with his or her extended family and community, a holistic approach to ethical consent is required. This concept of communitarism goes hand in hand with selflessly serving the needs of the family and community.

The following quote from the Canadian study illustrates the caregiving role of the family.[25] The excerpt also illustrates the influence of the notion of karmic cycle/fate on treatment decision making, and the family's involvement. It also exemplifies how, despite the concept of communitarianism and the involvement of the extended family, there are situations where the practical realities of work mean that the extended family cannot be presumed to provide care to their loved one.

> I didn't tell my sons for two weeks, then my daughter called me after two weeks and said "mummy, have you told your sons?," and I said, "no, daughter, why should I tell anyone, even my sons of what problem I have." My daughter then phoned my son and told him that in two weeks mummy is going to have her surgery. My son came out crying from his room and hugged me and said, "Mummy, you have such a big problem, and you didn't even tell us?" I said, "What was there to tell, whatever was in my karma will happen, if after giving pain god gives us happiness, even then whatever happens, happens, what would I get by shouting it out and crying?" He then called my other sons, who were at work and they all came home and were crying and I was consoling them. My sons said, "You are consoling us and you are suffering." I said "Son, if mother starts to cry, then what would happen to the children?" After the surgery, I had to stay at home alone since everyone has to work. Two weeks after the surgery, I got up and bathed by myself, cooked for myself, ate by myself because everybody was working.[26]

This example emphasizes the need for nurses to pay close attention to the detailed discharge assessment because the patient might be left alone to take care of themselves, even in an extended family.

Respect and the Profession of Nursing

> Abide in truth and contentment, O humble Siblings of Destiny.

> Hold tight to compassion and the Sanctuary of the True Guru.

> Know your soul, and know the Supreme Soul; associating with the Guru, you shall be emancipated.[27]

In research with South Asian women, ethical care was understood as the conjoining of respect and competency.[28] These two values of the health professional–client relationship can be understood as mapping back to the warrior and saint principles as the balance between the competent protector and compassionate healer. Sikh women being treated for cancer experienced respect as being friendly accepting one for whomever the person is being helpful and giving space to be. They stated that everyone is a human being, so therefore we have to be civil to each other, talk to each other with politeness, and treat each other well. This bears its roots from the Sikh code of conduct, or *Rehat Maryada,* which describes the relationship of Sikhs as being respectful of the other, regardless of gender. Fears of being in the "patient role" were alleviated as Sikh women felt their expectations of respect being granted during their relational experiences with health professionals who acknowledged their basic human emotions.[29] The following example describes Sikh woman's experiences of being vulnerable but felt that the health professionals' approach created a "safe" place in a strange environment while she was going for her first X-ray session:

> Respect is when any human being has come over to your home to visit; you should talk to them with politeness and kindness. You talk with love, and acknowledge them, regardless of who comes to your home. I always talk to everyone with respect because they are all human beings. I want others to speak to me in the same way as well. I am so afraid inside sometimes, especially when they did the x-ray the first time, but the nurses and therapists were very kind and stayed on both sides of me and told me that it was going to be all right. They told me not to be afraid and told me that they were together with me and that they were there for me.[30]

In some instances the patient may refer to the nurse as "daughter" or "son" or "sister" or "brother"; the nurse may refer to the patient as "auntie" or "uncle." Upon taking the *Amrit,* a Sikh commits to respecting one as daughter, sister, mother, son, brother, or father as appropriate to the age of the person, reflecting the universal and community connection and respect.

The importance of respect is underlined in two recent Canadian examples where nurses cut the beards of Sikh clients without taking into account the Sikh prohibition against cutting hair.[32] This prohibition relates to the historical sacrifice of Bhai Taru Singh, a Sikh martyr, who agreed to have his scalp removed rather than having his hair cut. This principle of sacrificing for humanity without giving up one's faith forms the identity of a Sikh, as *Kesh* (hair) is one of the five K's. By application, the Sikh patient will need an explanation for any medical procedures that might require cutting, trimming or shaving hair. It is crucial that the nurse seek prior permission by informing the Sikh patient or family in order to provide information and prepare the Sikh patient for what needs to be done, rather than assuming that cutting hair is acceptable. A patient's reluctance to certain medical procedures must be interpreted as a prompt to understand the moral code of conduct for the patient of Sikh faith.

Spiritual hero, who fights for the principle, is recognized.

He may be cut apart, piece-by-piece, but he never leaves the battlefield.[33]

The Sikh Individual Working as a Nurse

As an individual of Sikh faith, the nurse brings the concept of community and *seva* into the health professional–client relationship, especially when providing care for the patient who may need interpretation of language and more information for procedures. The Sikh nurse will also bring the principles of caring for elders and an understanding of how to interact respectfully, regardless of the patient's ethnicity as illustrated by the following excerpt from the study with South Asian in relationship with health professionals in a clinical setting.

The Indian nurse who is there she speaks to me in my own language and is very kind and calls me "aunty" and I feel good because it is respectful to me when she calls me "aunty" whereas the other nurses call me by my name which is the way that the other nurses and therapists call me because it is the normal way to do for them.[34]

In a different vein, Reimer-Kirkham describes the ambiguities of intra cultural interactions when nurses who spoke Punjabi were placed at a disadvantage and burdened with extra work when they were called upon to translate for Sikh patients.[35] Sometimes these nurses chose to downplay intra-group connections (e.g., as in the case of a nurse who chose not to reveal her ability to speak Punjabi to South Asian patients in order to avoid extra demands on her time).

Respect and Gender

Equality is very apparent in the Sikh scripture; the first Guru brought this notion into the foreground as one of the principles of the religion (as mentioned earlier in Table 13.1). During the *Amrit* ceremony, the Sikh is addressed as gender neutral and the *Rehat Maryada* (the Sikh Code of Conduct and conventions) guides men and women. Traditionally, women may prefer a female physician and vice versa for men when being examined; however, this is not a mere preference, but arises from modesty which is embedded into the Sikh woman/man's cultural and spiritual upbringing, as part of the social, ethical, and moral conduct of respect for the other woman/man who is not your spouse.

In cases of domestic and sexual violence, it is important for the nurse to be aware of the possible difference among Sikh women and children. Violence is not condoned in the religion as the equality and respect of women are primary tenets of the faith. In the cases of domestic violence, it is important to note the cultural and social implication of such situations. The role of the family may be critical and decisions will have to be made by the woman based on her needs and safety. The risk assessment will have to be considered in approaching the issue of questioning or assuming what the woman needs. It will be important to involve the women in any decisions that are required. Often, the community resources of community-based victim service workers and interpreters will play a critical role.

In sexual assault cases, it is not to be assumed that the woman will want her family or spouse informed without her consent. The implications of such decisions are often based on the woman's social, educational, and cultural beliefs. It has to be approached with safety of the woman as priority. The cultural belief that sexual assault will bring shame and blame to the woman and her family needs to be recognized. All women, irrespective of religious beliefs experience shame, blame, and guilt when subjected to such crimes.[36]

Concluding Comments

This chapter on Sikhism, nursing, and ethics has underscored the complex factors at play when English-speaking health care providers within the mainstream health care system provide health care to diverse ethnic populations, and how language is not the only barrier that most health care professionals as well as Sikh patients have to overcome. Although addressing the language barrier and use of interpreters are pivotal aspects of institutional health policies and guidelines, there are humane ways of providing respectful care for the individual. Recognizing the individual for his or her personal life experiences as someone who has not only mastered his or her own language along with an understanding of English, but is a person with his or her own values can foster respect within health professional–client relationships. This strategy of recognizing the individual with his or her own standpoint and acknowledging his or her social identity bestows respect for the individual's religion, social identity, location, and life experiences that he or she brings to the health care relationship. This respectful care allows individuals to be seen for who "they are" as human beings, not as stereotypes of a particular "other" ethnic group. The nurse shares humanity with the "other" people and creates respect by acknowledging the others' identity and personal life experiences, which will inform how they journey through the illness experience. Understanding the ways in which people's responses to health and illness are shaped by their religion, beliefs, and values can help health professionals adapt their practices to be more responsive to specific groups.

CONCLUSION

In conclusion, in the context of today's diverse societies, all nurses, regardless of their personal belief system, need to be self-aware and attuned to the influence of their own world view. The nurse's responsibility is to create a healing environment for the patient and the family by being critically conscious of any personal biases while respecting and accommodating the values and beliefs of the patient and family.

NOTES

1. Nayar, Kamala E. *The Sikh Diaspora in Vancouver: Three Generations Amid Tradition, Modernity, and Multiculturalism.* Toronto: University of Toronto Press, 2004.
2. Singh-Carlson, Savitri, Anne Neufeld, and Joanne Olson. "South Asian Immigrant Women's Experiences of Being Respected within Cancer Treatment Settings." *Canadian Oncology Nursing Journal* 20.4 (2010): 188–92.
3. British Broadcasting Corporation. "Religions. Sikhism." Web. 9 Aug. 2011. www.bbc.co.uk/religion/religions/sikhism/.
4. Siri Singh Sahib Bhai Sahib Harbhajan Singh Khalsa Yogiji. Originally published in *Beads of Truth.* 1.35 (Summer 1977). http://www.sikhdharma.org.
5. Ad Sri Guru Granth Sahib, M 1, p1087, cited in Singh, Jodh. "Ethics of the Sikhs." *Understanding Sikhism – The Research Journal, January-June* 7.1 (2005): 35–38.
6. Puri, Shamsher Singh. *Sikh Philosophy and Spiritual Life.* National Book Shop, USA: Delhi and Academy of Sikh Studies, 1999.
7. Ibid.
8. AGGS, Jap 13. 3, cited in Singh, Jodh. "Ethics of the Sikhs."
9. Singh, Gurbachan. *The Sikhs: Faith, Philosophy and Folk.* New Delhi, India: Lustre Press Pvt. Ltd., 1998.
10. Sikh Ragas. SikhiWiki. 2004. Web. 9 Aug. 2011. http://www.sikhiwiki.org/index.php/Sikh_Ragas.
11. Gurdwara – The Sikh Temple. Search Sikhism. nd. Web. 9 Aug. 2011. http://www.searchsikhism.com/temple.html.
12. Coward, Harold, Tejinder Sidhu, and Peter A. Singer. "Bioethics for Clinicians: 19 Hinduism and Sikhism." *Canadian Medical Association Journal* 163.9 (2000): 1167–1170.
13. No One is Illegal. "Report Back: National Days of Action in Support of Laibar Singh: No One Is Illegal." Feb. 08 2008. Available at http://noii-van.resist.ca/?cat=41.
14. Surrey Memorial Hospital Foundation. "South Asian Community Surpasses $2 Million Fundraising Goal." Media release November 2, 2009. Available from http://www.smhfoundation.com/cms/page1672.cfm.

15. Canadian Broadcasting Corporation. "B.C. Sikh Community Raises $1.5M for Haiti." Available from http://www.cbc.ca/news/canada/british-columbia/story/2010/01/22/bc-vancouver-surrey-sikh-haiti-donations.html#ixzz0pixHvYej.

16. Coward, Harold, Tejinder Sidhu, and Peter A. Singer. "Bioethics for Clinicians: 19 Hinduism and Sikhism."

17. Ibid.

18. Singh, Jodh. "Ethics of the Sikhs." *Siri Guru Granth Sahib Ji*, M 3: 1234.

19. Gurm, Balbir Kaur, Joanne Stephen, Gina Mackenzie, Richard Doll, Maria Cristina Barrotavena, and Susan Cadell. "Understanding Canadian Punjabi-speaking South Asian Women's Experience of Breast Cancer: A Qualitative Study." *International Journal of Nursing Studies* 45 (2008): 266–276. See also: Singh-Carlson, Savitri. "South Asian Immigrant Women's Perceptions of Respect within Health Professional-Client Relationships While Journeying through Cancer." Unpublished doctoral dissertation, University of Alberta, Edmonton, Alberta, Canada (2007). See also: Singh-Carlson, Savitri, Anne Neufeld, and Joanne Olson. "South Asian Immigrant Women's Experiences of Being Respected within Cancer Treatment Settings."

20. Singh-Carlson, Savitri. "South Asian Immigrant Women's Perceptions of Respect within Health Professional-Client Relationships While Journeying through Cancer." 91.

21. Gurm, Balbir Kaur, Joanne Stephen, Gina Mackenzie, Richard Doll, Maria Cristina Barrotavena, and Susan Cadell. "Understanding Canadian Punjabi-speaking South Asian Women's Experience of Breast Cancer: A Qualitative Study." See also: Singh-Carlson, Savitri. "South Asian Immigrant Women's Perceptions of Respect within Health Professional-Client Relationships While Journeying through Cancer." See also: Singh-Carlson, Savitri, Anne Neufeld, and Joanne Olson. "South Asian Immigrant Women's Experiences of Being Respected within Cancer Treatment Settings."

22. Singh-Carlson, Savitri. "Creating Informal Support within the Clinical Setting." *Canadian Oncology Nursing Journal* 19.3 (2009): 136.

23. Singh, Savitri W. "An Exploration of South Asian Women's Experiences Following Abnormal Pap Smear Results." Unpublished Masters Thesis, University of British Columbia, 2002.

24. Coward, Harold, Tejinder Sidhu, and Peter A. Singer. "Bioethics for Clinicians: 19 Hinduism and Sikhism."

25. Singh-Carlson, Savitri. "South Asian Immigrant Women's Perceptions of Respect within Health Professional-Client Relationships while Journeying through Cancer."

26. Ibid., 130

27. Singh, J. "Ethics of the Sikhs." *Siri Guru Granth Sahib Ji* 1030.

28. Singh-Carlson, Savitri, Anne Neufeld, and Joanne Olson. "South Asian Immigrant Women's Experiences of Being Respected within Cancer Treatment Settings."

29. Singh-Carlson, Savitri, Anne Neufeld, and Joanne Olson. "South Asian Immigrant Womens' Experiences of Being Respected within Cancer Treatment Settings."

30. Singh-Carlson, Savitri. "South Asian Immigrant Women's Perceptions of Respect within Health Professional-Client Relationships While Journeying through Cancer." 106.

31. Singh-Carlson, Savitri, Anne Neufeld, and Joanne Olson. "South Asian Immigrant Womens' Experiences of Being Respected within Cancer Treatment Settings."

32. Apology Issued after Nurse cuts Sikh's Beard. CBC.ca CBC, 24 Mar. 2010. Web. 9 Aug. 2011. http://www.cbc.ca/news/canada/british-columbia/story/2010/03/24/bc-sikh-beard-cut-fraser-health.html.

33. Singh, J. "Ethics of the Sikhs." *Siri Guru Granth Sahib Ji Kabir*, 1105.

34. Singh-Carlson, Savitri. "South Asian Immigrant Women's Perceptions of Respect within Health Professional-Client Relationships While Journeying through Cancer." 150.
35. Reimer-Kirkham, Sheryl. "The Politics of Belonging and Intercultural Health Care." *Western Journal of Nursing Research* 25.7 (2003): 762–780.
36. Detailed information on the short and long-term impact of sexual assault and domestic violence on women and the services are available at www.endingviolence.org.

14

Religions of Native Peoples and Nursing

Melania Calestani, Nereda White, Auntie Joan Hendricks,
and Donna Scemons

INTRODUCTION

This chapter takes an explicitly critical perspective to exploring the inter-
plays between culture, health, spirituality, and religion in relation to nursing
care. It considers the connections between health, ethics, and morality in
Aymara, American Indian/Dakota, and Aboriginal traditions. The three case
studies used are from different countries (Bolivia, United States of America,
and Australia) and are told in the voices of the three co-authors (Calestani,
Scemons, and White and Hendricks, respectively), yet they show many
common themes and provide a point of departure for further discussions
on the importance of knowing the local context of patients' lives. The three
traditions described in this chapter are considered from Orsi's concept of
lived religion, which means being "situated amid the ordinary concerns
of life at the junctures of self and culture, family and social world."[1]

These case studies encourage nurses to think about patients' self-
identity and to explore how religion should not be separated from social life,
being embedded in the many relationships in which patients are involved
(families, communities, natural world, and spirits). Professional nursing
practice has to take into consideration how patients' moralities may shape
ideas of health and illness. This realization may involve a redefinition of
nurses' role in health services delivery and requires reflexivity on the part of
nurses about the assumptions and values they carry.

BASIC CONCEPTS

Medical anthropologists usually distinguish between three "bodies" the personal, the social, and the political as socially constructed notions of the self, identity, and the social sphere.[2] It is therefore impossible not to take into consideration the historical and ongoing effects of colonization in our three case studies. Harris' model indicates the presence of two or more mutually exclusive knowledge systems, the model of the colonizers, and that of the colonized.[3] Harris explains that often this implies a juxtaposition or alternation of the systems, where both are accepted without a direct attempt to integration. In our three case studies, it emerged that this alternation of systems has an important impact on social justice and health disparities, implying ethical issues for the provision of health care and the role of health care professionals.

The concept of *cultural safety*, defined by Stout and Downey,[4] shows that nurses and indigenous people have been embedded in historically determined colonial power relations. Indigenous people often experienced these as a lack of trust and consequently as an emotional inability to access health services. Cultural safety tries to overcome this limit and finds expression in caring spaces that seek equality and are rights-oriented. The overarching goal is the health of indigenous people, but this cannot be achieved without an in-depth analysis of how spiritual and indigenous religious beliefs about health and illness may affect the role of health care providers.

Our three examples show that concepts such as health, spirituality, or ethics are seen as integrated into all aspects of life within indigenous traditions. Garvey, Towney, McPhee, Little, and Kerridge comment that:

> The terms "ethics" and "bioethics" are not evident within Aboriginal cultures because the ethical convictions that form these cultures cannot be dissociated from them and values are woven through the very fabric of Aboriginal cultures. In general terms, Aboriginal societies do not differentiate bioethics or the process of healthcare decision making from the values, narratives, and contexts that define and structure all dimensions of living.[5]

Diener and Suh define subjective well-being as "values people seek," emphasizing the importance of including people's ethical and evaluative judgments about their lives, about why it is worth living and what it means to be a person.[6] Taylor writes,

> People may see their identity as defined partly by some moral or spiritual commitment, as Catholic, or an anarchist. Or they may define it in part by the nation or tradition they belong to, as an American, say, or a Quebecois. What they are saying by this is not just that they are strongly attached to the

spiritual view or background; rather it is that this provides the frame within which they can determine where they stand on questions of what is good, or worthwhile, or admirable or of value. Put counterfactually, they are saying that were they to lose their commitment or identification, they would be at sea, as it were; they wouldn't know any more, for an important range of questions, what the significance of things was for them.[7]

Taylor continues "to know who you are is to be oriented in moral space."[8] This space is where there is a sense of what is good and what is bad, and what is worth doing or achieving. Well-being has to be about the way an individual exists and functions in relation to the world and to himself or herself.[9] Diener and Suh write about the importance of self-actualization and autonomy for the majority of individuals in North America.[10] They describe a highly independent adult as someone who is able to transcend the influences of others and society. This contrasts with our findings about Aymara, American Indian/Dakota, and Aboriginal people, where a person exists and functions in relation to others (humans and spirits). The community is responsible for the well-being of all its members and is the center of spiritual activity. Moralities include harmonious social relations with other human beings, and also with the natural world (land and sea), which is recognized as being alive; respect for and responsibility to the land is an important belief and a moral tie. Connectedness to people and connectedness to places are two important factors in the nurturing of the spirit within and maintaining the wellness of physical, mental, emotional, and spiritual spheres. The concepts of being healthy or unwell are understood within a system of harmony and balance; to be well, a person and his or her community must observe cultural and spiritual obligations. Illness is believed to be caused by spiritual forces such as grief, anger, conflicts with other human beings, or other unknown causes.

The case studies invite health care practitioners to consider the differences within the same ethnic group; assuming that all members of a tribe or an indigenous group share the same opinions and perceptions about the role of tradition or spirituality, or the same concepts of health and illness, would be wrong. Based on different community experiences, Dakota, Aboriginal, or Aymara individuals may be members of one of several Christian denominations. This does not preclude adherence to the practice of more traditional spirituality, but may in some cases involve a rejection of some practices. Members of a specific ethnic group find themselves participating at rituals and activities at times, withdrawing at other times, and carefully selecting which ones to embrace or avoid. The circumstances of different informants to our data varied even within the same ethnic group.

It is important that nurses are prepared to practice in a pluralistic society where perceptions of the self, illness, and social attitudes toward illness and disease can differ radically from their own. Moralities and spiritual orientations have also to be taken into account and cannot be separated from patients' everyday life and self-identity. When providing health care for people from native, aboriginal, or indigenous traditions, nurses have to take into consideration that beliefs about disease and its causes may be attributed to soul loss, spirit intrusion, sorcery, and natural and supernatural factors. In addition, patients may embrace an organized, usually Christian, religion together with tribal beliefs and practices, implying hybridism.

This hybridism can lead to religious and medical pluralism, which becomes very important for understanding individual and collective ethics and moralities, as well as what it means to be "a good person" and therefore to have "a good life." The decision-making process of nurses has to include a wider perspective on beliefs and values, becoming culturally and religiously sensitive and competent. These may lead to different views of and by health practitioners/nurses, redefining their role according to patients' needs. The role and perception of the local community of the patient also raise important reflections on the level of engagement that the community should or should not have in supporting its members when they are ill and sick. Holden and Littlewood argue that nurses could be seen like ethnographic fieldworkers.[11] The nurse must be immersed in understanding the patients' world and their religious beliefs to create a wider awareness of different patients' spiritual needs, showing awareness of their cosmological order and system of beliefs.

MEDICAL AND RELIGIOUS PLURALISM IN THE BOLIVIAN HIGHLANDS

M. Calestani

The first case study comes from ethnographic research carried out in the Bolivian highlands, focusing on two neighborhoods (urban Senkata and semi-urban Amachuma) of one of the most indigenous cities of Latin America, El Alto, populated largely by Aymara migrants from the countryside. There are 34 ethnic groups officially recognized in Bolivia. Quechua and Aymara are the larger language groups, although it is questionable how far linguistic markers in themselves represent distinctive and identifiable ethnic affiliations.

El Alto, at 4,000 m of altitude, is a place of medical and religious pluralism. Patients may experience difficulties of access to primary care centers and hospitals in the countryside, but in El Alto, Aymara migrants have the option to choose between Western medicine and traditional healing processes practiced by local shamans, known as *yatiri*. The people are mainly

Roman Catholic, with an increasing number converting to Pentecostal and Evangelical Protestantism. Inhabitants in El Alto also believe in the spiritual forces of the surrounding environment, *entorno*. They believe that each element of the dry plateau is alive; the snow-covered Andean peaks are *Achachilas* (God Mountains) and the earth itself is *Pachamama* (Mother Earth).

Well-being in El Alto and in the surrounding countryside is attributed to harmonious social relations, both with people and spirits. If a member of the household or of the community is ill, this affects the entire household and community, indicating many connections with the spiritual and religious spheres. The causes of various pathologies are unsolved tensions or conflicts among household or community members. Difficult relationships with spiritual forces can cause someone to be unwell. Those who have offended the God Mountains may experience illness of animals or household members as punishment.

The spirituality of El Alto's inhabitants has to be inclusive of all the multiple religious elements they are in contact with, because only in this way can they be fully protected, assuring their own, their household's, and the community's well-being; and avoiding the evil eye, often connected with jealousy both from humans and supernatural forces. *Suerte* (luck) guides health, including the different human spheres that are not limited to the body or the psyche.[12] It can be acquired through effort and work by asking for protection from supernatural forces. The process is extremely complex, requiring the full moral commitment of people who have to appease the spirits. Relations have to be continuously fed by the circulation of money and special offerings. Faith is another important ingredient. Money and offerings on their own are ineffective. It does not matter how ill someone is or how much someone lacks; what matters is the capacity to overcome a critical situation and to believe that the spiritual forces will help one to do so.

Supernatural forces are there to help people to overcome their difficulties, but they cannot do it for free. One has to pay respect by making material offerings. "The offerings made by people are going to be symbolically 'eaten' by supernatural forces through the burning of the objects offered. This allows one to enter into an empathic relationship with the objects as well as with the rest of one's community."[13] Hence, the process of consumption of sacred practices and objects is fundamental. This is considered as a kind of "culinary" pact based on "commensality" between people and gods. Individual and collective rituals and offerings are essential to promote and assure individual and collective health and well-being. These rituals often take place in sacred places and are a moral responsibility for the entire community.

During my fieldwork in the Bolivian highlands, I visited many sacred places. In particular, I spent much of my time in the Apachita de

Warakho Achachila, which is on the main road that goes to Oruro. This site belongs to the community of Amachuma and it becomes very busy during the month of August. This is the month of the *Pachamama*, the Mother Earth, and it is a time when beautiful as well as terrible things can happen, depending on how much respect one pays. At that time, the *Pachamama* "tiene más hambre" (is hungrier than usual) and the earth opens. This opening is neither completely positive nor completely negative; the offerings can enter more easily, but at the same time the evil can come out.[14] The outcome is always in the hands of people themselves. Some people believe that they might influence their *suerte* (luck) through their actions, and thus have an impact on their well-being.[15] This is the time when the culinary pact or commensality with the *Pachamama* is reconstituted.[16] For example, during the *Wilancha* (in Aymara, the literal translation of this word is *"hacer sangre"* [make blood]) ceremony a white llama is killed and offered to the *Pachamama*. This is followed by heavy social drinking of beer.

The opening of "a hole" in the earth is a powerful metaphor, which has been explained by Fernández Juárez as "a crossing of borders and limits" between opposites, such as health and illness, that can influence the conceptual stability of the Aymara world, affecting and upsetting the order attached to authority.[17] *Suerte* must be produced by putting a lot of effort into it and this process represents the only possible way of protecting the individual, the household, or the entire community from any sort of disturbance, disorder, distress, or illness.

Nevertheless, this practice and strategy to produce *suerte* is not shared by everyone. Some people, especially those who are Evangelical Christians, do not approve of these rituals and offerings to the *Pachamama*. One day in August 2004, while I was at the Apachita, a man approached me. He understood that I was not Bolivian and asked me where I came from. We started to talk about the rituals and the offerings that were taking place. He was against them and added:

> In this place there is something . . . a malevolent supernatural force belonging to the Devil . . . It is against God's Law . . . People visit this place with hopes . . . and their desires become true, but then they have to pay for what they have received. The Devil gives, but then he also takes everything away. Only God gives you forever . . . and stays forever. I don't do these kinds of rituals because I'm Protestant and we are different. It's not like the Catholic Church, which is like a prostitute. The Catholic Church accepts everything, even bad traditions.

Another time I went to visit two people who had recently opened a repair shop for electrical equipment in Senkata. While we were chatting about a personal experience I had with a *yatiri* (a local shaman), a woman with a broken black and white television entered the shop. She started to listen to us and looked as though she wanted to join in, therefore, I decided to include her in our conversation. "Madam, what do you think about *yatiri*?" She looked very happy about the question and replied that she did not believe in them and that she only believed in God. God was her protector and was giving her strength to overcome all the difficulties. "A *yatiri* is able to take away your partner. . . . They are all bad people. I don't trust them." She too belonged to a Protestant Church.

Evangelical conversions are fundamentally linked with a different conception of health and "the good life," which only happens post-conversion. Senkata residents often mentioned how their life had improved after they decided to become Evangelical Christian, especially with regard to their health; avoidance of alcohol has been a blessing for most of them, including the positive effects that non-participation in social drinking can have on economic stability.[18] This may have the effect of making more cash available to invest in children's education and in creating work opportunities. The people interviewed also expressed the benefits of conversion from a spiritual and moral perspective, saying that "they feel closer to the Lord."

Health and Religious Ethics: Identity and Hybridism

There are some differences between the many urban and semi-urban contexts of El Alto, often related to the effects of membership of different religious congregations and their different rules and views regarding community rituals and celebrations. For example, in the case of the *Warakho Apachita* (Amachuma sacred place), I saw some of the members of the Baptist Church from Amachuma visiting it (*Warakho Apachita*) during the month of August. The main community authority—the general secretary of the Trade Union, who belongs to the Baptist Church—also participated in some of the rituals in honor of the *Pachamama*. As mentioned in the previous section, this is not accepted by some Evangelical members. He was present at the closure ceremony (which is also a very important political and community event) of the festivities of the month of the *Pachamama*. Although he is very active in his church, he did not interpret his participation in the ceremony as disrespectful of his religious beliefs. He said that he had to participate for the sake of his community, which for him is the most important aspect of leading a good life. However, other evangelicals, especially from Senkata and those who belong to the Seventh Day Adventist congregation, see this as disrespectful, believing that it is the Devil that acts in the *Apachita*.

Roman Catholics generally believe that it is the *Pachamama* in conjunction with the *Achachilas* that offer protection and listen to people's desires for health, prosperity, and luck. They easily identify the *Pachamama* with the Virgin Mary and the *Achachilas* with the Saints. Therefore, they do not see their worship as something negative or malevolent, but as compatible with Catholic practice. Religious identities shift easily between different spiritual spheres. In Amachuma, conversions to evangelicalism have increased in recent years, especially among local administrative authorities (e.g., the general secretary of the Trade Union) who had a huge impact on other citizens' conversions. Amachuma is a good example of embracing different beliefs at different times, and of the existence of a certain degree of hybridism.

When I first arrived in Amachuma, it was a Sunday morning in the middle of December. The minibus left me in the unfinished main square, where the Town Hall and the Catholic Church were located. It was strangely silent and the church was closed. Then I heard some singing coming from a house; I discovered that this was the place where the Baptist Congregation of Amachuma was meeting.

The Catholic Church was always closed because there was no longer a priest in Amachuma. The priest lived in Senkata. Although Senkata and Ventilla were regularly attended by the priest, there was no time to reach Amachuma. By contrast, the Unión Bautista (Baptist Congregation) was open every Sunday and sometimes also in the middle of the week, offering religious courses to women and children. The pastor was a middle-aged woman from the United States of America. Her new house was being built at the entrance of the neighborhood. She had recently bought the land around her house from the Amachuma community with the idea of building a modern hospital where American doctors could work. "Why American doctors and not Bolivian?" I asked, and was told: "Well, she is American, and in the end, what is important is that we are going to have a hospital." On the other hand, Catholics had a different opinion. For instance, a Catholic Amachuma woman told me: "Yo no soy una mujer de hospital" (I am not a woman who goes to the hospital). In times of illness, she would only visit the local shaman, the *yatiri*.

This situation shows different orientations even within the same ethnic group and how people often negotiate their beliefs in order to achieve their well-being. Even in the case of health, there is a fundamental relation with faith and morality. Pentecostalism seems to stand to hospitals as Catholicism stands to local shamans. However, even in this case, people seem to shift their identities according to the different circumstances, trying to assure their personal as well as communal well-being by oscillating between different religious identities. Despite their religious affiliation to the Baptist Church, they proudly attend the rituals of the *Apachita*. It is important to participate in rituals to assure a reciprocal connection with the *Pachamama* and assure health and well-being for the entire community. Yet, it is also fundamental to become part of the Pentecostal congregation, so that the village can have a hospital. This religious pluralism is in accordance with a medical pluralism and shows how people have different orientations according to time and space.[19] It is impossible to outline a unique model for all Aymara people, as everybody aspires to different things and may have different values, as well. Well-being is socially and morally contextualized. There is a constant tension between different practices of sustained pluralism between rural and urban values, but also religious and medical practice. Values are never fixed and general formulations concerning well-being do not sufficiently take into account fluid social situations.[20,21]

A CASE STUDY FROM NORTH AMERICA

Donna Scemons

The following case provides particular information concerning some American Indian traditional, spiritual, or ethical concepts and time-honored Dakota tribal beliefs. Oral history, oral tradition, connectedness, and respect, including community and family, are presented from a traditional American Indian worldview with specific applications from the perspective of Dakota American Indians living in the United States of America. For American Indians, presenting such information may be criticized as intrinsically controversial because the "possession of knowledge does not confer the right to communicate that knowledge to outsiders."[22] The reference to outsiders herein is not intended as disrespectful; however, it includes those who are not American Indian, and thus it includes many individuals in professional nursing. The sum of what is offered here is presented with significant, careful deliberation, thought, and respect to and for all that American Indians and the Dakota People hold as sacred and true.

American Indian, Native American, Native, Injun, Indian, Indigenous, or Indigenous people are all expressions that represent the legacy of European contact with many of the original inhabitants of the United States of America. American Indian, according to the Health Resources and Services Administration, "refers to people descended from any of the original peoples of North and South America (including Central America) and who maintain tribal affiliation or community attachment."[23] The term has become the accepted delineation in the majority of health care records for every Native American receiving nursing care in any of the 50 states or U.S. territories. The inherent fallacy of these linguistic designations is the

grouping together of diverse human beings under one label that obliter-
ates more than 500 years of history,[24] disregards the complex cultural and
spiritual identities of more than 564 sovereign nations,[25,26] fails to account
for nearly half of American diversity,[27] and "implies a uniform culture and
healing system."[28] Some share certain beliefs, mores, and values; however,
every American Indian tribe and every person who identifies as a traditional
American Indian or Native American requires individual assessment of spirituality, ethics, religion, culture, and values. The terms traditional American
Indian, traditional Dakota, traditional Indian, or traditionalist are defined
thusly:

> . . . traditional, in an Indian sense is considered to mean multiple intercon-
> nections of emotional, physical, [mental], intellectual, and spiritual identity
> that combine to define expectations for the Indian way.[29]

Yet, for all who deal with American Indians in a health care setting, "it
is inaccurate to assume all members of one tribe-share opinions about matters such as the role of tradition [and] spirituality."[30] The terms American
Indian, Native American, Dakota People, First People, the People, or Peoples in the following are interchangeably used in reference to American
Indian People as a general referent and Dakota People as a more specific
linguistic reference. Understanding these various terms and their use in language must acknowledge the fact that before the coming of Europeans to
the Americas there were no such people as Indian, Injun, Indigenous, or
any of the multitudes of expressions meant to convey reference to the First
Peoples. *American Indian* is currently the federally accepted term and will
be used throughout the following as official designation for members of the
Oceti Sakowin, or *Seven Fireplaces*.[31]

Within the Oceti Sakowin are three linguistic groups or dialects:
Dakota, Nakota, and Lakota, who in the U.S. tribal system are federally referred to as the "Sioux."[32] Historically, each band inhabited adjoining lands
and members from each group moved freely among the various bands. The
Dakota were primarily a woodland tribe living in what was to become known
as Minnesota, whereas the Lakota inhabited areas along the Missouri river
and the Great Plains. Those People who spoke Nakota lived between the
Dakota and Lakota tribes along what is now the eastern border of South
Dakota.[33]

Historical geography has significant importance to American Indians
because a connection to the land is "intimately intertwined with native religion, values, culture, and lifestyle."[34] Deloria, a Standing Rock Sioux, explained ". . . the sacred lands remain as permanent fixtures in their [Indian]
cultural or religious understanding."[35] For many of European descent, a
sacred place has historical significance but rarely does the place "provide

a sense of permanency and rootedness that the Indian places represent."[36] The land is not seen through Euro American lenses implying ownership, rather as Laguna Pueblo author Paula Gunn Allen writes,

> The land is not really a place, separate from ourselves, where we act out the drama of our isolate destinies—the earth is not a mere source of survival, distant from the creatures it nurtures and from the spirit that breathes in us—the earth is being, as all creatures are also being; aware, palpable, intelligent, alive.[37]

To the First People, the land is seen as alive and connection to the land is at once one of respect but also one of responsibility; a recognition of ". . . sharing of a defined space."[38]

For professional nursing, an understanding of the self-identity of each patient coupled with at least a modicum of knowledge about the patient's culture and spirituality has become a necessary educational and self-reflective journey. During an encounter with a patient who chooses "American Indian" when asked about national origin or heritage, the nurse must acknowledge 500 years of historical oppression, subjugation, and attempted forced assimilation. Further query concerning what tribal group or groups the patient chooses to recognize for inclusion in the medical record is a final requirement. Inquiring about the patient's tribe or nation is a sign of respect.[39] Knowledge of how a patient self-identifies by tribal affiliation is the beginning of a patient–nurse relationship, as within tribal connections are embedded the concepts that include the patient's spiritual beliefs and ethical values.

From tribal affiliation and self-acknowledgment of belonging to the Dakota Nation, the nurse could reliably discern that the individual patient comes from a people who have a long and rich history of oral tradition.[40] This oral tradition is relied upon by most American Indians, including the Dakota to "convey ideas, feelings, culture, attitudes, and ways of life."[41] Spoken words are greatly appreciated in this tradition, representing a "sharing from the heart"[42] and a strong belief that, "If I do not speak with care, my words are wasted. If I do not listen with care, words are lost."[43]

Oral tradition does not simply mean that American Indian people talk and do not have written history or the ability to write. Ruoff explains this tradition, as "American Indians hold thought and word in great reverence. Breath, speech, and verbal art are so closely linked to each other that in many oral cultures they are often signified by the same word."[44]

This tradition reflects how information is gathered, then understood, and dispersed. Traditionally "old knowledge is valued,"[45] which is not to say that new knowledge is not sought. Oral tradition includes specific ceremonies, rituals, principles, and activities that are passed down through tribal elders. For an American Indian person, oral tradition is "a whole way of being."[46] One aspect of this tradition is storytelling, explained by Leslie Marmon Silko:

> I don't mean just sitting down and telling a once upon a time kind of story. I mean a whole way of seeing yourself, the people around you, your life, the place of your life in the bigger context, not just in terms of nature and location, but in terms of what has gone on before, what's happened to other people.[47]

The historical experience of "other people" is demonstrated through the art of storytelling as one of the mechanisms through which American Indians remember the history of the People, respect ancestors, and pass on spiritual, religious, and ethical values. The use of oral history is not the only method of communication employed by American Indians; however, to many traditional Indians orality is preferred over written methods. There may be distrust and suspicion of written words, as explained by Harjo and Bird:

> It is through writing in the colonizer's languages that our lands have been stolen, children taken away. We have been betrayed by those who first learned to write and speak the language of the occupier of our lands. Yet to speak well in our communities in whatever form is still respected.[48]

Voss, Douville, Soldier, and Twiss speak of the People being:

> . . . wary of the written word, for often the written word objectifies understandings and can be manipulated outside the relationship in which the understanding was shared. The written word can be exploited in ways that were not intended.[49]

As evidenced by these statements from American Indian authors, oral tradition and orality are the preferred mode of communication when presenting moral and ethical values, including spirituality and religion, for many *traditionals*.

Religion for an American Indian is "not separated out from the rest of social life . . . [its]beliefs and rituals-permeated everyday life."[50] Traditionalists do not build houses of worship, require a certain day or time to be spent in worship, nor do they evangelize. Rather than "have a religion," the Indian has a rich spiritual life devoted in part to finding and maintaining a balance through harmonious actions meant to demonstrate respect for all that Creator has fashioned. As Echo-Hawk and Foreward affirmed, spirituality has been and remains "a mystery to most Americans."[51] Perhaps one of the most important facts to acknowledge in any discussion of American Indian religion or spirituality is that there is no one religion or spiritual path acknowledged by this diverse cultural people. Each tribe and often the individuals in that tribe have personal beliefs that may be significantly different from other tribes or individuals.

Acknowledging the Dakota Indian person's spirituality and religion requires knowledge of what for a number of American Indians is a duality. Based on different community experiences, the Dakota person may be a member of one of several Christian religions. This does not preclude adherence to the practice of more traditional spirituality. Depending on the geographic region "historically subjected to Church rule or control,"[52] American Indians may consider themselves committed Catholics, Presbyterians, Methodists, Episcopalians,[53] or other Christian denominations while concomitantly maintaining belief in traditional practices, customs, ceremonies, and rituals. Having one foot in one tradition and the other foot in a moccasin creates this duality. Therefore, to ask an Indian "What is your religious affiliation?" is not as readily answered, as it might be for a person of Euro American descent. American Indian belief is that all is connected: the physical, the mental, the emotional, and the spiritual. "Some American Indians have converted to Christianity, some retain their American Indian spirituality, and some practice a mixture of both Christianity and American Indian spirituality."[54]

Dakota religion and spirituality are considered deep personal matters, about which one does not speak as long as one believes.[55] Eastman ascertains that the theology, religion, or spirituality of the Dakota are the last thing that any non-Indian person will be able to comprehend.[56] This latter statement may seem somewhat harsh, but Indian beliefs "cannot be compared to the religions brought [to the North American continent] from other nations."[57] In Dakota tradition, spirituality cannot be dissected away from the land or the relatedness of all things; life itself in all its forms is sacred. One example of this is the sense of community, where everyone is owed respect as imbued with life. An individual existing without the community is at once foreign and not well-understood by Dakota. This sense of community transcends the individual, the worldview of the Dakota is spirit filled and human beings are not considered superior to other life forms. A deep sense of unity with one's tribe through respecting kinship and family ties is a powerful force among American Indians and Dakota People.

Traditionally, there are no privileged groups among Dakota, rather respect is given to all. Those in the community deemed elders are revered for their spirituality, wisdom, life experience, and willingness to share with other community members.[58] The concept of sharing comes from a long tradition of generosity within the community and is an absolute value. Those who had the most are those who gave the most and "receiving was not stigmatized, needy people were seldom divided into the categories of deserving and non-deserving."[59] Sharing with all and caring for the less fortunate without stigma as a community value was at odds with the Protestant separatists who initially upheld that the poor required moral guidance and were generally indolent.[60] Interestingly, a perception of American Indians as ". . . helpless, hopeless, and doomed to inevitable destinies of drunkenness and poverty" has been a majority view since initial contact.[61]

This latter statement does not explain that ". . . most tribes maintain the view . . . the community is responsible for the well-being of its members."[62] During an illness, the community comes forward to make the sick individual feel nurtured and loved by all.[63] The importance and role of extended family for traditionalists is central in times of health as well as illness. Family members are central players during acute as well as chronic illnesses. In one study of chronically ill children, extended family caregivers were represented by "mothers, fathers, siblings, grandparents, aunts, uncles, and cousins."[64]

For the Dakota, the group is more important than the individual: ". . . interdependence is valued."[65] "Connections and close relationships between people are highly prized."[66] Cooperation among community members is thought to lead to and maintain group harmony. Balance and harmony are reflections of connectedness and a sense of relatedness; for many this is significant contrast to the Western concept of individualism. Although American Indians value each individual, the value comes as a member of the community. Based on this connectedness and sense of community, Dakota most often rely on consensus if decisions or solutions are required. Consensus may ". . . extend beyond the sphere of the traditional nuclear family,"[67] reflecting the community and connectedness.

At times, the community is seen as confusing to individuals outside of the group, for example, when Dakota refer to aunts and uncles as mother or father.[68] Traditionally, individual aunts and uncles participated in much the same manner as a mother or father would in a traditional Euro American family. An Indian family may be related to individuals from other clans, groups, or tribes from the community's perspective. This relatedness may not be through legal channels or actual birth into a family, although the community may refer to the individual, clan, or group as family. In a busy health care environment, referring to a mother, brother, aunt, or grandfather may be erroneously perceived as designating an associated biological or legal status. Consequently, the portrayal of a family member may lead to uncertainty on the part of health care providers.

The significance of community and family may lead to other inaccurate perceptions or actions by health care providers. A health care provider may solicit group members to participate in changing the health behaviors of a tribal or community member, yet Dakota have a strong aversion to interfering in another person's life or behavior.[69] This societal more emanates from a strong belief in the voluntary cooperation of each member of the tribe, group, or clan. Such belief is in part due to the consideration that each human being has a right to choose self-behavior at any particular point and relative to the situation. This is not to imply that behavior is never questioned by Dakota, rather it is reflective of respecting every individual's choice if it does not interfere with the overall goals or needs of the group. Consequently, many American Indians firmly believe that it is not any individual's right to interfere with the actions or activities of others. Such behavior is often not understood by those who believe in the doctrine of being one's brother's keeper. Good Tracks explains: ". . . when an Anglo is moved to be his brother's keeper and that brother is an Indian, then almost everything he says or does seems rude, ill-mannered, or hostile."[70] American Indians tend to view interference with another human being as at once authoritarian and also not the Indian way. The rights of every human being are respected and to interfere in another's behaviors or actions, even if the behaviors seem foolish, is to be disrespectful.

Dakota children are taught from earliest age to behave in a manner that is both modest and humble. A young Indian child learns that some behaviors are considered inappropriate, disrespectful, and likely to bring shame or loss of honor on themselves, family, clan, or community. For example, traditional American Indians consider talking about or bragging about one's accomplishments as disrespectful, ill-mannered, and lacking in sensitivity to those around them.[71] Dakota believe relationships with all things must be based on equality and respect.[72] In Dakota tradition, unlike many Western societal traditions, ". . . a great man must act like a servant, but live like a chief, looking up to the sun rather than the earth, content to have his feet touch the dirt, if his head was in the sky."[73]

While the idea of having one's feet in the dirt may be met with dismay among some cultures, to American Indians this reflects "the community view is inherent in the culture—the spirit of community neutralizes individual power—[and how] Native American people prefer to look at the community as a source of power and leadership."[74] For those of Euro American heritage, the concept of community as the source of power and leadership is an American Indian traditional belief that may be challenging to integrate. American Indians do not necessarily perceive the attainment of credentials and degrees as "signify[ing] power and status."[75] This does not preclude American Indian understanding of formal education or the effort required to attain credentials or degrees. Advanced formal education is viewed by many traditionalists as a journey undertaken by an individual as part of self-determination.[76] Values that are perceived as more important to American Indians are respect, generosity, sense of community, and connectedness. Finally, the information provided within this case study is intended to provide assistance to those professional nurses who provide care to members of the People in various health care settings. Remember to think and speak from your heart. *Mitakuye pidam-aya De yuonihan Yuhapi c'anet was'te Wopida unkenic'eyapi*, or in the dominant language: All my relatives. For this honor with a good heart, thank you.

A CASE STUDY FROM AUSTRALIA

Nereda White and Joan Hendricks

> For Aboriginal and Torres Strait people, health does not just entail the free-dom of the individual from sickness but requires support for health and interdependent relationships between families, communities, land, sea and spirit. The focus must be on spiritual, cultural, emotional and social well-being as well as physical health.[77]

Australia's population includes two Indigenous groups. The first group consists of the Aboriginal people who mainly inhabit the Australian main-land, Tasmania, and some islands off the coast of the Northern Territory and the state of Queensland. The second group includes the Torres Strait Islanders who live on the islands of the Torres Straits between Australia and Papua New Guinea, and in more recent years due to employment and edu-cation opportunities, reside in coastal towns and cities. From 2009 popula-tion figures, it is estimated there were a total number of 550,818 Indigenous Australians included in the total Australian population of approximately 21 million people (representing nearly 3% of the total population). The larg-est number (161,910) live in the state of New South Wales and 156,454 live in Queensland.[78]

This case study focuses on Aboriginal people's health and details the Aboriginal Health Centre on Stradbroke Island, located off the coast of Queensland near Brisbane. The use of *Indigenous* in this case study will include both Aboriginal people and Torres Strait Islanders.

Brief Overview of Australian Indigenous Health

Aboriginal people's current life chances are intrinsically linked to their past and present socioeconomic and cultural status in Australian society.[79] Australian Indigenous people continue to endure poor general health and for every key measure Indigenous Australians suffer greater health burdens. These disad-vantages begin at birth and continue throughout the lifespan. Mortality rates for Indigenous infants and children are two to three times higher than for the rest of the population, and 13% of Indigenous babies are of lower birth weight.

Indigenous people are more likely to be hospitalized. There is a greater prevalence of cardiovascular disease (leading cause of death), respiratory diseases (asthma), renal disease, and diabetes (especially Type 2). Life expectancy for both men and women is 17 years less than for other Australians, with Indigenous males 59 years compared with 77 years for non-Indigenous men and Indigenous females 65 years compared with 82 years for non-Indigenous women.[80]

The Indigenous age structure has implications for the health care of greater numbers of younger Indigenous people, but also highlights the reduced life expectancy of Indigenous Australians who may present end of lifespan conditions at a much earlier age. The median age at death in 2008 for Indigenous males was reported as being 49.0 years (South Australia) to 59.9 years (New South Wales).[81] Disparities also exist for Indigenous people's participation in the areas of education, employment, and access to adequate housing. Additionally, they suffer greater rates of incarceration. These disadvantages combine to be powerful determinants of contemporary health and well-being.

Dispossession and years of oppression have had long-term effects on Aboriginal people's physical, social, and emotional well-being, particularly for those people who were removed from their families. Their grief and loss are encapsulated in the following quote:

> We may go home, and we may reunite with our . . . (families), communities but we cannot relive the 20, 30, 40 years that we spent without their love and care, and they cannot undo the grief and mourning they felt when we were taken from them. We can go home for ourselves as Aboriginals, but this does not erase the attacks inflicted on our heart, minds, bodies and souls, by caretakers who thought their mission was to eliminate us as Aboriginals.[82]

This colonial legacy calls for a holistic approach to the health care of Indigenous Australians that addresses the current inequities that are faced in all areas of life.

Access to Resources and Culturally Appropriate Health Care

Although the majority live in cities, Indigenous people are "ten times more likely than non-Indigenous Australians to live in remote areas" where medical facilities and access to allied health care services are severely limited.[83] Service in some remote communities may be restricted to doctors and specialists flying in and out, and patients may be required to travel to major cities far from their communities for treatment. This, in turn, creates problems with the culture shock of being in an alien environment without the support of family. Eckerman et al. emphasize the impact on the individual and the "associated tension and anxiety of entering a new culture combined with the feelings of isolation, sensations of loss, confusion and powerlessness."[84] Being hospitalized can be a traumatic experience for anyone, but for Aboriginal people it may "cause them to withdraw from communicating and interacting with the health systems."[85]

In addition, families who are left behind suffer from the absence of significant members. For example, when women are required to travel to a city hospital to give birth, the family is often without the primary carer and unable to visit and bond with the new baby. There are many stories about Aboriginal people "pining for country" to the point that this has been believed to have contributed to their death (Authors' personal knowledge).

Available mainstream health services are not always utilized by Indigenous clients due to:

- lack of knowledge about the service and what it provides;
- lack of knowledge about health matters generally including understanding of their own health condition;
- distrust of health services due to a long history of poor relationships with government providers;
- feeling "shame" or embarrassment about speaking about health matters to a "white" person;
- issues such as preferring to speak to (or being treated by) same gender practitioner due to "women's business" or "men's business;"
- lack of culturally trained health care professionals; and
- language and communication difficulties (medical jargon; Standard Australian English [SAE]).

Language and communication are particular concerns for Aboriginal people for whom SAE may be a third or fourth language. Traditionally, there were over 250 languages, all with a number of dialects. The map of Aboriginal Australia published by the Australian Institute of Aboriginal and Torres Strait Islander Studies shows a division into nearly 700 language groups. Although colonization has resulted in significant language loss through the death of language speakers and forbidding people to speak their languages, there are still communities where traditional languages are spoken, as well as kriol/creole and Aboriginal English. This creates difficulties for Aboriginal and Torres Strait Islander people communicating with the outside world where SAE is the dominant language. The inability to be understood and communicate creates personal distress for patients in cross-cultural health care situations, thus impeding their treatment and recovery. Furthermore, the specific language of the medical world provides a significant obstacle to understanding and addressing health issues.

Training of Health Care Professionals

The appropriate training of health professionals is critical to enable the treatment of Aboriginal clients in culturally affirming ways and to enable practitioners to work together on health goals with Aboriginal communities. Aboriginal people are more likely to access health services where they feel welcomed by staff whom are not judgmental and who acknowledge the history of oppression that has led to many of the barriers currently faced by Aboriginal people. Eckerman et al. argue that

> . . . if we empathise, we try to understand—understand such factors as poverty, bad housing and unemployment, which create an unhealthy environment. We try to understand the effects of racism, what it does to a powerless minority, and we have a close look at the service we deliver and consider whether or not they suit the people's needs.[86]

Furthermore, it is vital for nurses to develop an understanding of the interplay between white race privilege and Indigenous disadvantage.[87] The growing body of writing about "whiteness" will help nurses to understand that by normalizing "whiteness," the privileges that one experiences as a member of a white group in Australian society perpetuates institutional racism.[88]

Spiritual Basis of Aboriginal Health: The Dreaming

Aboriginal spirituality is derived from *The Dreaming*, a spiritual concept, which is embedded in all aspects of daily life and is traditionally passed down the generations through the process of storytelling and enacted through law, kinship structures, and custodial obligations to the land and sea. The Dreaming tells of the journeys of Ancestral Beings who created the natural world and provides links with the past, present, and future. It is the natural world, especially the land or county to which a person belongs, which provides their links to their Dreaming.

> Dreaming relies on profoundly spiritual insights into the interrelations of land—the living spring of God's creation—family kinship and community. This interrelation of land, kinship and community is integral to human identity . . . This culture taught from early age that all living things matter. Land is the first teacher and its teachings are manifest in our deepest thinking.[89]

The Aboriginal concept of health is holistic, encompassing mental health and physical, cultural, and spiritual health. This holistic concept does not merely refer to the "whole body," but in fact is steeped in the harmonized interrelations that constitute cultural well-being. When the harmony of these interrelations is disrupted, Aboriginal ill health will persist.[90]

Connectedness to people and places of birth (referred to as "country") are two important factors in the nurturing of the spirit within and maintaining wellness. Rituals, celebrations, and ceremonies from birth to death are fine tuned to nature. The songs of the birds, the voice of the wind, the stillness of the billabongs, the landforms, and Dreaming tracks are constant reminders to respect and be still—to experience the fullness of the Dreaming and the presence of the sacred.[91]

There are significant cultural and community protocols relating to death, dying, and grieving. Aboriginal people believe life is a journey and that there is a time to come and a time to go. The pain of death of a loved one is quelled by the togetherness of community support for the immediate family and is regarded as "Sorry business" that affects not just the immediate family, but the whole community. It is common in many communities for all business to cease, to allow time for appropriate mourning practices. This practice can be challenging for outsiders wanting to provide services or conduct business. It is also the practice in some communities to refrain from speaking the name of the deceased person until the appropriate period of time has passed. Another belief associated with death is the warning to families through the appearance of an animal or bird.

Yulu-Burri-Ba Aboriginal Corporation for Community Health

North Stradbroke Island, known by its Aboriginal name Minjerriba, is located in Moreton Bay, 30 km south east of Brisbane, Queensland and belongs to the group of islands known collectively as Quandamooka (Moreton Bay). According to the 2001 census, North Stradbroke Island has a population of 2413, of whom 13.9% are Indigenous. It was first sighted by Captain James Cook in 1770 and permanent settlement of the island by Europeans began in 1825 when Amity Point was set up as Moreton Bay's first Pilot Station. At first, the local Aboriginal groups were welcoming to explorers and shipwrecked sailors but later, as the island received convicts and free settlers, there were often violent clashes between the locals and the newcomers. Today, Quandamooka (Moreton Bay) is the homeland of the three clan groups: the Nunukul, the Ngugi, and the Gorenpil, who are recognized as the people of the sand and waters Yulu-Burri-Ba (YBB). These three groups have descendants who have continued to maintain their identity on Minjerriba and a close affiliation with their traditional country of belonging.

The YBB Aboriginal Corporation for Community Health was established in 1990 under the auspice of North Stradbroke Island Aboriginal and Islander Housing Co-op. The Corporation is governed by a Board comprised of local community members. YBB provides a range of health services to the Indigenous population of North Stradbroke Island including: a general clinic, a massage therapy clinic, an optometry service for retinal screening and general eye testing, weekly diabetic clinics offering check on blood pressure, a methodone clinic, counseling service, and a Dental and Hearing Health Clinic. Professional staff includes doctors, registered nurses, and Aboriginal health workers, Counselors, a drug and alcohol worker, a dietician/nutritionist, optometrists, a maternal and child health nurse, and a hearing health team. YBB also provides home visit services for regular patients of the practice whose condition prevents them from physically attending the surgery and also provides transport as needed. The center's services are well-attended by the local Aboriginal population and also by some of the non-Aboriginal Stradbroke Island people. While the community is well-serviced during the day, there is concern about the lack of after hour services. This concern is compounded as access to mainland emergency services is by ferry, which does not operate a service from 8 p.m. until 6 a.m. Air sea emergency remains as the only alternative during these hours.

Through its services, YBB is an excellent example of the Aboriginal community taking control of their own health needs. This in its true sense is capacity building in community. Further information about the service can be found on its Web site: Web site: http://www.ybb.com.au

CONCLUSIONS

The chapter aims to encourage nurses toward a critical analysis of their own practice. All the contributions to the chapter bridge the disciplines of nursing/health studies, anthropology, and religious studies, and emphasize the importance of viewing the patient in the context of his/her family, community, culture, and religious affiliation. To enable appropriate care for Aymara, American Indian/Dakota, and Aboriginal people, there is an urgent need for nurses to have knowledge of the historical, colonial, and social processes that have resulted in social and health inequities for these groups. Also, understanding their spiritual dimensions and appreciating cultural difference may provide better health care services delivery. Hopefully, the experience of being hospitalized may be transformed from a traumatic one to a positive one, promoting the interaction of indigenous, American Indian, and Aboriginal people with their national health services. Importantly, the community of clients has to be involved in planning and evaluating health care services, interventions, and programs if they are to be effective.

All the case studies look at how members of different ethnic groups conceptualize health and illness, ethics and morality, sometimes in a panorama of everyday medical and religious pluralism. Their commitment to shared values and respect for the cosmological order is fundamental to achieve "the good life' and 'to be healthy." These definitions are morally constructed. Religious beliefs and practices also provide an important idiom for the expression of aspirations and the pursuit of ideals. Moreover, they also have a positive effect on emotional states, promoting solidarity, feelings of confidence, and a sense of full personhood and empowerment as various anthropologists have argued.[92] The case studies shed light on the role of beliefs and faith in therapy, providing an account of culturally "traditional" health treatments that are informed by religious beliefs.

NOTES

1. Orsi, Robert. "Is the Study of Lived Religion Irrelevant to the World We Live In?" Special Presidential Plenary Address, Society for the Scientific Study of Religion, Salt Lake City, November 2, 2002." *Journal for the Scientific Study of Religion* 42.2 (2003): 172.

2. Scheper-Hughes, Nancy and Margaret M. Lock. "The Mindful Body: A Prolegomenon to Future Work in Medical Anthropology." *Medical Anthropology Quarterly* 1 (1987): 6–41.

3. Harris, Olivia. "The Sources and Meanings of Money: Beyond the Market Paradigm in an Ayllu of Northern Potosí." *Ethnicity, Markets and Migration in the Andes: At the Crossroad of History and Anthropology.* Eds. Brooke Larson and Olivia Harris. London: Durham University Press, 1995.

4. Dion Stout, Madeleine, and Bernice Downey. "Nursing, Indigenous Peoples and Cultural Safety: So What? Now What?" *Contemporary Nurse* 2.2 (2006): 327–32.

5. Garvey, P. Towney, J. McPhee, M. Little, and I. Kerridge. "Is There an Aboriginal Bioethic?" *Journal of Medical Ethics* 30.6 (2004): 570–75. See also: Jonathan H. Ellerby, John McKenzie, Stanley McKay, Gilbert J. Gariépy, and Joseph M. Kaufert. "Bioethics for Clinicians:18. Aboriginal Cultures." *Canadian Medical Association Journal* 163.7 (2000): 845–50.

6. Diener, Edward, and Eun Kook Suh. *Culture and Subjective Well-Being.* Cambridge, MA: MIT Press, 2000.

7. Taylor, Charles. *Sources of the Self: The Making of the Modern Identity.* Cambridge, MA: Harvard University Press, Library of Congress, 1989. 27.

8. Ibid., 28.

9. Giorgi, L. Aspects of the Subjective Culture of Modernity: An Analysis of the European Value Survey (1981) on European Attitudes Towards Religion, Work, Politics and Well-Being, Phd Thesis. Anthropology Department, Cambridge: Cambridge University, 1990. 104.

10. Diener, Edward, and Eun Kook Suh. *Culture and Subjective Well-Being.*
11. Holden, Pat and Jenny Littlewood. *Anthropology and Nursing.* London: Routledge, 1991.
12. For a detailed discussion of the local meanings attributed to *suerte* see Calestani, Melania. "'Suerte' (Luck): Spirituality and Well-Being in El Alto, Bolivia." *Applied Research in Quality of Life* 4.1 (2009): 47–75.
13. Ibid.
14. Fernández Juárez, Gerardo. "El mundo 'abierto':agosto y Semana Santa en las celebraciones rituals aymaras." *Revista Española de Antropalogia Americana* 26 (1996): 205–29. 1996. Spanish.
15. Kessel, Juan van. "Tecnologia aymara: Un enfoque cultural" *La Cosmovision Aymara* En. Berg H. V. D. and Schiffers, N. (Comp.) La Paz: Hisbol-UCB, 1993, 187–19. Spanish. See also: Kessel, Juan van, and Dionisio Condori. *Criar la vida: Trabajo y tecnologia en el mundo andino.* Santiago de Chilie: Vivarium, 1992.
16. Fernández Juárez, Gerardo. "El mundo 'abierto':agosto y Semana Santa en las celebraciones rituals aymaras."
17. Ibid.
18. Alcohol used for libations is often drunk in large quantities in Catholic religious celebrations. There is a moral duty attached to the drinking of alcohol, the substance that connects human beings and spiritual forces.
19. Crandon-Malamud, Libbet. *From the Fat of Our Souls; Social Change, Political Process, and Medical Pluralism in Bolivia.* London, UK: University of California Press, 1993.
20. Sen, Amartya. *Development as Freedom.* New York: Alfred A. Knopf, 1999.
21. Nussbaum, Martha C. *Women and Human Development. The Capabilities Approach.* Cambridge: Cambridge University Press, 2000.
22. Smith, Andrea. "Spiritual Appropriation as Sexual Violence." *Wicazo Sa Review* 20.1 (2005): 108.
23. United States Census Bureau. *2000 Glossary.* Web. 13 Feb. 2010. http://www .census.gov/population/www/cen2000/censusatlas/pdf/16_Backmatter-Glossary.pdf.
24. Hodge, David R., Gordon E. Limb, and Terry L. Cross. "Moving From Colonization Toward Balance and Harmony: A Native American Perspective on Wellness." *Social Work* 54.3 (2009): 212.
25. US Department of the Interior: Bureau of Indian Affairs. *What We Do. Services Overview.* Web. 13 Feb. 2010. http://www.bia.gov/.
26. Bryan, Ralph T., Rebecca McLaughlin Schaefer, Laura DeBruyn, and Daniel D. Stier. "Public Health Legal Preparedness in Indian Country." *American Journal of Public Health* 99.4 (2009): 607. See also: Gone, Joseph P. "We Never was Happy Living like a Whiteman: Mental Health Disparities and the Postcolonial Predicament in American Indian Communities." *American Journal of Community Psychology* 40.3–4 (2007): 290. See also Fisher, Philip, A., and Thomas J. Ball, "Tribal Participatory Research: Mechanisms of a Collaborative Model." *American Journal of Community Psychology* 32.3–4 (2003): 210.
27. Hodgkinson, Harold L. "The Demographics of American Indians: One Percent of the People; Fifty Percent of the Diversity." *Washington D.C. Institute for Educational Leadership.* 31. 1990. See also: Yurkovich, Eleanor E. "Working with American Indians Toward Educational Success." *Journal of Nursing Education* 40.6 (2001): 260.
28. Cohen, Ken Bear Hawk. "Native American Medicine." *Alternative Therapies* 4.6 (1998): 45.

29. Montgomery, Diane, Marie L. Mivillle, Carrie Winterowd, Beth Jeffries, and Matthew F. Baysden. "American Indian College Students: An Exploration into Resiliency Factors Revealed through Personal Stories." *Cultural Diversity and Ethnic Minority Psychology* 6.4 (2000): 388.

30. Duran, Bonnie, Ted Jojola, Nathania T. Tsosie, and Nina Wallerstein. "Assessment, Program Planning, and Evaluation in Indian Country." American Indians and Alaska Native Populations. *Indian Country Toward a Postcolonial Practice of Indigenous Planning.* Web. 13 Feb. 2010. http://depts.washington.edu/depth/print/Assessment2C_Program_Planning2C_and_Evaluation_in_Indian_Country__Toward_a_Postcolonial_Practice_of_Indigenous_Planning.pdf.

31. Whelan, Mary K. "Dakota Indian Economics and the Nineteenth-Century Fur Trade." *Ethnohistory* 40.2 (1993): 147–48. See also: Powers, William K. "Wiping the Tears: Lakota Religion in the Twenty-first Century." *Native Religions and Cultures of North America.* Ed. Sullivan, Lawrence E. New York: The Continuum International Publishing Group, Inc. (2000): 104.

32. Ibid.

33. Ibid.

34. Weaver, Hilary N. "Indigenous People in a Multicultural Society: Unique Issues for Human Services." *Social Work* 43.3 (1998): 208.

35. Deloria, Vine Jr. *God is Red.* 3rd ed. Golden, CO: Fulcrum Publishing, 2003. 66.

36. Ibid.

37. Allen, Paula Gunn. *The Sacred Hoop: Recovering the Feminine in American Indian Traditions.* Boston, MA: Beacon Press, 1992: 119. Print.

38. Meli, Franco. "Images of the Sacred in Native American Literature." *Native Religions and Cultures of North America.* Ed. Sullivan, Lawrence E. New York: The Continuum International Publishing Group, Inc. 2000. 209.

39. Weaver, Hilary N. "Indigenous People in a Multicultural Society: Unique Issues for Human Services." *Social Work* 43.3 (1998): 208.

40. Rich, Elizabeth. "'Remember Wounded Knee': AIM's use of Metonymy in 21st Century Protest." *College Literature* 31.3 (2004): 83.

41. Marashio, Paul. "Enlighten My Mind: Examining the Learning Process through Native Americans' Ways." *Journal of American Indian Education* 21.2 (1982): 2–10. Web. 13 Feb. 2010. http://jaie.asu.edu/v21/V21S2enl.html.

42. Salois, Emily Matt, Patricia A. Holkup, Toni Tripp-Reimer, and Clarann Weinert. "Research as Covenant." *Western Journal of Nursing Research* 28.5 (2006): 509.

43. Momaday, N. Scott. *The Names.* New York: Harper & Row, 1976. 200–01.

44. Rouff, LaVonne Brown. *American Indian Literatures: An Introduction, Bibliographic Review and Selected Bibliography.* New York: MLA. 1990. 6–7.

45. Moss, Margaret, Lorayne Tibbetts, Susan J. Henly, Barbara J. Dahlen, Beverly Patchell, and Roxanne Struthers. "Strengthening American Indian Nurse Scientist Training Through Tradition: Partnering with Elders." *Journal of Cultural Nursing* 12.2 (2005): 51.

46. Allen, Paula Gunn. *The Sacred Hoop: Recovering the Feminine in American Indian Traditions.* 11.

47. Barnes, Kim. "Leslie Marmon Silko Interview." *The Journal of Ethnic Studies* 13.4 (1986): 86.

48. Harjo, Joy and Gloria Bird. *Reinventing the Enemy's Language: Contemporary Native Women's Writings of North America.* New York: W.W. Norton & Company, 1997. 86.

49. Voss, Richard W., Victor Douville, Alex Little Soldier, and Gayla Twiss. "Tribal and Shamanic-Based Social Work Practice": A Lakota Perspective. *Social Work* 44.3 (1999): 228.

50. Demaille, Raymond J. "Lakota Belief and Ritual in the Nineteenth Century." *Sioux Indian Religion: Traditions and Innovations.* Eds. Raymond J Demaille, and Douglas R. Parks. Norman, OK: University of Oklahoma Press, 1987. 27.

51. Echo-Hawk, Walter R. Forward. *Encyclopedia of Native American Religions: An Introduction.* Eds. Arlene Hirshfelder and Paulette Molin. New York: Facts on File, Inc, 2002.

52. Burhansstipanov, Linda and Walter Hollow. "Native American Cultural Aspects of Oncology Nursing Care." *Seminars in Oncology Nursing* 17.3 (2001): 211.

53. Bowden, Henry Warner. *American Indians and Christian Missions: Studies in Cultural Conflict.* Chicago, IL: The University of Chicago Press, 1981.

54. Flowers, Deborah L. "Culturally Competent Nursing Care for American Indian Clients in a Critical Care Setting." *Critical Care Nurse* 25.1 (2005): 46.

55. Barnes, Kim. "Leslie Marmon Silko Interview." *The Journal of Ethnic Studies.* 13.4. (1986): 86.

56. Eastman, Charles Alexander. *The Soul of the Indian and Other Writings.* 2nd ed. Novato, CA: New World Library, 1993. 6.

57. Giago, Tim A. "Spirituality Comes from the Heart, Not from a Book." *American Indian Religions: An Interdisciplinary Journal* 1.1 (Winter 1994): 98.

58. Fuller-Thompson, Esme and Meredith Minkler. "American Indian/Alaskan Native Grandparents Raising Grandchildren: Findings from the Census 2000 Supplementary Survey." *Social Work* 50.2 (2005): 132.

59. Hetzel, Theodore B. "We Can Learn from American Indians." *Journal of American Indian Education* 4.3 (1965): 2. Web. 13 Feb. 2010. http://jaie.asu.edu/v4/V4S3lear .html

60. Williams, Edith Ellison and Florence Ellison. "Culturally Informed Social Work Practice with American Indian Clients: Guidelines for Non-Indian Social Workers." *Social Work* 41.2 (1996): 148.

61. Ibid.

62. Gross, Emma R. "Deconstructing Politically Correct Practice Literature: The American Indian Case." *Social Work* 40.2 (1995): 207.

63. Dwyer, Kathy. "Culturally Appropriate Consumer-directed Care: The American Indian Choices Project." *Generations* 24.3 (2000): 91.

64. Hetzel, Theodore B. "We Can Learn from American Indians." *Journal of American Indian Education* 4.3 (1965): 2. Web. 13 Feb. 2010.

65. Weaver, Hilary N. "Indigenous People in a Multicultural Society: Unique Issues for Human Services." *Social Work* 43.3 (1998): 204.

66. Garwick, Ann and Sally Auger. "What do Providers Need to Know about American Indian Culture? Recommendations from Urban Indian Family Caregivers." *Families, Systems & Health* 18.2 (2000): 182.

67. Weaver, Hilary N. "Indigenous People in a Multicultural Society: Unique Issues for Human Services." Social Work 43.3 (1998): 204.

68. Office of Minority Health and Bureau of Primary Health Care. "The Provider's Guide to Quality & Culture: American Indians and Alaska Natives-Health Disparities Overview." 5. Web. 13 Feb. 2010. http://erc.msh.org/mainpage.cfm?file=7.3.0.htm &module=provider&language=English

69. Jones, Loring. "The Distinctive Characteristics and Needs of Domestic Violence Victims in a Native American Community." *Journal of Family Violence* 28 (2008): 115.

70. Everett, Frances, Noble Proctor and Betty Cartmell. "Providing Psychological Services to American Indian Children and Families." *Professional Psychology: Research and Practice* 14.5 (1983): 596.

71. Good Tracks, Jimm G. "Native American Noninterference." *Social Casework* 18 (Nov. 1973): 30.

72. Everett, Frances, Noble Proctor and Betty Cartmell. "Providing Psychological Services to American Indian Children and Families." 597.

73. Malan, Vernone D. "The Value System of the Dakota Indians: Harmony with Nature, Kinship, and Animism." *Journal of American Indian Education* 3.1 (1963): 2. Web. 13 Feb. 2010. http://jaie.asu.edu/v3/V3S1valu.html

74. Simms, Muriel. "Impressions of Leadership through a Native Woman's Eyes." *Urban Education* 35. 5 (2000): 638.

75. Malan, Vernone D. "The Value System of the Dakota Indians: Harmony with Nature, Kinship, and Animism." 3.

76. Everett, Frances, Noble Proctor and Betty Cartmell. "Providing Psychological Services to American Indian Children and Families." 592.

77. Burgess, Christopher, Fay Johnston, Helen Berry, Joseph McDonnell, Dean Yibarbuk, Charlie Gunabarra, Albert Mileran, and Ross Bailie. "Healthy Country, Healthy People: The Relationship between Indigenous Health Status and Caring for Country." *Medical Journal of Australia* 190.10 (2009): 567–72.

78. Australian Bureau of Statistics. *Experimental Estimates and Projections, Aboriginal and Torres Strait Islander Australians 1991 to 2002.* Canberra: Australian Bureau of Statistics, 2009.

79. Eckermann, Anne-Marie, Toni Dowd, Ena Chong, Lynette Nixon, Roy Gray, and Sally Johnson. *Binan Goonj: Bridging Cultures in Aboriginal Health.* 2nd ed. Sydney: Elsevier, 2006.

80. Goold, Sally. "Transcultural Nursing: Can We Meet the Challenge of Caring for the Australian Indigenous Person?" *Journal of Transcultural Nursing* 12 (2001): 95.

81. Thomson, Neil, Andrea MacRae, Jane Burns, Michelle Catto, Olivier Debuyst, Ineke Krom, Christine Potter, Kathy Ride, Sasha Stumpers, and Belinda Urquhart. "Overview of Australian Indigenous Health Status, December 2009." *Australian Indigenous Health Info Net"* 2009. Perth: Western Australia. Web. 15 March 2010. http://www.healthinfonet.ecu.edu.au/health-facts/overviews

82. HREOC. *Bringing Them Home: A Guide to the Findings and Recommendations of the National Inquiry into the Separation of Aboriginal and Torres Strait Islander Children from their Families.* Australia: HREOC, 1997. 3.

83. Thomson, Neil, Andrea MacRae, Jane Burns, Michelle Catto, Olivier Debuyst, Ineke Krom, Christine Potter, Kathy Ride, Sasha Stumpers and Belinda Urquhart. "Overview of Australian Indigenous Health Status, December 2009."

84. Eckermann, Anne-Marie, Toni Dowd, Ena Chong, Lynette Nixon, Roy Gray, and Sally Johnson. *Binan Goonj: Bridging Cultures in Aboriginal Health.* 94.

85. Ibid., 107.

86. Ibid., 138.

87. Fredericks, B. "Which Way? Educating for Nursing Aboriginal and Torres Strait Islander Peoples." *Contemporary Nurse Journal* 23.1 (2006): 87–99.

88. Eckermann, Anne-Marie, Toni Dowd, Ena Chong, Lynette Nixon, Roy Gray, and Sally Johnson. *Binan Goonj: Bridging Cultures in Aboriginal Health.* 170. For further readings on whiteness, see the works of Aileen Moreton-Robinson.

89. Hendricks, Joan. Epilogue: Indigenous and Christian: An Australian Perspective. *Foundations of Christian Faith: An Introduction for Students.* Eds. Damien Casey, Gerard Hall and Anne Hunt. Southbank, Vic: Social Science Press, 2004. 171.

90. Swan, Pat and Beverly Raphael. "Ways Forward: National A&TSI Mental Health Policy." *National Consultancy Report.* Canberra AGPS, 1995.

91. Hendricks, Joan. *"Welcome to Country"* Quandamooka Bayside Indigenous Health Forum. North Stradbroke Island: North Stradbroke Island Housing Co-op Dunwich, 2009. Speech.

92. Barbalet, J. M. *Emotion, Social Theory and Social Structure.* Cambridge: Cambridge University Press, 2001. See also: Turner, Victor. Liminality and communitas. *A Reader in the Anthropology of Religion.* Ed. Michael Lambek. London: Blackwell, 2002. See also: Gillian Bandelow and Simon J. Williams. Ed. *Emotions in Social Life: Critical Themes and Contemporary Issues.* New York: Routledge, 1997.

15

Emergent Nonreligious Spiritualities

Sonya Sharma, Sheryl Reimer-Kirkham, and Marsha D. Fowler

The religious and spiritual landscape of many countries has seen considerable change in the last decade, with secularism rooted in the public sphere of many Western societies; with global patterns of migration resulting in societies that are more religiously pluralistic than ever, often with strong adherence to religions such as Islam, Hinduism, Sikhism, Buddhism, and Christianity; and with an increasing proportion of citizens not affiliating with any religious or spiritual community. A related societal trend that has taken particular forms in nursing theory, and that carries significant ramifications for nursing practice and health care services delivery, is that of emergent nonreligious spiritualities. By emergent nonreligious spiritualities, we are referring to the ever-growing phenomenon in modern Western society of the sacralization of nature, the self, and everyday life.[1] Such a conceptualization of spirituality is a less organized phenomenon but has some key expressions that will be discussed.

In this chapter, we explore implications for nurses and nursing ethics introduced by emergent nonreligious spiritualities. We begin by providing background to the discussion with an overview of the social context in which emergent spiritualities are born and, although there is great variation within personalized expressions of emergent spiritualities, we identify some philosophic underpinnings associated with this genre of spiritual beliefs and practices. For nursing, emergent spiritualities are implicit and influential in much of its' current spirituality discourses, although nursing scholars tend not to locate themselves explicitly within the tradition of "emergent" or "alternative" spiritualities. Therefore, our approach in this chapter has been to infer this location, not for the sake of pigeon-holing or essentializing, but to (a) extract, from current writings in spirituality and nursing, direction for the care of patients and families who themselves hold to emergent spiritualities; (b) provide insight into what nursing practice from the stance of emergent spiritualities might look like, for the sake of enhancing workplace relationships, and fostering self-reflection and insight; and (c) as with other works in this collection, examine the intersections of emergent spirituality, ethics, and nursing, addressing the question of how ethics might be lived out with reference to health-related decisions and nursing practice.

LOCATING EMERGENT SPIRITUALITIES

The contemporary development of emergent nonreligious spiritualities, also known as alternative, new, or progressive spiritualities, lies within the context of the social phenomenon of secularization. Many sociologists of religion agree that secularization is the decline of the importance of religion not only in "the operation of nonreligious institutions like the state and the economy," but also in the "social standing of religious roles and institutions" and the extent to which people engage in traditionally tied religious practices and beliefs.[2]

Societies in the West, and Europe in particular, have certainly seen a secularization of the public sphere, including in the contexts of academia, public education, government, and health care. This phenomenon has caused many to ponder the importance of religion and spirituality, and some have continued to predict their eventual irrelevance. Despite such predictions, perhaps a better description of what has occurred is that religion, spirituality, and secularization are not separate from each other but shape and inform one another and intersect in complex and sometimes contradictory ways. More so, religion and spirituality are not restricted to sacred places of worship and belief, but are omnipresent in everyday life. While significant is the decline in church attendance, so is the growth and widespread interest in spirituality. Although many may not attend church, synagogue, mosque, or temple, many want to believe in something more, whether from within or beyond themselves.

Theorists and sociologists of religion have remarked on the changing nature of religion and spirituality, a cultural transformation marked by "a reaction against outer authority such as that found in the churches to more inward forms of authority rooted in the inner life of the individual."[3] It is what Heelas and Woodhead refer to as the "subjective turn."[4] Canadian sociologist of religion Bibby concurs that even in the midst of the reduced national influence of Catholic and Protestant religious groups, many continue to be deeply spiritual.[5] Thus, there has been a "return to sacralization, the relocation of the sacred in a new individual and holistic manner."[6] The growth of holistic spirituality since the 1960s has influenced the sacralization of the subjective life.[7] God is located within oneself, and through the subjective life, spiritual practices are honed and generated.[8] Secularization has not meant the disappearance of religion and spirituality, but its redefinition and reorganization.[9]

Such transformations of religious and spiritual practices in Western society have, in part, been affected by the women's rights movement during the 1960s. Not only were the conventional gendered constructions of religious traditions challenged, specifically traditional Christianity in the West, but also religious change in Western Europe and North America has been "strongly influenced by long-term and largely unexamined changes in women's lives."[10] The shift in social patterns such as women's employment outside of the home, the demand for equal status, and the right to make decisions about their own lives altered women's patterns of religiosity.[11] Brown argues that women's abandonment of traditional forms of religion is a key to understanding larger patterns of religious and spiritual pluralism.[12] As a result of changes to various aspects of women's lives spurred on by feminism, many formed new spiritual collectives that affirmed their voices and roles. There has since been a proliferation of distinct groups, including Wiccans, Ecofeminists, Goddess Feminists, and Neo-Pagan groups.[13]

In recent years, other social patterns, like global migration, have meant an increase in the diversity in religious affiliations and spiritual practices and new forms of syncretization. Increased immigration from India, Asia, the Middle East, and Africa to historically Christian-dominant nations has created growing Muslim, Buddhist, Sikh, and Hindu communities.[14]

These diasporic communities in the context of globalization tend to retain strong ties to their religion.[15] Although a decline has been noted in mainline Protestant and Catholic forms of Christianity in the West, other Christian strands, particularly evangelical and charismatic groups, have grown.[16] The growth of newcomers to North America has had an impact on the development of religious and spiritual pluralism, often resulting in instances of religious and spiritual syncretism as well as contextualization. For decades now, the traditional Euro-North American Christian understanding of the nature of God has been changing as a result of the effervescent input of Christian and non-Christian theologies from outside the West, including those from India, Africa, Latin America, and Asia.[17] There are also numerous instances of people who might best be described as "fusers," those who, for example, represent new forms of spiritualized Christianity, bringing together Christian modes of belief with Neo-Paganism, Hindu yogic practices, and/or Buddhist forms of meditation, to name a few.[18] Such fusions are individualized: some are syncretic fusions of content and some are fusions of practices that leave preexisting beliefs untouched.

Some level of syncretization occurs in virtually every religion where divergent belief structures are combined, often heterogeneously and without reconciliation. In modern contexts, syncretization may also occur between religious beliefs and specific nonreligious cultural values. Niebuhr discussed the elision of Christian faith and American culture in a way that is so commingled that they become inseparable.[19] A Christian evangelical emphasis on the non-Biblical American value of radical individualism serves as one example. *Syncretization* differs from *contextualization* or *inculturation* in that contextualization does not challenge the basic beliefs or structures. Instead, contextualization of a religion imports into the cultus system of religious beliefs and rituals indigenous forms of music, prayer, piety, and so forth. Historically, religions that colonized, missionized, conquered, or burst forth have shown some syncretization with existing indigenous or dominant religions before or as they gained ascendency. Where two cultures met or perhaps collided, religious ideas would be exchanged and customarily those of the dominant culture would prevail. For example, the Roman Empire commandeered the gods of other conquered cultures, fusing them with or remaking them into Roman gods. The Romans imported the Anatolian goddess Cybele and the Celtic God Sucellus. Christianity, too, has a history of permitting prior "old beliefs" and practices to persist where they did not overtly conflict with Christianity or could be remade as Christian. To illustrate, the pre-Christian "green man," a leafy male face associated with death and spring renewal, serves as an architectural adornment to cathedrals in north England. As another example, Regla de Ocha Santería is a system of beliefs that merges the Yoruba religion, brought by enslaved peoples transported to the Carribean, with Roman Catholic and Native American traditions.

Such historical and contemporary social shifts have culminated in attempts to define what religion and spirituality mean to society today. Modernity, urbanization, and global migration have caused many scholars to consider how these occurrences have affected the phenomena of religion and spirituality. In a time characterized by the crossover of cultures, races, and faith traditions, where forms of spirituality and religiosity are consistently challenged, negotiated, and generated, defining the many ways that people live out their relationship to the divine or to the sacred is particularly difficult. There are many definitions of each, with religion often thought of as institutional, bureaucratic, social, inflexible, authoritarian, and bound by history and hierarchy, and spirituality, as "personal, unique, self-validating, authentic, and authoritative . . . emphasizing individual experience."[20] At one point, spirituality might have been considered as that which religious institutions like the church, synagogue, mosque, or temple defined, but now many wish to define spirituality as that which originates in the personal, making it difficult to give one definition that applies to all who live out spiritual lives. Undoubtedly, the developing processes of individualization and secularization have therefore been crucial to the varied conceptions and forms of religiosity and spirituality and their continued presence in Western societies. Religion and spirituality, thus, need to also be thought of as historically specific and dependent on historical processes and geocultural contexts.[21]

In considering these numerous social patterns, one of the areas in which there has been a proliferation of interest in spirituality is the nursing profession. For more than a decade, there has been a growing and new attention to the spirit in nursing. Spirituality, for many nurses, gives a way, conceptually and clinically, to contextualize illness, suffering, death, and healing.[22] Many health care professionals recognize that with illness there may be personal questions about the meaning of illness and suffering, and thus an imperative to address not just physical ailments but also matters of faith and spirituality. The body is increasingly considered in its wholeness, not in discrete parts. Spirituality is now more accepted in theory and practice, as a contributor to health and well-being.[23]

Interestingly, a new line of work related to healing has emerged simultaneously, in which women provide alternate forms of caring. Alongside women's work of care in nursing, there has been a preponderance of women in holistic spirituality. This has been for many women a way in which they have found subjective fulfillment. While men find purpose and advancement in numerous domains like business, entertainment, academia, and medicine, many of these doors still remain closed to women. Woodhead contends that women have found purpose-filled lives in industries that focus on beauty and alternate forms of health and well-being. The explosive growth of such forms of work and life for women over the past decades in many instances correlates with the increased emphasis on spirituality.[24] Women's distancing from traditional religions and the conventional roles espoused by these means women have been able to find for themselves, in the realm of holistic spirituality, financial independence, new forms of identity, spiritual communities, and practices.[25]

THE NATURE OF EMERGENT SPIRITUALITIES

In considering these numerous changes to religion and spirituality, spiritual persons are often more interested in ethical guidelines and spiritual disciplines than in doctrines, resulting in a universal trend away from hierarchical, regional, patriarchal, and institutional religion.[26] The movement toward a partial de-institutionalization of religion and spirituality has meant a reorganization of how religion and spirituality are lived and

practiced. The field is diverse with numerous religious and spiritual practices and approaches in the West. Emergent nonreligious spiritualities
moreover share commonalities that are situated in Western traditions that
are fascinated with the inner life of the self, and nature as a source of
beauty and meaning.[27] Even though they can be difficult to place on alternative spiritualities such as these, "they do not have roots in any particular
religion, but are principally rooted if not always solely in modern Western
culture."[28]

Robinson characterizes emergent spiritualities—what he refers to as
the "New Age Movement"—with the following themes: asserting freedom
of spirituality from patriarchy, institutions, and authorities; tolerance for a
great range of spirituality with all free to choose their own spiritual path;
spirituality as concerned with the "other worldly," often stressing the mystical or magical; spirituality as antirational and embracing of feelings and
experience; the interconnectedness of all forms of life.[29] Although terms
such as "emergent" and "New Age" connote novelty, the movement *also*
recaptures ancient traditions, for example, paganism, Druidism, both real
and conjectural.

In identifying people who practice emergent spirituality, it is important to get a sense of how they live, their approach to life, which can reveal
their personal ethics and customs. Many people who practice such forms of
spirituality might be in addition to meditation classes, retreating to scenic
landscapes to practice yoga or contemplate the psyche or self, to experience
the spiritual. Significant to such spiritual practices is the intertwinement of
nature and self. In people's everyday worlds, we see, for example, a rising interest in home and community gardens, the growing prominence of organic
and local food movements, and environmental initiatives related to recy-
cling, composting, and carbon footprints. The ever-growing importance of
well-being consists of eating well, communing with others, living a healthy
lifestyle, and taking care of the environment in which one lives.[30] These
aspects have become embedded and widely evident in film and television
shows; web sites; magazines at the supermarket; food products on stores
shelves; whole sections devoted to mind, body, and spirit at bookstores;
organic and local food served at local cafes and restaurants; offices with
spaces in which one can be quiet; classrooms teaching meditation to young
people; and school cafeterias reinventing their menus to reflect a healthy
holistic lifestyle. These practices can be eclectic and compatible with or
supportive of earth-centered spiritualities, ecology movements, feminism,
and seeker movements as well as with traditional religions. Though these
spiritual practices are not necessarily linked to traditional theology or religion, and in some cases to historical evidence, their moral groundings are
not free-floating or completely relativist, but coalesce with anti-patriarchal,
anti-capitalist, earth-centred, and social justice commitments.[31] Health

choices are now linked to global ecology, health and well-being linked to a larger, holistic natural order.

Because this type of spirituality emerges from modern western culture, it inevitably intersects with social class and race. Class is related to power inequalities structured by income, education, family background, and location. It is also concerned with relationships, identities, boundaries, and those distinctions we make between others and ourselves. Class "can be explicit or hidden, conscious or unconscious . . . Class factors into how we vote, what kinds of bread we eat, and even how we worship and live our religion," or spirituality.[32] Carette and King argue that within many Western societies, religion has taken a backseat to a new capitalist spirituality seen in the proliferation of self-help literature and products that emphasize the individual and that channel spiritualized forms of Western and Eastern religions.[33] With a critical eye to how spirituality is often considered neutral ground, they view modern practices and understandings of spirituality as underscored by values that often promote consumerism and corporate capitalism. This results in the commoditization of spirituality, which has the capacity to be available only to those who can afford it.

Although intended as inclusive, emergent spirituality discourses—particularly where a sharp distinction is made between spirituality and religion—have been questioned as perpetuating White Euro Christian privilege and taking on a racializing dimension.[34] Henery notes that ethnic minorities who adhere to non-Christian religions are deemed as religious first, then spiritual.[35] When the "spiritual-but-not-religious" binary is operationalized, they are automatically placed in the non-favored half of the binary, thus reinscribing social relations of "other." As explained by Wong and Vinsky: "if the racialized ethnic 'other' is religious and culturally bound by traditions and doctrines, the Western 'self' is spiritual, free and independent in their personal quest of the 'Ultimate'. The ordering of social relations between the 'spiritual' Western 'self' and the 'religious' ethnic 'other' is produced."[36] A further problem arises with the Western propensity to view all religious traditions as part of the spiritual marketplace where individuals can choose freely to adopt various practices and beliefs (for example, chanting, indigenous spiritualities, yoga) that are divorced from their historical and contextual roots,[37] a process that may diminish and expropriate complex and long-standing belief systems. The distancing of spirituality from historical roots may thus pose consternation for people of marginalized and racialized communities who fight to have their traditions and histories recognized within dominant society.[38] The point to be made here is that of the complexities and multiplicities involved in spiritual and religious identities, and the need to create inclusive spaces for the full range of expressions and affiliations, a goal that must be reflected in nursing's approaches to spirituality and religion.

EMERGENT SPIRITUALITIES, NURSING, AND ETHICS

Trends of emergent spirituality are threaded through contemporary nursing theory and practice, although not typically positioned or articulated as "emergent," or "alternative." When spirituality discourses in nursing are examined more closely, the qualities associated with emergent spiritualities are apparent. Themes of holism, ecology, pantheism, eclectic mixing of various spiritual traditions, and personalized ontologies of spirituality are relatively common in nursing spirituality discourses. Given that individualized and subjective admixing or syncretization is a feature of alternative spiritualities, we include in our discussion nursing literature that may well demonstrate remnants of admixt Christian, Eastern, indigenous and other theologies and philosophies of religion.

Several typologies of spirituality and nursing have been developed that provide structure to our interest in explicating the implications of emergent spiritualities for nursing.[39] Pesut's typology organizes spirituality discourses within nursing as theist, humanist, and monist.[40] McSherry and Cash articulate a typology, deriving from different branches of philosophy that includes theistic, religious, phenomenological, existential, and mystical descriptors for conceptions of spirituality within nursing.[41] Tinley and Kinney take a similar approach of classifying spirituality discourse within nursing according to three philosophic paradigms: empiricism, interpretivism, and poststructuralism.[42] Emergent nonreligious spiritualities map on to these typologies as existential and mystical;[43] interpretivist/poststructural;[44] and monist.[45] Taking guidance from these typologies, theoretical examples of emergent spiritualities would include Watson's postmodern nursing and caring theory; Parse's Theory of Human Becoming; Barnum's discussion of New Age nursing; and the holistic nursing movement.[46]

A shared underlying assumption is that humanity is part of an indivisible universal consciousness extending beyond space, time, and the human body.[47] In the language of the holistic nursing movement also referred to as integral nursing: "an integral understanding recognizes the wholeness of humanity and the world that is open, dynamic, interdependent, fluid, and continuously interacting with changing variables that can lead to greater complexity and order."[48] Persons are deemed primarily spiritual rather than biopsychosocial beings.[49] Health is seen as balance, integration, harmony, right relationship, and the betterment of well-being, not just the absence of disease.[50] Spirituality is understood as integrative energy, with emphasis on immanence the divine within the individual and the everyday and interconnectedness.[51] Nursing practice and health-related decisions strives to be contextual and ecological. Nursing practice informed by emergent spiritualities is described as carrying emphases on aesthetic knowing, intuition, and creativity; caring and relationship-centered nursing; and as healing-oriented.[52] Broadly speaking, nurses working within this paradigm bring together bodywork and soul work, what Barnum referred to as the scientific model, or "doing," and the New Age paradigm, or "being."[53]

These theoretical expressions of emergent spiritualities result in an approach to ethics that is highly contextual, with an emphasis on "lived ethics" —ethics as a way of being rather than as a way of knowing, with discrete frameworks for ethical decision making.[54] Spohn explains:

> "Lived spirituality," analogous to morality, refers to the practice of transformative, affective, practical and holistic disciplines that seek to connect the person with reality's deepest meanings . . . Reflective spirituality, analogous to ethics, stands for the second-order interpretation and communication of this dimension of experience as experience. It employs theological, historical-contextual, artistic, anthropological and hermeneutical methods to analyze lived experience.[55]

As the foundations of ethics, and bioethics in particular, were distanced from religious and theological traditions in the 1960s and 1970s, the trend was to locate ethics in a rationalist model of principalism.[56] Using allegedly neutral, secular, or philosophical language, the move legitimated ethics in the domain of biomedicine and positioned bioethics as influential in regulating sometimes through legislation the fields of medicine and health care research.[57] Such approaches to bioethics, and now health care and nursing ethics, are increasingly criticized, with calls for alternative ethical systems influenced by feminist, indigenous, and other contemporary theories, as well as an examination of the cultural and philosophical situatedness of contemporary bioethics. Feminists Gilligan[58] and Noddings,[59] for example, laid the groundwork for care ethics—*ethics of care*—that have developed as a promising alternative to dominant moral approaches.[60] A further ethical theme prominent in emergent spiritualities is that of *ecological ethics*, in which dichotomies between human and nonhuman life forms are countered, and the concern is how to treat the entire natural world based on the premise that nature, which includes humanity, is the ultimate source of all value.[61] Lynch,[62] a sociologist of religion, challenges those who equate emergent spiritualities with social trends toward demoralization, noting that there have been shifts in sources of moral authority, but that emergent spiritualities are neither free-floating nor completely relativistic. Rather, new spiritualities coalesce around *social ethics* that are non-patriarchal, earth-centered, and committed to social justice. Indeed, Lynch explains that many advocates of progressive spiritualities "resist the demoralizing effects of a rationalized, dehumanized, capitalist system."[63] Prozesky expands on this position, with an assertion that spiritually enriched ethics, such as those characteristic of emergent spiritualities, provide greater moral and spiritual cohesion than secular, humanist, or religious ethics.[64]

There are varying degrees to which caring ethics, ecological ethics, and social ethics are emphasized within those nursing theories most characteristic of emergent spiritualities. Burkhardt and Keegan, for example, define holistic ethics under the umbrella of holistic nursing as

> the basic underlying concept of the unity and integral wholeness of all people and of all nature, which is identified and pursued by finding unity and wholeness within one's self and within humanity. In this framework, acts are not performed for the sake of law, precedent, or social norms, but rather from a desire to do good freely to witness, identify, and contribute to unity.[65]

Holistic ethics embraces and strives for fusion between self and others, flowing to a cosmic ecology. From this perspective, all events and ethical decisions become part of the unfolding of a harmonious order and a realization of potentials. Watson puts forward the ethic of caring as the first principle or ultimate moral foundation for nurses.[66] These theories result in ethical approaches that are not focused on rational decision making through the application of universal principles, but instead a focus on the context that lifts the human spirit.[67] Watson articulates a further distinction, where nurses from traditional stances perform actions out of a sense of duty or moral obligation, nurses from an emergent standpoint do so out of a "higher sense of spirit of self."[68]

IMPLICATIONS FOR ETHICAL NURSING PRACTICE

Our interest in this chapter is to provide theoretical and analytical foundations that can guide nurses in understanding patients who align with emergent spiritualities; or who themselves practice from the perspective of emergent spiritualities.[69] In this last section, we explore practice-relevant implications of emergent spiritualities for nursing ethics, focusing on self-knowledge for nurses and patient-focused ethics.

As with all religious and spiritual identities, it is incumbent upon the nurse to be highly self-aware to avoid coercion, such as that which might result from assuming universally shared views of spirituality as integrative, personal, energy-based, and apart from religion and imposing those views. Self-awareness is also necessary in regard to one's own particularistic views that could prevent the nurse from hearing what the patient is saying or cause nurses to see what they are already looking for. Generally, nurses in this tradition are likely to strive for an awareness of the interconnectedness of individuals to the human and global community, tending to the health of the ecosystem. It is not uncommon for nurses practicing emergent spiritualities to view themselves as instruments of healing, while recognizing that the person is the authority on his or her own health experience. They focus on practices of self-care, intentionality, presence, mindfulness, and therapeutic use of self as key for facilitation of healing in self and others.[70] "Soul care" tends to be elevated over "bodily care" as primary function of the nurse within emergent or monist nursing theories.[71]

Because of this difference in focus, nursing within emergent spiritualities tends toward a different moral horizon. Barnum explains:

> In a New Age paradigm, rights and equity often dissolve into broad perspectives, possibly involving reincarnation and ultimate soul growth. A nurse operating in this paradigm may feel that there is not adequate knowledge to make any judgments concerning what is fair or equitable. Her principles arise from other sources. A nurse holding a New Age ideology might find the problem of scarcity beside the point. She might argue that prolonging or enhancing life is not itself an important goal. She might hold that solving these problems could obstruct the soul development of persons who have elected to experience lives cut short at a young age or lives lived in difficult situations. Indeed, she might consider the markers of life, death, and comfort to be inconsequential in the longer view of a soul's development over various lifetimes.[72]

Barnum's particular interpretation of emergent spirituality ethics points toward potential conflict in religious-moral values in situations where the nurse and the patient do not share the same worldview. Barnum elaborates:

> Patients and nurses may have radically different expectations. Patients expect nurses will take care of them when they are ill . . . If a nurse were introduced to the patient as a professional who is there to expand his consciousness or put his soul back in harmony, many patients might be confused.[73]

A similar example illustrating such conflict comes from a study where a Christian male told of coming to consciousness following an accident and being horrified by a nurse at his bedside, initiating therapeutic touch.[74] The professional codes of ethics of both the Canadian and American nurses' associations provide clear statements of the nurse's accountability to patients, respecting the values and beliefs they hold. Nurses have the responsibility to affirm the values of the patient in their nursing care, to guard against coercion, to ensure patient confidentiality, to reflect on the influence of their own spiritual selves, and to serve the needs of a diverse society.[75]

A similar degree of self-awareness and patient-focus is required in the case where it is the patient, not the nurse, holding to emergent spirituality. McSherry notes that the postmodern forms of emergent spirituality are very subjective, containing an infinite number of descriptors that may be

> phenomenological and existentially determined such as meaning and pur-
> pose in life, creativity, and relationships . . . . Nurses in practice may experi-
> ence difficulty in attending to patients whose spiritual needs arise out of such
> a definition because they may be subjective making them hard to address.[76]

This remark underlines the importance of nurses following the cues of patients in determining what might be meaningful for them. Patients who hold to emergent spiritualities may well integrate a range of nontraditional healing modalities, along with more traditional allopathic medical interventions. For example, some patients have decorated their hospital bedsides with artifacts such as special fabric and crystals that represent forms of spirituality and healing to them. Nursing practices that may be welcomed to encompass emergent spiritualities are being present, fostering mindfulness, self-nurturing activities, and creation of and participation in healing rituals.[77] Emergent spiritualities celebrate life, and birth is therefore viewed as sacred and empowering.[78] Because of a commonly held belief in some form of reincarnation, death tends to be viewed as a transition within a continuing process of existence. Death is accepted as a natural part of life and many wish to know they are dying so that they may consciously prepare for it.

Ethical practice as a way-of-being that centers on awareness of self and other, developing meaning through critical hermeneutic inquiry and dialogue, and generating creative responses to the ethical dilemma best typifies an ethics of emergent spirituality.[79] Emphasis is placed on moral development of those involved in "making meaning" as well as the development of the involved community what Robinson refers to as a "community of care." He cautions against individualistic applications of spirituality to ethics:

> Spirituality cannot be seen simply as individualistic, with the person choos-
> ing to take what they want from "religious experience." It is about making
> sense of and responding to the communities of which we are a part, from
> local to global, from family to environment.[80]

Because spirituality is embedded in moral responsibility, and is a part of and responsive to the person's social and physical context, it is relation-centered, rather than individual-centered. From such a stance, it is not the task of the health care community to solve ethical dilemmas for patients, or to medicalize spirituality with terms such as "spiritual distress" or "spiritual pain."[81] Rather, the care community provides an environment in which the patient can make sense of his or her experience as lived in relationship, and this may well involve connecting to existing values and beliefs. Where the care community also continually reflects on its meaning, it is better able to resist dehumanizing conditions (for example, unbalanced rationalism or managerialism) and respond to each other in hope, moral imagination, and transformation.[82] Ethics of care, ecological ethics, and social ethics are reflected in this vision.

CONCLUDING COMMENTS

Emergent spiritualities are increasingly common in today's postmodern societies and are strongly influencing the nursing profession. These spiritualities open up possibilities for engagement with non-patriarchal, ecological, feminist, and relational ethical dialogues, and thus are a great contribution to nursing, health, and health care services. Because emergent spiritualities tend to represent a personal, individual worldview rather than a shared view, a nurse's self-awareness and an affirmation of the patient's meaning systems are of utmost importance.

NOTES

1. Lynch, Gordon. *The New Spirituality: An Introduction to Progressive Belief in the Twenty-first Century*. London: I. B. Tauris, 2007.
2. Bruce, Steve. *God is Dead: Secularization in the West*. Oxford: Blackwell, 2002.
3. Woodhead, Linda. "Why So Many Women in Holistic Spirituality? A Puzzle Revisited." *A Sociology of Spirituality*. Eds. Kieran C. Flanagan and Peter C. Jupp. Aldershot, Hampshire, UK: Ashgate, 2007. 115–25.
4. Heelas, Paul, and Linda Woodhead. *The Spiritual Revolution: Why Religion is Giving Way to Spirituality*. Oxford, UK: Blackwell, 2005.
5. Bibby, Reginald. "Canada's Mythical Religious Mosaic: Some Census Findings." *Journal for the Scientific Study of Religion* 39.2 (2000): 235–39.
6. Vincett, Giselle, Sonya Sharma, and Kristin Aune. "Women, Religion and Secularization in the West: One Size Does Not Fit All." *Women and Religion in the West: Challenging Secularization*. Eds. Giselle Vincett, Sonya Sharma, and Kristin Aune. Aldershot, Hampshire, UK: Ashgate, 2008. 1–13.
7. Woodhead, Linda. "Why So Many Women in Holistic Spirituality? A Puzzle Revisited." *A Sociology of Spirituality*. Eds. Kieran C. Flanagan and Peter C. Jupp. Aldershot, Hampshire, UK: Ashgate, 2007. 115–25.
8. Heelas, Paul and Linda Woodhead. *The Spiritual Revolution: Why Religion is Giving Way to Spirituality*.
9. Gökariksel, Banu. "Beyond the Officially Sacred: Religion, Secularism, and the Body in the Production of Subjectivity." *Social & Cultural Geography* 10.6 (2009): 657–74.

10. See for example Mary Daly's. *Beyond God the Father.* Boston: Beacon Press, 1985. Also see Marler, Penny Long. "Religious Change in the West: Watch the Women." *Women and Religion in the West: Challenging Secularization.* Eds. Giselle Vincett, Sonya Sharma, and Kristin Aune. Aldershot, Hampshire, UK: Ashgate, 2008. 23–56.

11. Marler, Penny Long. "Religious Change in the West: Watch the Women." 23–56. See also: Woodhead, Linda. "'Because I'm Worth It': Religion and Women's Changing Lives." *Women and Religion in the West: Challenging Secularization.* Eds. Giselle Vincett, Sonya Sharma, and Kristin Aune. Aldershot, Hampshire, UK: Ashgate, 2008. 147–61. See also: Brown, Callum. *The Death of Christian Britain.* London: Routledge, 2001.

12. Brown, Callum. *The Death of Christian Britain.* London: Routledge, 2001.

13. Anderson, Leona M., and Pamela Dickey Young, eds. *Women and Religious Traditions.* Toronto: Oxford University Press, 2004.

14. Levey, Geoffrey B. and Tariq Modood. *Secularism, Religion and Multicultural Citizenship.* Cambridge: Cambridge University Press, 2009.

15. Reimer-Kirkham, Sheryl, and Sonya Sharma. "Adding Religion to Gender, Race, and Class: Seeking New Insights on Intersectionality in Health Care Contexts." *Intersectionality-Type Health Research in Canada.* Ed. O. Hankivsky. Vancouver, B.C.: University of British Columbia Press, 2011. 112-127.

16. Martin, David. "Secularisation and the Future of Christianity." *Journal of Contemporary Religion* 20.2 (2005): 145–60.

17. Cox, Harvey. *The Future of Faith.* New York: Harper Collins Publishers, 2009.

18. Vincett, Giselle. "The Fusers: New Forms of Spiritualized Christianity." *Women and Religion in the West: Challenging Secularization.* Eds. Giselle Vincett, Sonya Sharma, and Kristin Aune. Aldershot, Hampshire, UK: Ashgate, 2008. 133–45.

19. Niebuhr, H. Richard. *Christ and Culture.* New York: Harper Torchbooks, 1951. 83–15.

20. Anderson, Leona M., and Pamela Dickey Young, eds. *Women and Religious Traditions.* Toronto: Oxford University Press, 2004. 219.

21. See Asad, Talal. *Genealogies of Religion: Discipline and Reasons of Power in Christianity and Islam.* Baltimore, MD: Johns Hopkins University Press, 1993. See also: Asad, Talal. *Formations of the Secular: Christianity, Islam, Modernity.* Stanford, CA: Stanford University Press, 2003.

22. Holmes, Peter R. "Spirituality: Some Disciplinary Perspectives." *A Sociology of Spirituality.* Eds. Kieran C. Flanagan and Peter C. Jupp. Aldershot, Hampshire, UK: Ashgate, 2007. 23–42.

23. McSherry, Wilfred. "Making Sense of Spirituality in Nursing and Health Care." 2nd ed. Philadelphia, PA: Jessica Kingsley Publishers, 2006. See also: Orchard, Helen C. ed. *Spirituality in Health Care Contexts.* London, UK: Jessica Kingsley Publishers, 2001. See also: Koenig, Harold G. "Religion, Spirituality and Medicine: A Rebuttal to Skeptics." *International Journal of Psychiatry in Religion* 29.2 (1999): 123–31.

24. Woodhead, Linda. "Why so Many Women in Holistic Spirituality? A Puzzle Revisited." 115–25.

25. Ibid.

26. Cox, Harvey. *The Future of Faith.* New York: HarperCollins Publishers, 2009.

27. Lynch, Gordon. *The New Spirituality: An Introduction to Progressive Belief in the Twenty-first Century.* London: I. B. Tauris, 2007. 124.

28. Partridge, Chris. "Introduction." *Encyclopedia of New Religions: New Religious Movements, Sects and Alternative Spiritualities*. Ed. Chris Partridge. Oxford, UK: Lion Publishing, 2004. 23.

29. Robinson, Simon. *Spirituality, Ethics, and Care*. London, UK: Jessica Kingsley Publishers, 2008.

30. Lynch, Gordon. *The New Spirituality: An Introduction to Progressive Belief in the Twenty-first Century*.

31. Ibid.

32. McCloud, Sean. *Divine Hierarchies: Class in American Religion and Religious Studies*. Chapel Hill, NC: University of North Carolina Press, 2007. 2.

33. Carrette, Jeremy, and Richard King. *Selling of Spirituality: The Silent Takeover of Religion*. New York: Routledge, 2005.

34. For further discussion see: Wong, Yuk-Lin Renita and Jana Vinsky. "Speaking from the Margins: A Critical Reflection on the 'Spiritual-but-not-Religious' Discourse in Social Work." *British Journal of Social Work* 39 (2009): 1343–59; Henery, Neil. "The Reality of Visions: Contemporary Theories of Spirituality in Social Work." *British Journal of Social Work* 33 (2003): 1105–13; and Joshi, Kyatri. "The racialization of Hinduism, Islam, and Sikhism in the United States." *Equity and Excellence in Education* 39.3 (2006): 211–26.

35. Henery, Neil. "The Reality of Visions: Contemporary Theories of Spirituality in Social Work." *British Journal of Social Work* 33 (2003): 1105–13.

36. Wong, Yuk-Lin Renita and Jana Vinsky. "Speaking from the Margins: A Critical Reflection on the 'Spiritual-but-not-Religious' Discourse in Social Work." 11.

37. Carrette, Jeremy, and Richard King. *Selling of Spirituality: The Silent Takeover of Religion*.

38. Wong, Yuk-Lin Renita and Jana Vinsky. "Speaking from the Margins: A Critical Reflection on the 'Spiritual-but-not-Religious' Discourse in Social Work."

39. Other such typologies have been created outside of nursing. See: Fenwick, Tara, and Leona English. Dimensions of spirituality. A framework for adult educators. *Journal of Adult Theological Education*, 1.1 (2004). See also: Twigg, N., and S. Parayitam. "Spirit at Work: Spiritual Typologies as Theory Builders." *Journal of Organizational Culture, Communications and Conflict* 10.2 (2006): 117-133. Twigg and Parayitam 2006 map spirituality/religion on a quadrant of transcendence and connectedness, with emergent or "new age/popular" falling in the quadrant of low transcendence and high connectedness.

40. Pesut, Barbara. "A Philosophic Analysis of the Spiritual in Nursing Literature." Diss. University of British Columbia, Vancouver, B.C., 2005.

41. McSherry, Wilfred and Keith Cash. "The Language of Spirituality: An Emerging Typology." *International Journal of Nursing Studies* 41.2 (2004): 151–61.

42. Tinley, Susan, and Anita Y. Kinney. "Three Philosophical Approaches to the Study of Spirituality." *Advances in Nursing Science* 30.1 (2007): 71–80.

43. McSherry, Wilfred, and Keith Cash. "The Language of Spirituality: An Emerging Typology." 151–61.

44. Tinley, Susan, and Anita Y. Kinney. "Three Philosophical Approaches to the Study of Spirituality." 71–80.

45. Pesut, Barbara. "A Philosophic Analysis of the Spiritual in Nursing Literature."

46. Watson, Jean. *Nursing: Human Science and Human Care: A Theory of Nursing*. Sudbury, MA: Jones & Bartlett, 1999. See also: Parse, Rosemary. *ManLiving-Health: A Theory of Nursing*. New York: Wiley, 1981. And: Barnum, Barbara. *Spirituality in*

Nursing: From Traditional to New Age. 2nd ed. New York: Springer, 2006. See for example, Dossey, Barbara M., and Lynn Keegan. *Holistic Nursing: A Handbook for Practice*. 5th ed. Sudbury, MA: Jones & Bartlett, 2009.

47. Pesut, Barbara. "A Philosophic Analysis of the Spiritual in Nursing Literature." 49.
48. Dossey, B. M. "Integral and Holistic Nursing: Local to Global." *Holistic Nursing: A Handbook for Practice*. 5th ed. Eds. Barbara M.Dossey, and Lynn Keegan. Sudbury, MA: Jones & Bartlett, 2009. 40.
49. See Barnum, B. *Spirituality in Nursing: From Traditional to New Age*. 2nd ed.
50. Mariano, C. "Holistic Nursing: Scope and Standards of Practice." *Holistic Nursing: A Handbook for Practice*. 5th ed. Eds. Barbara M. Dossey, and Lynn Keegan. Sudbury, MA: Jones & Bartlett, 2009. 47–74.
51. Lauver, D. "Commonalities in Women's Spiritualities and Women's Health." *Advances in Nursing Science* 22.3 (2000): 76–88. See also: Twigg, Nicholas W., and Satyanarayana Parayitam. "Spirit at Work: Spiritual Typologies as Theory Builders." *Journal of Organizational Culture, Communications and Conflict* 10.2 (2006): 117–33.
52. Keegan, Lynn. "The Art of Holistic Nursing and the Human Health Experience." *Holistic Nursing: A Handbook for Practice*. 5th ed. Eds. Barbara M. Dossey, and Lynn Keegan. Sudbury, MA: Jones & Bartlett, 2009. 101–12. And: Mariano, Carla. "Holistic Nursing: Scope and Standards of Practice." 47–74.
53. Barnum, Barbara S. *Spirituality in Nursing: From Traditional to New Age*. 2nd ed.
54. Bruce, A. "Opening Conversations: Dilemmas and Possibilities of Spirituality and Spiritual Care." *Realities of Canadian Nursing: Professional, Practice, and Power Issues*. 3rd ed. Eds. M. McIntyre, and C. McDonald. Toronto: Lippincott, 2010. 455–69.
55. Spohn, W. "Spirituality and Ethics: Exploring the Connections." *Theological Studies* 58.1 (1997): 109–23.
56. Fowler, Marsha. "Religion, Bioethics, and Nursing Practice." *Nursing Ethics* 16.4 (2009): 393–05. Also: Sowle Cahill, Lisa. "Theology's Role in Public Bioethics." *Handbook of Bioethics and Religion*. Ed. David Guinn. New York: Oxford University Press, 2006. 37–57.
57. Guinn, David, ed. *Handbook of Bioethics and Religion*. New York: Oxford University Press, 2006.
58. Gilligan, Carol. *In a Different Voice: Psychological Theory and Women's Development*. Harvard, MA: Harvard University Press, 1982.
59. Noddings, Nell. *Caring: A Feminine Approach to Ethics and Moral Education*. Berkeley, CA: University of California Press, 1986.
60. Held, Virginia. *The Ethics of Care: Personal, Political, and Global*. Oxford, UK: Oxford University Press, 2006.
61. Curry, Patrick. *Ecological Ethics: An Introduction*. Cambridge, UK: Polity Press, 2006.
62. Lynch, Gordon. *The New Spirituality: An Introduction to Progressive Belief in the Twenty-first Century*.
63. Ibid., 155.
64. Prozesky, M. "'Everything that Rises Must Converge': Some Ideas for an Ethical Spirituality and a Spiritually-Enriched Ethic." *Spirituality and Society in the New Millennium*. Ed. Ursula King. Brighton, UK: Sussex Academic Press, 2001. 179–91.
65. Burkhardt, Margaret, and Lynn Keegan. "Holistic Ethics." *Holistic Nursing: A Handbook for Practice*. 5th ed. Eds. Barbara M. Dossey, and Lynn Keegan. Sudbury, MA: Jones & Bartlett, 2009. 125.

66. Watson, Jean. *Caring Science as Sacred Science.* Philadelphia, PA: F.A. Davis, 2005.

67. Barnum, Barbara. *Spirituality in Nursing: From Traditional to New Age.* 2nd ed. Also: Pesut, Barbara. "A Philosophic Analysis of the Spiritual in Nursing Literature."

68. Barnum, Barbara. *Spirituality in Nursing: From Traditional to New Age.* 2nd ed. 188.

69. We offer but brief general comments here, given that many sources exist that provide more specific direction for nursing practice. See: Watson, Jean. *Caring Science as Sacred Science.* See also: Barnum, Barbara. *Spirituality in Nursing: From Traditional to New Age.* 2nd ed.; Dossey, Barbara M. and Lynn Keegan. *Holistic Nursing: A Handbook for Practice.* 5th ed.

70. Mariano, C. "Holistic Nursing: Scope and Standards of Practice." 47–74.

71. Pesut, Barbara. "A Philosophic Analysis of the Spiritual in Nursing Literature."

72. Barnum, Barbara. *Spirituality in Nursing: From Traditional to New Age.* 2nd ed. 190.

73. Ibid., 124.

74. Pesut, Barbara, and Sheryl Reimer-Kirkham. "Situated clinical encounters in the negotiation of religious and spiritual plurality: A critical ethnography." *International Journal of Nursing Studies* 47.7 (2010): 815-825.

75. Pesut, Barbara. "A Philosophic Analysis of the Spiritual in Nursing Literature."

76. McSherry, Wilfred. *The Meaning of Spirituality and Spiritual Care within Nursing and Health Care Practice.* London, UK: Quay Books, 2007. 37.

77. Lauver, D. "Commonalities in Women's Spiritualities and Women's Health."

78. National Health Service for Education of Scotland. *A Multi-Faith Resource for Healthcare Staff.* Glasgow, UK: NHS Scotland, 2006.

79. Robinson, Simon. *Spirituality, Ethics, and Care.*

80. Ibid., 192.

81. Robinson, Simon. *Spirituality, Ethics, and Care.*

82. Ibid.

16

Religion and Patient Care

Elizabeth Johnston Taylor

A nurse's initial mental image of religion may be that of Jehovah's Witness patient refusing to receive a blood product. Or it may be of a Christian Scientist who refuses medical advice, or a Jewish or Christian Sabbatarian who prefers to not have surgery on Saturday. This chapter goes beyond those images to how religious beliefs can influence patient responses to health challenges. This will be done by exploring religious interpretations of illness, and by reviewing the literature that shows associations between religious coping (RC) and adjustment, and religiosity and decision making. This literature will reveal how religious beliefs have an impact on patients in much more subtle ways than those images to which nurses are drawn. The chapter also explores the interplay of religious practices and health, and what religious care patients want and get. The chapter will conclude by identifying implications this evidence provides for clinical nursing practice.

Some caveats about the use of the concept of religion in the literature are necessary. Much of the pertinent literature on these topics mix or join the terms spirituality and religion. For example, a researcher may describe "spiritual practices," but then identify prayer or a faith in God as the indicator of these practices. Effort is given to delimit the literature reviewed in this chapter to that which is described as involving religion or religiosity. Also, when studying religion among recipients of health care, researchers use a variety of measures to indicate the concept. For example, religion may be the frequency of attendance at religious services, religious affiliation, intrinsic or extrinsic religiosity (i.e., a lived, internalized religion vs. a religion used for some personal gain), a more subjective "faith" component of spiritual well-being, or some other aspect of religion. Thus, it is important to consider the way religion is empirically indicated when examining this complex arena of religion in health research. (For more on measurement of religious concepts, please see Chapter 18.)

RELIGIOUS BELIEFS AND ILLNESS

Religious Interpretations of Illness and Suffering

"Suffering is a spiritual phenomenon, an event that strikes at the faith we can have in life."[1] Yet, much of the health care research exploring meanings patients give to suffering despiritualizes it, describing it with psychological theory and terms. Although many researchers have recognized the spiritual nature of meaning-making,[2–4] they typically refrain from more than a nod of acknowledgement about the religious faith that may influence the process.

Empirical Perspectives

Numerous studies suggest finding positive meaning is associated with various indicators of quality of life or adjustment to illness.[5–8] However, some inconsistencies in this body of research may be explained by inadequate measures that reflect conceptualizations of meaning-making that are too broad.[9,10] That is, there is a difference between understanding and construing benefit, seeking and finding meaning (whether it is a sense of understanding or construing a benefit). Likewise, Park and Folkman theorized that there is a difference between global meanings (i.e., assumptions about the world and fundamental commitments and goals persons have—beliefs and purpose religions can provide) and situational meanings (e.g., why the illness, why this person).[11] It is hypothesized that distress is caused when situational meanings challenge global meanings, when one's assumptions about the world are shattered.[12] Conversely, adjustment occurs when one is able to refine or reconstruct global meaning. Sherman and colleagues observe that when they measured meaning among 73 British breast cancer survivors with scales that measured each of these types of meaning-making experience, each was associated with different psychological outcomes.[13] Most significant, however, was that the strongest predictor overall for well-being was positive global meaning. Although these findings ought to be taken with caution due to limited sample size, they do raise awareness of the need to further explore the meanings–especially global meanings—ascribed to illness with more finesse.

These scientific observations corroborate what Mohrmann, Healey, and Childress described over a decade ago about those who believe in God when their beliefs are challenged by suffering.[14] Mohrmann and colleagues suggest three ways in which persons resolve their struggle to make sense of suffering in relation to God:

> You can change what you believe about God, or even whether you believe, in order to devise a way to make sense of the inescapable reality of the suffering and to recreate some kind of order. Or, you can change what you believe about the suffering, even about its reality, so that you make it fit somehow with what you still believe about God. Or, of course, you can do a little of each.[15]

A patient, for example, who is diagnosed with a severely debilitating disease may decide God does not exist, or that God is uninvolved or unconcerned about her welfare. More likely, however, this client may wonder what she did to deserve the disease, or she may opt to construe benefit and believe that the disease is a blessing in some way.

Patient Theological Perspectives

Whereas earlier chapters have discussed global meanings from diverse theological perspectives, this chapter will explore patients' lay theologies for illness and suffering. A dated, yet timely, clinical study of patients with pain presenting to an outpatient clinic identified 11 interpretations for suffering.[16] Most of these categories of lay interpretations can involve religious thinking. The most overt religious interpretations include the following:

- Punishment (e.g., "I am sick because I sinned and disobeyed God.")
- Testing (e.g., "My illness is a test of my faith. Although God doesn't give us more than we can bear, I resent being tested.")
- Resignation to the will of God (e.g., "It's God's will. I can't figure out why, but God let it happen for some reason—maybe.")
- Acceptance of the human condition (e.g., "I have a purpose for living until the end comes. While I hope for a miracle, I realize that I may experience a lot of suffering.")
- Personal growth (e.g., "God is trying to teach me something through this suffering.")
- Divine perspective (e.g., "This disability isn't God's will; but God does give it meaning. As I reflect, I see it as a blessing in disguise.")
- Redemption (e.g., "I can actually rejoice in my suffering, because I am understanding and sharing in Christ's suffering, life and death").

These interpretations likely reflect the worldview of investigator Foley, a Roman Catholic psychologist, and the American culture of the informants. There is evidence, however, from studies of patients in other countries that endorses several of these interpretations.

Many of these studies are influenced by the categorization of meanings offered over 30 years ago by Canadian psychiatrist Lipowski.[17–19] Of Lipowski's eight categories of meaning for illness (i.e., illness as challenge, enemy, punishment, weakness, relief, strategy, irreparable loss, and as value [thought to be a superior way to cope]), several studies link some of these with religious connotations. The meanings most often linked with religious beliefs are challenge, value, and punishment.

Challenge and Value. Although "challenge" was conceived to refer to an active approach to illness whereby the patient strives to master the demands of illness, and "value" was proposed to describe the approach to illness whereby the patient is able to assign some intrinsic worth to the illness, in reality patients often see these two meanings as interrelated.[20] Examples of values (or described in many studies as construed benefits, positive meanings, transformation, or stress-related growth) are feeling closer to God, observing one's faith being stronger, gaining renewed appreciation for life, improving relationships with family and friends, reprioritizing what is really important in life.[21] A majority of patients report these interpretations as part of their response to illness. In an English sample, 62% viewed illness as a "challenge,"[22] whereas only 33% deemed it such in a Swedish study—yet still the most reported meaning.[23] "Value" is reported less often as an interpretation, hovering around 10% in these three studies and 38% in a study of advanced cancer patients when conceptualized as transformation.[24] Studies that explore relationships between these categories and health outcomes find that those who ascribe positive values and see their illness as a challenge generally have healthier psychological well-being.[25–27]

Punishment, Enemy, and Weakness. In contrast, interpreting illness as a punishment has been found to link with negative health outcomes.[28,29] Punishment as an interpretation of illness can refer to Divine retribution or consequence for past wrongdoing.[30] It is an ancient explanation for suffering, a projection of human behavior to the gods—or God.[31] When measuring the frequency of this interpretation, most researchers have found 10% or fewer to utilize this meaning,[32–34] although some have observed higher percentages (e.g., 17%[35], 22%[36]) when studying it as negative coping. It is unknown, however, how social desirability—or even the desire to look good to oneself—might influence study participants' responses.

Occasionally, patients may explain illness as enemy with religious beliefs. That is, evil or demonic forces are thought to cause the illness or misfortune affecting health. For example, "the devil caused the cancer" was ascribed by 6 of 68 advanced cancer patients.[37] In a similar vein, religious forms of weakness can be ascribed to explain illness. For example, Wittink,

Joo, Lewis, and Barg found that older African Americans believed a "loss of faith" contributed to persons becoming depressed.[38] A sample of mostly Baptist African Americans with HIV noted 27% believed their illness was caused by sin (32% were "unsure").[39]

Summary

This review of literature about patient meanings of illness shows how religious beliefs not only overtly influence how a patient explains the cause of illness or tragedy, but also finds understanding and possibly benefit for that illness or tragedy. The impact of global meanings—often the assumptions and purpose that a religion gives a patient—more than situational meanings, on adjustment and well-being highlights the importance of understanding patients' religious beliefs.

Cognitive Religious Coping

Coping involves appraising an event, determining how harmful to self the event is and what one can do about it.[40] Thus, religious coping (RC) involves relying on or reframing religious meanings, and consequently implementing actions reflective of these cognitive meanings. Although health researchers have described and measured RC among patients for a few decades, it is since the late 1990s that the concept has evolved to differentiate between positive and negative RC. This advancement was led by psychologist Pargament, who developed a lengthy measure for RC, the RCOPE.[41] The RCOPE items reflect the assumption that religion functions to provide persons with religious methods of coping, and includes both potential positive and negative aspects of these functions:

- To find meaning via various reappraisals (e.g., redefining God's power to influence the stressor, or viewing the stressor as an act of the Devil);
- To gain control (e.g., collaborating with, actively surrendering, or passively deferring to God);
- To gain comfort or closeness to God (e.g., by seeking support from God, pursuing religious activities to distract oneself from the stressor or to seek purification, or being discontented in relationship with God);
- To gain intimacy with others or closeness to God (e.g., making effort to connect with a faith community, help others in a spiritual way, being dissatisfied with relationships in the faith community); and
- To experience spiritual transformation (e.g., looking for conversion or religious direction or forgiveness).

Mixed methods studies of "religious/spiritual" coping in school-aged children and adolescents also suggest similar, if less mature, use of religious thinking to adapt to illness.[42,43]

Because of the importance of negative RCs in predicting poor health, it is helpful to review what are the negative RCs. Pargament and colleagues label these as: punishing God reappraisal (e.g., "Wondered what I did for God to punish me"); demonic reappraisal (e.g., "Decided the devil made this happen"); reappraisal of God's power (e.g., "Realized that God cannot answer all my prayers"); passive religious deferral (e.g., "Didn't do much, just expected God to solve my problems for me"); and pleading for direction intercession (e.g., "Prayed for a miracle").[44] In initial testing of the RCOPE with college students and hospitalized patients, it was observed that although both samples used more positive RCs than negative RCs, negative RCs were still predictive of adjustment (negative adjustment, of course).

Myriad studies have investigated RC.[45] A meta-analysis of 49 investigations (with over 100 effect sizes to allow comparisons) exploring the relationship between RC and psychological adjustment to stress concluded that, in general, positive RC was associated with adjustment. Conversely, negative RC was associated with poor adjustment.[46] A landmark study (conducted in the "Bible Belt" of the United States) of 577 consecutive hospitalized older adult patients found that the sicker and more disabled the patients, the more they used RC.[47] Although RC was related positively to physical health outcomes, it was more strongly related to mental health indicators and spiritual growth. The most common positive RCs were seeking support from God, actively surrendering the problem to God, and confessing and asking forgiveness, whereas the negative RCs that most strongly predicted poor physical health included punishing God reappraisals, spiritual discontent, and pleading for direct intercession.

Negative Religious Coping: A Closer Look

These findings and those of others' continue to build strong evidence that religious struggle, doubt, feeling abandoned or punished by God, and negative RC in general typically contribute to poor outcomes.[48–52] Negative RC not only impacts psychological well-being, but affects physical outcomes such as immune function[53,54] and mortality,[55] as well.

Not only has negative RC been explored among patients in relation to psychological and physical well-being, it has also been studied some among family caregivers. For example, Herrera, Lee, Nanyonjo, Laufman, and Torres-Vigil find that negative RC among Latino family carers of elders predicted greater depression.[56] Mickley and fellow researchers observe in a sample of 92 family carers of hospice patients that negative RCs predicted negative mental and spiritual health outcomes.[57]

Summary

Together, the considerable evidence about RC—whether it be positive or negative—provides further support for the contention that religious beliefs do affect how patients and family carers adapt to health-related stress. These beliefs that constitute a form of coping, in turn affect physical, mental, and spiritual health outcomes. This evidence calls nurses to support positive RC, and consider how to address the deleterious effects of negative RC.

Religiosity and Decision Making

Religious beliefs not only provide a patient with explanations and meaning and ways of cognitively coping, but also guidance. One's religious beliefs can guide decision making by providing "an interpretive framework that helps to move forward in the face of overwhelming and intelligible circumstances."[58] The growing body of evidence linking religious belief with health care decision making describes the influence of beliefs on varied decisions, from those related to pregnancy and genetic testing[59,60] to cancer and HIV treatment.[61-63] Most of the research, however, illuminates how beliefs impact end-of-life–related decisions, such as those around resuscitation and prolongation of life[64-66] and advanced directives and elder care planning.[67-69]

Although religious belief is recognized by many patients as influential, it is typically not the most salient factor thought to influence a decision.[70] Indeed, in response to a question about the importance of "faith in God" as a factor in deciding whether to pursue chemotherapy or supportive care, both 100 lung cancer patients and their family carers ranked this factor second, after oncologist's recommendation. Hence, religious belief ranked higher than ability to cure, side effects, and family and family doctor input.[71] Likewise, 48% of 79 persons with HIV recognized that their spiritual beliefs (most having to do with the control of power of "God/Higher Power") influenced their decision making about receiving antiretroviral therapy.[72] Although such embedded beliefs will inevitably influence a decision about health, it is sometimes not overt or recognized.

Associated Negative Outcomes

A closer look at this health-related decision-making research reveals, just as with what religious meanings are ascribed and what RC strategies are used, that the outcomes of decisions influenced by religious belief can be negative, as well as positive.[73-75] For example, in a study of 345 advanced cancer patients, Phelps and colleagues observed that patients using positive RC were three times more likely to be put on a ventilator at the end of life (in spite of statistically controlling for numerous possible confounding factors) and were less likely to have made any type of advanced directive.[76] Kremer and colleagues' interviews with 79 persons positive for HIV/AIDS

(63% of whom were African American or Latino—populations known to self-report high religiosity) revealed that a "belief in God/Higher Power controls health" led to a 4.75 times increased likelihood for the person to refuse antiretroviral treatment.[77] Another study of HIV patients showed that those who believed their diagnosis was a punishment or result of sin were more likely to delay treatment.[78]

The dynamic that explains this linkage between religiosity and what may be considered negative outcomes is likely complex. Is it that highly religious patients hold life to be more sacred and consequently hold on to it more tightly? Or are there psychological mechanisms such as escape or avoidance coping using religious beliefs, such as "leaving it all to God," that explain? Several studies provide hints that may support such hypotheses. To support the first hypothesis, some studies indicate that religious persons are more willing to take risks to prolong life.[79,80] Several studies support the second possible explanation.[81–85] These studies intimate that a passive style of decision making where patients abdicate control over the health challenge to God, tend to also then want all life-prolonging measures used. For example, in a qualitative study of 26 mothers of high-risk infants that included an audit of the respective charts, it was observed that while most mothers' religious beliefs guided decision making about resuscitation, those who did not overtly make a decision and "left things in God's hands" were also those who staff noted "want everything done."[86] In a series of psychological experiments with college students, Vess and colleagues conclude that when individuals who are strong in "fundamentalist" beliefs become more aware of their mortality, their beliefs strengthen, and they are more likely to make decisions that are congruent with their belief that faith alone is the best option.[87] Indeed, the evidence reveals an interplay between religious belief and psychological coping styles to influence decision making.

Associated Positive Outcomes

Conversely, however, religious beliefs can be associated with positive outcomes. In the two studies of HIV patients cited above,[88,89] it was found that those with positive religious beliefs were more adherent to taking their medication and keeping their medical appointments, and had better symptom management compared with those who denied religious beliefs. Balboni and colleagues found that those with positive RC who received spiritual support from their health care team were less likely to pursue aggressive end-of-life care and to accept hospice care.[90] Qualitative research indicates also how religion is often perceived by patients making serious decisions about health care as not only a way to find guidance, but also a means for support from God and faith community, and a source for comfort, peace, and solace amidst the agony of trying to choose what is right.[91–93]

Summary

This review supports the contention that religious belief can strongly influence health care decision making. It also begins to show the complexity of the relationship. Although some studies highlight some positive aspects and outcomes of religious belief on decision making (e.g., adherence to treatment, support and comfort), others show possible negative outcomes (e.g., delayed treatment seeking, increased use of life-prolonging interventions at the end of life). A bird's eye view of this literature suggests that the religious beliefs that produce negative outcomes may do so by offering negative meanings (e.g., illness as sin or punishment) and utilizing negative RC (e.g., deferring decision "to God"). Such beliefs allow passivity or place the locus of control completely with God.[94,95] Religion and coping styles clearly interplay in the process of decision making.

RELIGIOUS PRACTICES IN RESPONSE TO ILLNESS

Nurses encounter religious practices among sick and well persons. Patient dietary proscriptions, religious artifacts at the bedside, and other religious practices may have health implications that a nurse should address. For example, a Muslim commencing the Hajj, a pilgrimage to Mecca, would be well advised by his nurse regarding immunizations, dehydration, and communicable disease prevention.[96] A parent whose child is circumcised should be instructed about hygiene and signs of complications. Religious practices can have health implications. However, this section will briefly explore how religious practices, especially prayer, are often a response to health challenges.

When a challenge to health occurs, the religious person typically relies on practices or rituals of his or her tradition to find comfort or guidance. For some, religious practices that may have accumulated some "cobwebs" may get dusted off for use during illness or tragedy. Or, illness may require a modification of a religious practice. For example, a newly diagnosed patient may decide to start attending religious services more, or a chronically ill person may rely on televised services to fill the void that an inability to attend brings. Many Christians whose condition is serious may ask clergy or leaders in the faith community to administer a ritual anointing. Some religious persons may simply want to continue their religious devotional practices, such as meditation, prayer, reading or reciting of holy Scripture or inspirational literature. Some patients may perform rituals prescribed to them by a religious leader or healer, or go on a pilgrimage in search of healing. Some may wash or drink "holy water" such as Zimbabweans trying to care their diabetes.[97] For religious patients facing death, the need for forgiveness and "preparing to meet one's Maker" become pressing. Many diverse rituals influenced by culture and religion surround the dying and bereavement process (e.g., Hindu chants, burial preparation by fellow believers among Jews and Muslims, creating a calm environment for the dying Buddhist). In various ways, the religious believer facing a health challenge may engage in religious practices as a mean for pursuing healing or health, or a good death and afterlife.

Prevalence

In Western cultures where Abrahamic faiths predominate, prayer is the most frequently reported spiritual practice for times of health or illness. Gallup polling of Americans over the past several decades shows that roughly 9 of 10 believe in prayer.[98] More recently, a Parade poll ($N = 1,051$) reported 51% prayed every day.[99] This poll also reported respondents prayed most for guidance and direction (51%) and comfort and hope (67%). When asked what they typically prayed for, 53% said good health, to get through a crisis (65%), and for the wellness of others (72%). Similarly, a survey of American cancer survivors found that most of them (69%) had prayed for their health.[100] Being black and being female are often noted to be associated with use of prayer.[101,102]

Many studies measuring the frequency of various complementary and alternative therapies (CATs) include an item about "spiritual therapies" or "spiritual or faith healing." While prayer is often found to be one of the most frequently used CATs, the category of spiritual/faith healing is also fairly prevalent.[103] Studies representing a diversity of adults samples have documented rates of spiritual therapies or healing to be 6% to 56%.[104–106] A systematic review of research on the prevalence of CATs used by children with cancer found nine studies where the prevalence of faith healing (excluding prayer) was assessed; the prevalence ranged from 3% to 30% across these studies.[107] In concert, these studies indicate that spiritual or faith healing (religious practices to petition the divine for healing) are sought out by many patients.

Prayer

Given prayer is a frequent aspect of living with illness or tragedy, it is worth further discussion. The literature describes both personal private prayer as well as intercessory prayer for the sick. In intercessory prayer, one person "intercedes with God" on behalf of another person. The notion of intercessory praying for the cure or physical improvement of patients (an "intervention"), however, has received considerable attention and research

funding during the past few decades. A Cochrane review of the 10 existent clinical trials (involving 7,646 patients) led Roberts and colleagues to
conclude:

> These findings are equivocal and, although some of the results of individual
> studies suggest a positive effect of intercessory prayer, the majority do not
> and the evidence does not support a recommendation either in favor or
> against the use of intercessory prayer.[108]

Such unsupportive evidence for intercessory prayer may disillusion some.
The observations of Bishop provide a balanced perspective for this by reiterating what is prayer. Prayer is:

> . . . a human response to serious human questions—questions that every
> human has likely asked, or will likely ask when faced with serious illness. . . .
> If it does not work as defined by science, it still works by fulfilling its role
> in helping a patient to seek meaning in the face of existential crises. . . .
> (p. 1407)[109]

Or as a panel of Anglican ethicists observed: "In prayer, God is peti-
tioned, not controlled; God trusted, not tested."[110]

Although intercessory prayer may not cure patients, how does praying privately affect patient emotional well-being? A critical review of
26 research studies exploring how personal prayer affects health outcomes
was conducted by Hollywell and Walker.[111] These nurses observed that
prayer (typically measured by its frequency) was usually associated with
positive health outcomes (often inversely related to anxiety and depression).
This association was particularly true for those who already had a religious
faith and regularly experienced prayer. Likewise, they noted research that
documents pleading, bargaining, and passive prayers (like wishful thinking)
as associated with negative health outcomes.

Although prayer is generally a helpful and comforting religious ritual,
it is important to consider the possible challenges that illness can have on
praying. Nurse researchers interviewing patients about how illness affected
praying identified the following: drugs befuddle the mind, making thought-
filled prayer difficult; the fatigue, pain, and other symptoms of illness make
it hard to concentrate on prayer or attend religious services where communal prayers are experienced; hospitalization brings interruptions, and lack
of privacy and quiet time for prayer; the uncertainties and fears of illness
enter the prayer experience, often increasing the intensity and frequency of
praying, as well as changing the content and type of prayer; and illness can
bring to the surface spiritual doubts or distress about the nature of God and
prayer.[112,113] Indeed, Taylor and colleagues identify several spiritual pains

related to praying that persons with cancer described.[114] These included doubts about whether prayer was efficacious, whether God was able to respond, whether they were praying in the "right" way, and whether they were worthy or good enough to pray or receive an "answer" to prayer.

Summary

Prayer as well as other religious practices can become enormously important for those seeking the Divine during health challenges. Religious rituals, as methods for bridging the gap between humanity and the Divine, allow persons to find comfort and guidance. Other religious practices may be pursued not only for health-related reasons, but also for spiritual reasons (e.g., "to get right with God"), as a health challenge often reminds mortals of their mortality and their yearning for immortality. Using prayer as an exemplar of religious practice, this section has highlighted the potential positive and potential negative outcomes of religious practice for persons with illness.

SUPPORTING PATIENT RELIGIOSITY

Although many patients report that their faith or religiosity has increased subsequent to an illness—indeed, a significant spiritual transformation may occur—this is not true for others.[115–117] It is possible that sudden attention to religiosity may be a function of how the illness is appraised, particularly if it is viewed as life-threatening. However, it is also possible that increased religiosity with a diagnosis may be merely a perception, rather than a reality. A British study of 202 breast cancer patients and control group of 110 healthy women found that although the patients reported an increase in religious faith and practice, there was no measureable difference between patient and control group religiosity.[118] Regardless, the religious patient may want to receive religious support. This section will review the limited literature that describes what patients desire in terms of religious support during times of illness, what support is given in health care institutions, and the outcomes of such support.

Patient Preferences

Patient preferences for religious support in a health care context will reflect what they perceive as their religious needs. Although many studies have documented what are patient spiritual needs, none have specifically or directly explored religious needs. Yet, within the vast literature describing patient spiritual needs, there invariably is recognition of religious needs.[119–122]

Religious needs typically identified include support of clergy and religious rituals (e.g., prayer and worship practices), as well as the more vague spiritual needs which religions typically support (e.g., finding hope, meaning, and peace). Needs can also include doubts about faith, questioning beliefs, revitalizing a relationship with God, seeking forgiveness with God and others, searching for religious explanation and meaning for illness and death, reinventing religious practices so that they are doable and meaningful in the context of illness, and so forth.[123,124] Two studies ranking importance of multiple physical and emotional concerns at end of life have found being at peace to rank second.[125,126]

In studies assessing the prevalence of religious needs of patients, the question is always asked with the concepts of religious and spiritual together—if the term religious is even used. With understanding of this limitation, it is still informative to note the frequency of patient identified "religious/spiritual concerns" in the few studies that offer such a glimpse. Several substantial studies of persons with cancer have overtly quantified patients' perceptions of spiritual/religious need.[127–130] These researchers have observed that 42%[131] to 73%[132] of patients endorse that they experience at least one spiritual/religious need. Alcorn and colleagues noted that 51% (of 68 advanced cancer patients) responded with four or more religious/spiritual concerns; they found there was no difference in the number or reported concerns by whether the patient self-identified spirituality/religion as important.[133] Moadel and colleagues reported 29% of cancer patients indicating at least five spiritual/existential needs[134]; they observed ethnicity to be the best predictor of high spiritual needs (with Hispanics experiencing 60%, African Americans 49%, and whites 31%).[135] Another study of cancer patients and their family carers measured no statistical differences between these groups on the importance of numerous spiritual needs.[136] This study found that frequency of religious services attendance, length of time since diagnosis, being female, living with others, and being an inpatient all were associated with increased report of spiritual/religious need. These findings, although limited to American oncology samples, suggest spiritual/existential/religious needs are common for these seriously ill persons and their families.

Although patients (at least cancer patients) frequently report spiritual/religious concerns or needs, little is known as to what assistance they would like for these needs. A few studies offering insight can be patched together to begin to form an answer. In Astrow and colleagues' study, of those who expressed a spiritual need (73% of 369 cancer patients), the most common resource requested was "formal religious assistance," which 35% identified.[137] A survey mailed to 592 Japanese bereaved family members, which inquired about the appropriateness of religious care for terminally ill, identified several types of religious care the religious respondents recommended be available: music (e.g., hymns); "good and cheerful tales;" encouraging words; religious events (e.g., mass); and pastoral care visits.[138] These Japanese families also noted that hospitals should offer freedom of choice for religious care and have staff be involved in religious care as well.

While quite a few studies have inquired of patients about how they would like a physician to support spiritual/religious needs, few have explored if and how patients want nurses to provide religious or spiritual support. Although some cancer patients and family caregivers are enthusiastic about receiving some forms of spiritual care from nurses, others do not want it.[139] Patients with a serious or life-threatening condition, patients who are religious, and patients who perceive they have some relationship with the clinician are especially receptive to nurses supporting their spiritual health.[140–142] Some types of spiritual care from a nurse are more welcomed than others; generally, interventions that were less intimate, commonly used, and not overtly religious were most welcomed. For example, a nurse talking with a patient about problems with praying, encouraging self-expression through art, or supporting a patient with making sense of a dream were ranked low for nurse-provided spiritual care. In contrast, this sample of cancer patients and family carers alike ranked allowing a patient quiet time, space, and private prayer as the most desirable nurse-provided spiritual care.[143]

Summary

These research findings begin to show that many, but not all, seriously ill patients may recognize a spiritual/religious concern. This literature also suggests that the types of religious support patients and their families want vary. It is likely, however, that particularly intimate and unusual methods for providing religious support are perceived as inappropriate. This underscores research findings that show that a respectful nurse–patient relationship should be a requisite for religious/spiritual care.

The State of Religious Care

The above literature offers evidence about what religious support patients may desire. But what religious support is given to patients today in health care contexts? Although the evidence is extremely skimpy, a few studies offer a glimpse on the state of religious care in health care. In a systematic review of research (i.e., 57 pertinent studies) about the unmet supportive care needs of persons with cancer, Harrison, Young, Price, Butow, and Solomon found only two that quantified unmet spiritual needs, concluding that spiritual needs were unmet for 14% to 51% of patients.[144] Subsequently, Balboni and colleagues asked Texan and New England cancer patients about the spiritual support they received.[145] Of these 343 patients,

60% reported that they had received spiritual support from the medical system not at all or to a small extent. Only 11% felt completely supported. Likewise, 45% indicated that they received spiritual support from a religious community not at all or to a small extent. Visits from clergy (44%) and hospital chaplains (46%) were reported. For this sample, spiritual support, including religious support from clergy or a religious community, was often absent. Findings from another large study of American cancer patients provide a contrast. Astrow and colleagues find that although 82% reported having spiritual needs met, only 9% perceived that a staff member had asked about spiritual or religious needs.[146] These few studies show there is wide variation (i.e., 11% to 82%) among patients as far as perception of spiritual/religious needs being met during times of illness. Not only is there plenty of room for improving religious support, but also for further evidence about what patients perceive and want as far as religious support.

Outcomes of Religious Care

Again, there is a paucity of evidence to provide information about how supporting patient religiosity has an impact on patient condition. The existent evidence, however, shows there is great potential for religious support to contribute to significant positive clinical outcomes. An intervention study investigating the outcomes of oncologists including a spiritual/religious assessment during patient visits showed that 76% (of 118) felt the physician's inquiry was somewhat or very helpful. This study, using an experimental design, also observed that those who received the intervention of an inquiry about their spiritual/religious state were less depressed and had a higher quality of life than those who did not receive the intervention.[147] Balboni and colleagues' findings also show that when health care teams work in an interdisciplinary way to provide spiritual/religious support (instead of leaving it just for the spiritual care experts), significant outcomes occur: Advanced cancer patients are about three times more likely to accept hospice care and experience greater quality of life (28% improvement on average).[148] Although from only two studies, this evidence provides impetus for nurses to become more involved in exploring how best to support patient religiosity.

PATIENT RELIGIOUS BELIEFS AND PRACTICES: CLINICAL IMPLICATIONS

Although the evidence linking religious beliefs and practices with interpretations for illness, coping, and decision making in health-related contexts offers significant directions for nursing practice, specific evidence for guiding nurses to support patient religiosity is minimal. To fully appreciate the literature reviewed, it is vital to consider some of the implications for clinical nursing practice supported by this empirical evidence.

- Although potentially powerful, the impact of religiosity on health is often subtle and indirect. It is easily unobserved and neglected by health care professionals. Indeed, patients may not even recognize how their religious beliefs influence their response to illness. Religiosity may be a "white elephant" in health care. This suggests that nurses need to be proactive about assessing and supporting religious beliefs and practices for patients. Nursing literature about spiritual assessment offers suggestions on how nurses can approach this assessment without offending patients, given the socially taboo nature of the topic.[149]
- Positive religious beliefs are generally associated with positive health. That is, positive global meanings for illness and tragedy offered by religion, if unshattered, appear to greatly aid patients. Likewise, positive RC contributes to a healthy adjustment. Supporting positive religious belief, therefore, is an appropriate goal for nurses as long as the forms of support are within the purview and ability of the nurse. Therefore, in situations where the impact of religious belief on coping and decision making are necessary to explore, nurses ought to promote positive health outcomes by encouraging a patient to identify helpful religious beliefs and discuss how those beliefs can be respected.
- This literature also recognizes the negative health outcomes of unhelpful religious belief (e.g., illness as punishment or spiritual weakness, and passive abdication to God for decision making). Suppressing doubt and other religious struggles is not conducive to health.[150] Therefore, when a nurse hears a patient express religious struggle or pain such as described by researchers as negative RC, a red flag should go up for the health care team. Such struggle is likely best addressed by a spiritual care expert who can gently help the patient to examine the fallacies behind negative religious thinking. Therefore, a nurse facilitating a referral to a trained chaplain, clergy, spiritual director, or mental health professional who appreciates the role of religion may be the appropriate intervention. To hear such religious struggle, however, likely requires a nurse who creates a trusting nurse–patient relationship and who does not emotionally or physically run away from such pain.[151]
- White identifies various religious beliefs affecting decisions that would have negative health consequences, and suggests that such belief would magnify the burden of illness.[152] Examples of these deleterious beliefs would include thinking the illness or tragedy is punishment, reflects a lack of faith, or is a way to deepen religious commitment. Likewise, believing that one needs only to have faith in a miracle or that only

prayer can heal (i.e., abdicating one's role in managing the illness), or even reframing suffering as redemptive, can be harmful ways of thinking. Yet, as with various forms of denial, these religious beliefs offer patients a defense mechanism. As a defense mechanism, they should only be addressed by an expert and with much caution! However, when negative meanings and causal explanations ascribed to an illness are religious, the treatment needs to address this religious thinking.[153]

- The evidence of one fairly strong study suggests that it is a multidisciplinary approach to religious support that affects positive outcomes, not a solo approach by a spiritual care expert.[154] Also, several studies indicate that some (especially religious and dying patients), but not all, want nonspiritual care expert members of their health care team to inquire about and support their religiosity. Nurses need to gain some level of skill to assess and address religious beliefs and practices vis-à-vis health. Nurses need to remember that spiritual and religious care must occur in the context of a multidisciplinary team. Patients' religious concerns that impact health should be discussed with appropriate team members. The nurse (as well as the spiritual care expert) is never the patient's "savior" who heals all diseases.

- The evidence on RC shows how religious beliefs influence not only adults, but also children and adolescents. Indeed, religion is not just for old people. Nurses will do well to remember to assess religion's impact on health for all patients, regardless of their age. Although research often shows women and persons from minority cultures (e.g., African Americans, Latinos, immigrants) to self-report greater religiosity, religion is obviously a phenomenon that crosses all cultures. However, knowing this can suggest to nurses that certain populations may be more amenable than others to receiving religious support.

- Religious practices are engaged by patients to seek comfort, guidance, health, or a good death and afterlife. If a patient is unable to continue a practice, this may be very distressing. Nurses can discuss with the patient and/or their family or clergy ways that the practice can be adapted so it can be continued. For example, a Muslim patient who cannot perform the ritual washing prior to prayer may accept instead the "cleansing" of submerging hands in sand or rubbing the hands on a clean stone. A Christian who is used to a colloquial prayer that requires thinking may be distressed when medicines befuddle the mind; such a patient can be introduced to an image (e.g., icon, flower), a guided imagery, or other method for praying to experience God's presence.[155]

Prayer is a particularly important religious practice. Given the evidence about the potential negative as well as positive outcomes of prayer experience during times of illness, it behooves nurses to approach the topic of prayer. Hollywell and Walker recommend that patients first be assessed regarding their religious faith and experience of prayer, and that nurses should not indiscriminately recommend to patients that they need to pray.[156] Such assessment would do well to determine if prayer is an undeveloped practice used only in times of extremis and if negative types of prayer are used.

- Although this literature review did not directly include research about spiritual responses, there is evidence that it is positive religiosity in combination with high spirituality that is particularly predictive of positive health outcomes.[157–159] This profile of positive religiosity and high spirituality likely overlaps with what sociologist Allport described as intrinsic religiosity several decades ago.[160] It is a religion that is lived, rather than used. It is a religion that is integrated congruently within one's life, rather than used to gain something. It is a religiosity that, by nature, produces a healthy spirituality.

    Thus, it is inadequate and simplistic to think that the goal for nurses is to facilitate cure of patients' irrational religious beliefs and enactment of healthful religious practices. The nurse can support positive religiosity and spirituality, but ultimately healthful religious experience is not something a nurse can make happen. The goal of nursing in this regard may best be to place the patient in an environment where worship can occur, however, that is experienced by the client. That is not necessarily a physical sacred space, but also (mostly) an interpersonal relationship where an awareness of the sacred can occur.

CONCLUSION

This chapter has reviewed recent research from various health-related fields to describe how religious beliefs and practices affect a patient's response to a health challenge. Although research over the past few decades has provided considerable evidence indicating, in general, a positive relationship between religiosity and health, recent improvements in the measurement and conceptualization of religiosity have allowed progress in understanding this relationship. Continued development, however, is needed. Most notable is the increased understanding about how religious beliefs can, in effect, be negative or positive. As yet, the research regards all devoutly religious persons as a single category. No attempt has, as yet, been made, to separate, for example, those who are conservative in religious belief from those who are progressive, to see if correlations exist in terms of positive versus negative RC. Religious thinking influences how one makes sense of illness, copes with the illness, and consequently makes decisions about how to treat the health condition.

The easily conjectured hypothesis appears to be supported: Negative beliefs are associated with negative outcomes and positive beliefs are linked to positive outcomes.

Although there is considerable evidence to suggest the importance of understanding and supporting healthful religious experience, there is much less evidence that can more directly inform nursing practice. Research from both patient and professional perspectives needs to investigate: What religious support do patients want or benefit from nurses? What are appropriate and effective ways that nurses can assess and address negative religious thinking and coping? What, if any, requisites should be in place prior to a nurse addressing religious concerns? How should nurses work in a multidisciplinary team to promote spiritual/ religious health for patients? (e.g., when is it appropriate to document religious beliefs?) What are the outcomes of nurse-provided religious support? (On patients? On nurses? On the health care organization?) Indeed, there is a paucity of nursing research addressing such questions as these, and only a few studies describe the client perspective rather than the nurse viewpoint. In addition to empirical evidence, there is also need for ethical analysis about the nature of the nurse–patient relationship in the context of religious support.

Although there is little direct evidence for nursing care in this regard, there is substantial evidence that religion is a significant contributor to meaning, coping, and decision making related to health. Therefore, nurses ought to recognize and strive to support positive, healthful religious beliefs and practices of patients.

NOTES

1. Van Hooft, Stan. "The Meanings of Suffering." *Hastings Center Report* 28.5 (1998): 13–20.
2. Ferrell, Betty. R., Stephany Smith, Gloria Juarez, et al. "Meaning of Illness and Spirituality in Ovarian Cancer Survivors." *Oncology Nursing Forum* 30.2 (2003): 249–257.
3. Taylor, Elizabeth J. "Transformation of Tragedy Among Women Surviving Breast Cancer." *Oncology Nursing Forum* 27.7 (2000): 781–788.
4. Bussing, Arndt, Thomas Ostermann, and Edmund Neugebauer, et al. "Adaptive Coping Strategies in Patients with Chronic Pain Conditions and their Interpretation of Disease." *BMC Public Health* 10 (2010): 507- [epub ahead of print].
5. Downe-Wamboldt, Barbara, Lorna Butler, and Lynn Coulter. "The Relationship between Meaning of Illness, Social Support, Coping Strategies, and Quality of Life for Lung Cancer Patients and their Family Members." *Cancer Nursing* 29.2 (2006): 111–119.

6. Sarna, Linda, Jean Brown, Mary Cooley, et al. "Quality of Life and Meaning of Illness of Women with Lung Cancer." *Oncology Nursing Forum* 32.1 (2005): E9–19.
7. Farber, Eugene, Hamid Mirsalimi, Karen Williams, et al. "Meaning of Illness and Psychological Adjustment to HIV/AIDS." *Psychosomatic* 44.6 (2003): 485–491.
8. Bussing et al. 507.
9. Fjelland, Joyce, Cecilia Barron, and Martha Foxall. "A Review of Instruments Measuring two Aspects of Meaning: Search for Meaning and Meaning of Illness." *Journal of Advanced Nursing* 62.4 (2008): 394–406.
10. Sherman, Allen, Stephanie Simonton, Umaira Latif, et al. "Effects of Global Meaning and Illness-Specific Meaning on Health Outcomes among Breast Cancer Patients." *Journal of Behavioral Medicine* 33.5 (2010): 364–377.
11. Park, Crystal, and Susan Folkman. "Meaning in the Context of Stress and Coping." *Review of General Psychology* 2 (1997): 115–144.
12. Janoff-Bulman, Ronnie. *Shattered Assumptions: Towards a New Psychology of Trauma*. New York: Free Press, 1992.
13. Sherman, et al. 364–377.
14. Mohrmann, Margaret, D. E. Healey, and M. D. Childress. "Suffering's Witness: The Problem of Evil in Medical Practice." *Second Opinion* 3 (2000): 55–70.
15. Mohrmann, Healey, Childress. 60.
16. Foley, Daniel Patrick. "Eleven Interpretations of Personal Suffering." *Journal of Religion and Health* 27 (1988): 321–328.
17. Wallberg, Birgitta, Helena Michelson, Marianne Nystedt, et al. "The Meaning of Breast Cancer." *Acta Oncologica* 42.1 (2003): 30–35.
18. Bussing, Arndt, and Julia Fischer. "Interpretation of Illness in Cancer Survivors is Associated with Health-Related Variables and Adaptive Coping Styles." *BMC Womens Health* 9 (2009): 2.
19. Caress, Ann-Louise, Karen Luker, and R. Glynn Owen. "A Descriptive Study of Meaning of Illness in Chronic Renal Disease." *Journal of Advanced Nursing* 33.6 (2001): 716–727.
20. Caress, Luker, Owen. 716–727.
21. Taylor. 781–788.
22. Caress, Luker, Owen. 716–727.
23. Wallberg, Michaelson, Nystedt. 30–35.
24. Alcorn, Sara, Michael Balboni, Holly Prigerson, et al. "'If God Wanted me Yesterday, I Wouldn't be here Today': Religious and Spiritual Themes in Patients' Experiences of Advanced Cancer." *Journal of Palliative Medicine* 13.5 (2010): 581–588.
25. Bussing and Fischer. 2.
26. Taylor. 781–788.
27. Sherman, et al. 364–377.
28. Pargament, Kenneth, Harold Koenig, and Lisa Perez. "The Many Methods of Religious Coping: Development and Validation of the RCOPE." *Journal of Clinical Psychology* 56.4 (2000): 519–543.
29. Parsons, Sharon, Peter Cruise, W. M. Davenport, et al. "Religious Beliefs, Practices and Treatment Adherence among Individuals with HIV in the Southern United States." *AIDS Patient Care and STDs* 20.2 (2006): 97–111.
30. Caress, Luker, Owen. 716–727.
31. Van Hooft. 13–20.
32. Caress, Luker, Owen. 716–727.
33. Bussing and Fischer. 2.

34. Wallberg, et al. 30–35.
35. Pendleton, Sara, Kristina Cavalli, Kenneth Pargament, et al. "Religious Coping in Cystic Fibrosis." *Pediatrics* 109.1 (2002): E8.
36. Alcorn, et al. 581–588.
37. Ibid.
38. Wittink, Marsha, Jin Hui Joo, Lisa Lewis, et al. "Losing Faith and Using Faith: Older African Americans Discuss Spirituality, Religious Activities, and Depression." *Journal of General Internal Medicine* 24.3 (2009): 402–407.
39. Parson, et al. 97–111.
40. Park and Folkman. 115–144.
41. Pargament, et al. (2000): 519–543.
42. Pendleton, et al. E8.
43. Cotton, Sian, Daniel Grossoehme, Susan Rosenthal, et al. Religious/spiritual coping in adolescents with sickle cell disease: A pilot study. *Journal of Pediatric Hematology and Oncology* 31.5 (2009): 313–318.
44. Pargament, et al. 2000: 519–543.
45. Pargament, Kenneth. *The Psychology of Religion and Coping: Theory, Research, and Practice.* New York: Guildford Press, 1997.
46. Ano, Gene, and Erin Vasconcelles. "Religious Coping and Psychological Adjustment to Stress: A Meta-Analysis." *Journal of Clinical Psychology* 61.4 (2005): 461–480.
47. Koenig, Harold, Kenneth Pargament, and Julie Nielsen. "Religious Coping and Health Status in Medically ill Hospitalized Older Adults." *Journal of Nervous & Mental Disease* 186.9 (1998): 513–521.
48. McConnell, Kelly, Kenneth Pargament, Christopher Ellison, et al. "Examining the Links between Spiritual Struggles and Symptoms of Psychopathology in a National Sample." *Journal of Clinical Psychology* 62.12 (2006): 1469–1484.
49. Park, Crystal, Donald Edmondson, Amy Hale-Smith, et al. "Religiousness/Spirituality and Health Behaviors in Younger Adult Cancer Survivors: Does Faith Promote a Healthier Lifestyle?" *Journal of Behavioral Medicine* 32.6 (2009): 582–591.
50. Ai, Amy, Kenneth Pargament, Ziad Kronfol, et al. "Pathways to Postoperative Hostility in Cardiac Patients: Mediation of Coping, Spiritual Struggle and Interleukin-6." *Journal of Health Psychology* 15.2 (2010): 186–195.
51. Edmondson, Donald, Crystal Park, Stephanie Chaudoir, et al. "Death without God: Religious Struggle, Death Concerns, and Depression in the Terminally Ill." *Psychological Science* 19.8 (2008): 754–758.
52. Pargament, Kenneth, Harold Koenig, Nalini Tarakeshwar, et al. "Religious Struggle as a Predictor of Mortality among Medically Ill Elderly Patients: A 2-Year Longitudinal Study." *Archives of Internal Medicine* 161.15 (2001): 1881–1885.
53. Ai, et al. 186–195.
54. Trevino, Kelly, Kenneth Pargament, Sian Cotton, et al. "Religious Coping and Physical, Psychological, Social, and Spiritual Outcomes in Patients with HIV/AIDS: Cross-Sectional and Longitudinal Findings." *AIDS and Behavior* 14.2 (2010): 379–389.
55. Pargament, et al. (2001): 1881–1885.
56. Herrera, Angelica, Jerry Lee, Rebecca Nanyonjo, et al. "Religious Coping and Caregiver Well-Being in Mexican-American Families." *Aging and Mental Health* 13.1 (2009): 84–91.
57. Mickley, Jacqueline, Kenneth Pargament, C. R. Brant, et al. "God and the Search for Meaning among Hospice Caregivers." *Hospice Journal* 13.4 (1998): 1–17.

58. White, M. T. Making Sense of Genetic Uncertainty: The Role of Religion and Spirituality." *American Journal of Medical Genetics, Part C, Seminars in Medical Genetics 151C*.1 (2009): 68–76. 75.

59. Ibid.

60. Jesse, D. Elizabeth, Chantel Schoneboom, and Amy Blanchard. "The Effect of Faith or Spirituality in Pregnancy: A Content Analysis." *Journal of Holistic Nursing* 25.3 (2007): 151–158.

61. Silvestri, Gerard, Sommer Knittig, James Zoller, et al. "Importance of Faith on Medical Decisions Regarding Cancer Care." *Journal of Clinical Oncology* 21.7 (2003):1379–1382.

62. Kremer, Heidemarie, and Gail Ironson. "Everything Changed: Spiritual Transformation in People with HIV." *International Journal of Psychiatry in Medicine* 39.3 (2009): 243–262.

63. Phelps, Andrea, Paul Maciejewski, Matthew Nilsson, et al. "Religious Coping and use of Intensive Life-Prolonging Care Near Death in Patients with Advanced Cancer." *Journal of the American Medical Association* 301.11 (2009): 1140–1147.

64. Hexen, K., C. Mollen, K. Carroll, et al. "How Parents of Children Receiving Pediatric Palliative Care use Religion, Spirituality, or Life Philosophy in Tough Times." *Journal of Palliative Medicine* 14 (2011): 39–44.

65. Palen Lopez, Ruth. "Doing What's Best: Decisions by Families of Acutely Ill Nursing Home Residents." *Western Journal of Nursing Research* 31.5 (2009): 613–626.

66. Vess, Matthew, Jamie Arndt, Cathy Cox, et al. "Exploring the Existential Function of Religion: The Effect of Religious Fundamentalism and Mortality Salience on Faith-Based Medical Refusals." *Journal of Personality & Social Psychology* 97.2 (2009): 334–350.

67. Cohen, Marya, Jessica McCannon, Susan Edgeman-Levitan, et al. "Exploring Attitudes Toward Advance Care Directives in two Diverse Settings." *Journal of Palliative Medicine* 13.12 (2010): 1427–1432.

68. Ai, Amy, Crystal Park, and Marshall Shearer. "Spiritual and Religious Involvement Relate to End-of-Life Decision-making in Patients Undergoing Coronary Bypass Graft Surgery." *International Journal of Psychiatry in Medicine* 38.1 (2008):113–132.

69. Elliott, Barbara, Charles Gessert, and Cynthia Peden-McAlpine. "Decision Making by Families of Older Adults with Advanced Cognitive Impairment: Spirituality and Meaning." *Journal of Gerontological Nursing* 33.8 (2007): 49–55.

70. White. 1881–1885.

71. Silvestri, et al. 1379–1382.

72. Kremer, Heidemarie, Gail Ironson, and Martina Porr. "Spiritual and Mind-Body Beliefs as Barriers and Motivators to HIV-Treatment Decision-Making and Medication Adherence? A Qualitative Study." *AIDS Patient Care and STDs* 23.2 (2009): 127–134.

73. Hexen, et al. 39–44.

74. White. 1881–1885.

75. Vess, et al. 334–350.

76. Phelps, et al. 1140–1147.

77. Kremer, et al. 127–134.

78. Parsons, et al. 97–111.

79. Lam, Hugh, Samuel Wong, Flora Liu, et al. "Attitudes Toward Neonatal Intensive Care Treatment of Preterm Infants with a High Risk of Developing Long-Term Disabilities." *Pediatrics* 123.6 (2009): 1501–1208.

80. Van Ness, Peter, Virginia Towle, John O'Leary, et al. "Religion, Risk, and Medical Decision Making at the end of Life." *Journal of Aging & Health* 20.5 (2008): 545–549.
81. Matlock, Dan, Carolyn Nowels, and David Bekelman. "Patient Perspectives on Decision Making in Heart Failure." *Journal of Cardiac Failure* 16.10 (2010): 823–826.
82. Vess, 334–350.
83. Lam, et al. 1501–1208.
84. Boss, Renee, Nancy Hutton, Leslie Sulpar, et al. "Values Parents Apply to Decision-Making Regarding Delivery Room Resuscitation for High-Risk Newborns." *Pediatrics* 122.3 (2008): 583–589.
85. Kremer, et al. 127–134.
86. Boss, et al. 583–589.
87. Vess, et al. 334–350.
88. Parsons, et al. 97–111.
89. Kremer, et al. 581–588.
90. Balboni, Tracy, Mary Elizabeth Paulk, Michael J. Balboni, et al. "Provision of Spiritual Care to Patients with Advanced Cancer: Associations with Medical Care and Quality of Life Near Death. *Journal of Clinical Oncology* 28.3 (2010): 445–452.
91. White. 581–588.
92. Hexen, et al. 581–588.
93. Taylor and Outlaw, 2002.
94. Matlock, et al. 823–826.
95. Kremer, et al. 581–588.
96. Ahmed, Qanta, Yaseen Arabi, and Ziad Memish. "Health Risks at the Hajj." *The Lancet* 367.9515 (2006): 1008–1015.
97. Hjelm, Katarina, and Esther Mufunda. "Zimbabwean Diabetics' Beliefs about Health and Illness: An Interview Study." *BMC International Health and Human Rights* 10.7 (2010): doi: 10.1186/1472-698X-10-7.
98. Gallup, George. H., Jr., *Religion in America*. Princeton, NJ: Princeton Religion Research Center, 1996.
99. "Spirituality Poll Results." *Parade*. 2010. Web. 8 Feb. 2011.
100. Ross, Louie, Ingrid Hall, Temeika Fairley, et al. "Prayer and Self-Reported Health among Cancer Survivors in the United States, National Health Survey, 2002." *Journal of Alternative & Complementary Medicine* 14.8 (2008): 931–938.
101. Gillum, Frank, and Derek Griffith. Prayer and Spiritual Practices for Health Reasons among American Adults: The Role of Race and Ethnicity." *Journal of Religion and Health* 49.3 (2009): 283–295.
102. Ross, et al.
103. Taylor, Elizabeth J. "Spiritual Complementary Therapies in Cancer Care." *Seminars in Oncology Nursing* 21.3 (2005): 159–163.
104. Callahan, Leigh, Elizabeth Wiley-Exley, Thelma Mielenz, et al. "Use of Complementary and Alternative Medicine Among Patients with Arthritis." *Prevention of Chronic Disease*, 6.2 (2009): A44.
105. Amin, Mohammed, F. Glynn, S. Rowley, et al. "Complementary Medicine use in Patients with Head and Neck Cancer in Ireland." *European Archives of Otorhinolaryngology* 267.8 (2010): 1291–1297.
106. Molassiotis, Alex, P. Fernadez-Ortega, D. Pud, et al. "Use of Complementary and Alternative Medicine in Cancer Patients: A European Survey." *Annals of Oncology* 16.4 (2005): 655–663.

107. Bishop, Felicity, Phillip Prescott, Yean Koon Chan, et al. "Prevalence of Complementary Medicine use in Pediatric Cancer: A Systematic Review." *Pediatrics* 125.4 (2010): 768–776.
108. Roberts, L., Ahmed, I., Hall, S., and Davison A. "Intercessory Prayer for the Alleviation of Ill Health." *Cochrane Database of Systematic Reviews* 2 (2009): CD000368.
109. Bishop, Jeffrey P. "Prayer, Science, and the Moral Life of Medicine." *Archives of Internal Medicine* 163.12 (2003): 1405–1408. 1407.
110. Cohen, et al. 2000, 43.
111. Hollywell, Claire, and Jan Walker. "Private Prayer as a Suitable Intervention for Hospitalized Patients: A Critical Review of the Literature." *Journal of Clinical Nursing* 18.5 (2008): 637–651.
112. Taylor, Elizabeth J., Outlaw, Frieda, Theresa Bernardo, et al. "Spiritual Conflicts of Cancer Patients who pray." *Psycho-Oncology* 8 (1999): 386–394.
113. Hawley, Georgina, and Vera Irurita. "Seeking Comfort through Prayer." *International Journal of Nursing Practice* 4.1 (1998): 9–18.
114. Taylor and Outlaw. 386–394.
115. Campbell, James, Dong Phil Yoon, and Brick Johnstone. "Determining Relationships between Physical Health and Spiritual Experience, Religious Practices, and Congregational Support in a Heterogeneous Medical Sample." *Journal of Religion and Health* 49.1 (2010): 3–17.
116. Alcorn, et al. 581–588.
117. Kremer and Ironson. 243–262.
118. Thuné-Boyle, I. C., J. Stygall, M. R. Keshtgar, et al. "The Impact of a Breast Cancer Diagnosis on Religious/Spiritual Beliefs and Practices in the UK." *Journal of Religion and Health* 50.2 (2011): 203–218 [epub ahead of print].
119. Howell, Doris, and K. Brazil. "Reaching Common Ground: A Patient-Family-Based Conceptual Framework of Quality EOL Care." *Journal of Palliative Care* 21.1 (2005): 19–26.
120. Bussing, Arndt, Hans-Joachim Balzat, and Peter Heusser. "Spiritual needs of Patients with Chronic Pain Diseases and Cancer – Validation of the Spiritual Needs Questionnaire." *European Journal of Medical Research* 15.6 (2010): 266–273.
121. Moadel, Alyson, Carole Morgan, Anne Fatone, et al. "Seeking Meaning and Hope: Self-Reported Spiritual and Existential Needs among an Ethnically-Diverse Cancer Patient Population. *Psycho-Oncology* 8.5 (1999): 378–385.
122. Alcorn, et al. 581–588.
123. Taylor, Elizabeth J. "Prevalence of Spiritual Needs among Cancer Patients and Family Caregivers." *Oncology Nursing Forum* 33.4 (2006): 729–735.
124. Alcorn, et al. 581–588.
125. Bonin-Scaon, Sylvie. "End of Life Preferences: A Theory Driven Inventory." *International Journal of Aging and Human Development* 68.1 (2009): 1–26.
126. Steinhauser, Karen. E., Nicholas Christakis, Elizabeth Clipp, et al. "Factors Considered Important at the End of Life by Patients, Family, Physicians, and Other Care Providers." *Journal of the American Medical Association* 284.19 (2000): 2476–2482.
127. Taylor. (2006): 729–735.
128. Moadel, Alyson, Carole Morgan, and Janice Dutcher. "Psychosocial Needs Assessment among an Underserved, Ethnically Diverse Cancer Patient Population." *Cancer* 109.2 *Supplement* (2007): 446–454.
129. Alcorn, et al. 581–588.

130. Astrow, Alan, Ann Wexler, Kenneth Texeira, et al. "Is Failure to Meet Spiritual Needs Associated with Cancer Patients' Perceptions of Quality of Care and their Satisfaction with Care?" *Journal of Clinical Oncology* 25.36 (2007): 5753–5757.

131. Moadel, et al. 2007.

132. Astrow, et al. 5733–5757.

133. Astrow, et al. 5733–5757.

134. Moadel, et al. (1999): 378–385.

135. Moadel, et al. (2007): 446–454.

136. Taylor. (2006): 729–735.

137. Astrow, et al. 5733–5757.

138. Okamoto, Takuya, Michiyo Ando, Tatsuya Morita, et al. "Religious Care Required for Japanese Terminally ill Patients with Cancer from the Perspective of Bereaved Family Members." *American Journal of Hospice & Palliative Care* 27.1 (2010): 50–54.

139. Taylor, Elizabeth J., and Iris Mamier. "Spiritual Care Nursing: What Cancer Patients and Family Caregivers Want." *Journal of Advanced Nursing* 49.3 (2005): 260–267.

140. Taylor, Elizabeth J. "Client Perspectives about Nurse Requisites for Spiritual Caregiving." *Applied Nursing Research* 20.1 (2007): 44–46.

141. Taylor. (2006): 729–735.

142. Taylor and Mamier. 260–267.

143. Taylor and Mamier. 260–267.

144. Harrison, James D., Jane Young, Melanie Price, et al. "What are the Unmet Supportive Care Needs of People with Cancer? A Systematic Review." *Supportive Care in Cancer* 17.8 (2009): 1117–1128.

145. Balboni, et al. 445–452.

146. Astrow, et al. 5753–5757.

147. Kristeller, Jean, M. Rhodes, Larry Cripe, et al. "Oncologist Assisted Spiritual Intervention Study (OASIS): Patient Acceptability and Initial Evidence of Effects." *International Journal of Psychiatry in Medicine* 35.4 (2005): 329–347.

148. Balboni, et al. 445–452.

149. Taylor, Elizabeth J. "Spiritual Assessment." Eds. Betty Ferrell and Nessa Coyle. *Textbook of Palliative Nursing Care* 3rd ed. New York: Oxford University Press, 2010.

150. Krause, Neal, and Christopher Ellison. "The Doubting Process: A Longitudinal Study of the Precipitants and Consequences of Religious Doubt." *Journal for the Scientific Study of Religion* 48.2 (2009): 293–312.

151. Taylor, Elizabeth J. *What do I say? Talking with Patients about Spirituality.* Philadelphia, PA: Templeton Press, 2007.

152. White. 581–588.

153. Wittink, et al. 402–407.

154. Balboni, et al. 445–452.

155. Taylor, Elizabeth J. "Prayer's Clinical Issues and Implications." *Holistic Nursing Practice* 17.4 (2003): 179–188.

156. Hollywell and Walker. 637–651.

157. Bussing, Ostermann, and Neugebauer. 266–273.

158. Lawler-Row, Kathleen, and Jeff Elliott. "The Role of Religious Activity and Spirituality in the Health and Well-Being of Older Adults." *Journal of Health Psychology* 14.1 (2009): 43–52.

159. Yanez, Betina, Donald Edmondson, Annette Stanton, et al. "Facets of Spirituality as Predictors of Adjustment to Cancer: Relative Contributions of Having Faith and Finding Meaning." *Journal of Consulting & Clinical Psychology* 77.4 (2009): 730–741.

160. Sherman, et al. 364–377.

17

The Nurse as a Religious Person

Elizabeth Johnston Taylor and Marsha D. Fowler

Everyone has a worldview—a way of explaining reality—that is in part received and in part self-constructed. This worldview inevitably walks with the nurse to the bedside. This chapter will explore how the worldviews of nurses have an impact on their nursing care. The focus is on those nurses who affiliate with a particular religion, but similar points could well be made about the influence of secular, atheist, or nonreligious spiritual worldviews.

To begin, we will imagine how nurses of diverse religious traditions might possibly draw upon somewhat typical features or approaches of the religion to care for an anxious patient, each in her or his religiously unique way. This will highlight the importance of recognizing a nurse's religiosity. After reviewing literature that suggests how the religiosity of nurses does influence their practice of nursing, recommendations for how personal religiosity may or may not be appropriately brought to the bedside will be presented.

A NURSE'S RELIGION AT THE BEDSIDE

Vignettes

Lynn is a 48-year-old woman who knows she is dying of breast cancer. Nights are particularly distressing for Lynn, as that is when her friends and family sleep, and she is left to face the angst of her physical pain and mortality alone and without distraction. She queries her nurse, Leslie, one night: "I'm really having a hard time sleeping. What can I do so I'm not so anxious?" What will Lynn's nurse offer to ameliorate her distress?

If Lynn's nurse is paralyzed by the idea of dying and unable to be present to Lynn in her suffering, this nurse will likely prescribe a sedative or anti-anxiety drug. And stay out of Lynn's room. But let us assume that Lynn's nurse is a well-trained palliative care nurse who is comfortable attending to dying patients. What will this nurse offer?

If nurse Leslie is Buddhist, her repertoire of ways to address stress will likely include meditation techniques. She may suggest to Lynn that it could be helpful if she were to clear her mind of all distracting thoughts and meditate on an object of spiritual or religious significance, or on something from nature (e.g., a flower). Leslie may help Lynn to become aware and grateful for her gentle, regular breathing. She might suggest one of her favorite CDs with chants for focusing. Leslie might also share a written meditation about loving kindness with Lynn, or offer her a mantra on which to focus (e.g., "May I take care of myself with joy"). As Leslie talks with Lynn about her anxiousness and fear of dying, it is possible that in an attempt to comfort, Leslie will project her views about suffering and life after death. That is, she may suggest Lynn's anxieties reflect her attachments to the present life. By releasing these attachments, she could lessen her suffering. And indeed, doing so will put her in good stead for the rebirth after death—a rebirth that brings her nearer to Enlightenment.

If nurse Leslie, however, is a Seventh-day Adventist (SDA) Christian, her approach to helping Lynn will contrast. The SDA Leslie may offer a colloquial prayer, petitioning God to ease Lynn's anxieties and fears. If this Leslie converses with Lynn about her anxieties regarding dying, Leslie might share her beliefs about death and the afterlife. That is, death is like sleep; the next thing Lynn will see after "falling asleep in Jesus" will be a resurrection that occurs with the glorious advent of Jesus. Thereafter, all who want to live with God (i.e., those judged righteous, having accepted Jesus' grace) will go to heaven and enjoy eternal life free of suffering.

To provide a further contrast, consider Leslie, RN as a Roman Catholic. Catholic Leslie may pray colloquially, but may just as well offer a silent prayer or memorized or read form of prayer. She may also encourage Lynn to pray to Archangel Michael, the patron saint for the sick. In lieu of lighting a novena candle (fire regulations), Leslie may have a prayer card to give to Lynn with this angel's picture on it as a reminder of Michael's intercession on her behalf. If Lynn and Leslie have any dialogue about what death and afterlife are like, Leslie's beliefs will likely influence her remarks. For Leslie, death allows the soul to leave the dead body. The soul is evaluated in an initial judgment, which determines whether the life lived worthies it for heaven, purgatory, or hell. Purgatory is a temporary existence that allows suffering to cleanse one of sin, and readies one for heaven. Nurse Leslie will likely wish for Lynn an opportunity to confess her sins (perhaps formally to a priest) before her death.

These vignettes are not meant to essentialize any religious tradition but rather, for the purposes of discussion, to raise the issue that some typical features of a religion, as understood by the layperson nurse may well affect nursing care as well as perspectives on the nursing enterprise itself. Although different "Leslies" even within one religious tradition will have varying interpretations of their religion and approaches to comforting Lynn, this scenario vividly portrays how a nurse's worldview can influence his or her attempts to care. Even for spiritual nurses who do not formally affiliate with a religion, the religious lens that their family or society gives may have an impact on their care.

Should Nurses' Religiosity Be at the Bedside?

But ought a nurse's religious beliefs and practices be found at the bedside? As an editorial in the *British Journal of Nursing* stated:

> While respecting nurses' right to faith, I strongly believe that nurses have to—like teachers and the police—divide themselves from their faith in the conduct of their duties. Most do so admirably. To proselytize, or even just share, their faith with patients, many of whom are in a very vulnerable position, not only smacks to me of arrogance, but contradicts the treasured, inclusive, non-judgmental heart of nursing.[1]

Pollard's recommendation in this editorial assumes that nurses can divide themselves from their faith. But can they? There also seems to be an assumption that any sharing of faith constitutes proselytizing. But does it?

To answer these questions, it is helpful to consider how a nonreligious nurse might assist Lynn. Imagine that self-professed atheist and humanist Leslie is Lynn's nurse. This Leslie might draw from an arsenal of empirical evidence that indicates massage, aromatherapy, music, active listening, and pharmacologic agents can all be used to lessen anxiety. (Of course, the religious Leslies can do the same.) In the conversation that might ensue, Leslie would find comfort in remembering that medical therapeutics often cure disease and possibly project her confident reliance on science to Lynn. Or, if embracing Lynn's death as imminent, Leslie may have in her nursing care plan for Lynn the goal of making meaning for her life and death—a meaningfulness that does not require a supportive religious framework. Leslie might also interject questions to encourage Lynn to examine the reasons for her anxiety and possibly share skepticism about any ideations regarding an afterlife.

These contrasting "Leslies" all have a system of beliefs—whether a personally collected cluster of values or a codified religious worldview—that have an influence on their responses to patients. Regardless of how aware of these beliefs the nurse is, if the nurse is to behave in a professional context in a manner that is authentic to self—congruent with privately held beliefs, then these beliefs will motivate and shape to some degree the care that is given. Ironically, it is the nurse who is least aware of the influence of private religious (or nonreligious philosophical) beliefs who is most likely to impose these beliefs inappropriately during patient care. This is because the lack of awareness impedes the ability to bracket these beliefs when ethical care may demand it.

Therefore, we argue that it is inappropriate and disrespectful to expect nurses to divide themselves from their religiosity. To do so is to amputate an essential part of their being, and a part of their being that likely prompts their desire to be a nurse. No. The question is not whether nurses should bring their religion to the bedside (they cannot help but do so), but rather the manner in which they should bring their religion to the bedside. It is a question not of ought but how.

LITERATURE REVIEW

Nurse Religiosity

There is no study documenting the religiosity of a nurse population. A few studies about how nurses think about and practice spiritual care do superficially inquire about participants' religiosity. Given the topic for these studies about nursing spiritual care, it is likely that nurses for whom spirituality or religion is rather important comprise these samples.

Claiming a representative sample based on comparison with non-participants, one study of Arizonan nurses in a state university hospital queried them regarding a wide assortment of opinions and practices about spiritual care.[2] Of the 299 survey respondents, 42% self-reported that they were "religious" while 41% stated they were "spiritual but not religious." (Grant and colleagues cite a comparable polling of Americans that showed 30% reported they were "spiritual but not religious.") What is fascinating is that many of these nurses, in or out of religion, described nursing as a "calling" and were willing to provide the same services of a hospital chaplain if they received time and training. Religious nurses, unsurprisingly, were more agreeable about providing this spiritual care (37% vs. 28%).

Other American studies investigating nurse perspectives on spiritual care that assess study participant religiosity suggest that these nurses who are interested enough to participate are predominantly Christian (roughly 90%), with roughly 40% to 50% being Roman Catholic and the other half

Protestant.[3–6] When nurses are asked to self-report spirituality and religiosity, their spirituality is found to be higher or similar to religiosity.[7,8] A few studies document about half of the nurses attending religious services regularly or viewing them as moderately or very important.[9–11]

Pesut and Reimer-Kirkham's ethnographic study describes how the spiritual and religious identities of various health care professionals significantly influence their interactions with patients around spirituality.[12] In discussing their findings, these nurse researchers observed that these Canadian clinicians' religious or spiritual identities were varied, dynamic, and complex. For example, some participants fused aspects of different religious traditions to compose their own identity. Others resonated with the "spiritual but not religious" identity, while still being influenced by earlier religious experience. As these scholars noted, "there were no spiritualities from nowhere."[13]

A survey of all Flemish palliative care nurses' ($N = 415$) religious and ideological views and practices observed them to be interested in religious issues and likely to believe in a transcendent power.[14] These researchers clustered the nurses' religiosity as follows: church-goers (29%), atheists/agnostics (18%), doubters (18%), religious but not church-goers (18%), and devout church-goers (17%). Combining the three religious groups shows 55% of these nurses to self-report as religious, comparable with Flemish society at large.

A study of Israeli oncology nurses (96% Jewish) measured intrinsic and extrinsic religiosity, spiritual well-being, as well as attitudes toward spiritual care.[15] Among the Jewish nurses, 58% self-identified as "secular" while 21% perceived themselves as "traditional" and 21% were "religious." Although these categories were not used in the subsequent path analysis, the religiosity (especially intrinsic) was observed to contribute indirectly to spiritual care attitude.

Unfortunately, this paltry body of data regarding the religiosity of nurses is too limited in scope and method to provide a base for strong generalization. It is likely that nurses simply reflect the religious diversity of the societies in which they live. As with societal trends, nurses often see themselves more as spiritual than religious. This relatively recent phenomenon suggests individuals desire the essence of religion but without its institutional forms.

Relationships Between Nurse Religiosity and Nursing Care

Although we know little about the specifics of nurses' religiosity, it is logical to assume that whatever religiosity shapes a nurse will impact her or his work. Some evidence in this regard suggests that not only does nurses' religiosity have an impact on the nursing care they deliver, but the experience of giving nursing care can have an impact on nurse religiosity. Theoretical and empirical literature exploring this interrelatedness follows.

Theory

From a philosophical perspective, Cusveller addresses the question of whether religious nurses should allow religious commitments to influence their nursing care.[16] Cusveller raised several pertinent questions: Do nurses' moral and religious commitments stay in the private realm and never enter health care? Can a nurse really divide commitments? Does nursing "professionalism" really require a neutral moral or religious stance? Is neutrality possible? How is nursing care implemented and evaluated when there are no systems of meaning (philosophy, worldview, or religion) whereby to judge it? After all, science only goes so far in providing answers to what is right, what is well-being, what should be the goal of care, and so forth.

A nurse needs "control beliefs," beliefs that can guide decisions about what nursing actions to take or not take when universally accepted facts for guiding practice are nonexistent. Cusveller posits that religious beliefs offer religious nurses control beliefs. Cusveller concludes with the following guidance for how the commitments of religious nurses should affect their practice:

> Just as scholars cannot rid themselves of their particular points of view, but have to discuss them in order to develop the best possible theories, so nurses have to bring their particular points of view to nursing and [sic] to discuss them in order to provide the best possible care. Moral, philosophical and religious convictions are not just bias, although they may be, but they can also have a positive function. Where there is no universally accepted set of fundamental principles, be it Christian, scientific or professional, nurses may enter the practice of nursing as religious committed nurses.[17]

Note that Cusveller does not suggest that religious beliefs supersede universally accepted nursing dogma. Thus, rather than sterilizing themselves of religious beliefs while at the bedside, religious nurses can appreciate the control beliefs their religion's gift to them. Indeed, it is a matter of morality that the nurse maintains integrity, respecting his or her identity and living respectfully with those beliefs.[18]

Indeed, the notion of value neutrality is an illusion. Ethicist Pellegrino portrays how a clinician's decision making is inevitably influenced by personal and professional values.[19] For example, a nurse teaching a diabetic likely believes that a certain diet and lifestyle is conducive to health, that health should be a high priority for people and society, that teaching the individual is more important than teaching the family, and so forth. Pellegrino disagrees with ethicists who argue the clinician can put aside or alter personal values when a professional role is better filled by doing so (e.g., assist with terminating fetal life when it is against the clinician's beliefs). To do so would be "moral schizophrenia"; it is impossible and fails to respect the autonomy and dignity of the clinician. Pellegrino suggests that the ethical approach when there is such a clash in values making care impossible should involve: (a) informing the patient of the reasons for why the clinician is removing him or herself from caring, and (b) assisting the patient to find a clinician who will be supportive. The process for informing a patient of a nurse's removal from care activities, of course, should be respectful and not take advantage of the patient's vulnerability.

Bjarnason applies physician Daniel Foster's reasoning for why doctors must consider religion in routine patient care to the work of nurses.[20] In addition to accepting that many patients' responses to illness are influenced by their religious beliefs and that illness often brings to the surface religious issues, Foster recognizes that clinicians' decisions about how to care for patients is influenced by their own religious beliefs. Although Bjarnason cites a handful of studies about medical doctors' treatment decisions as being associated with religious beliefs, there is a paucity of research to show how nurses' caring is influenced by religiosity. A fourth reason for addressing religion among clinicians, according to Foster, is that patients typically place the clinician in the role of secular "priest" (or "priestess" as Bjarnason applies it to nurses). It is not unusual for nurses to receive "confession" from a patient. Such confessions may be of wrongs committed (e.g., sexual indiscretions) or of realizations of the consequences for medical decisions that the patient made while uninformed or under coercion (e.g., to be coded).

Meux and Rooda offer a conceptual model for "religio-specific nursing practice."[21] This model acknowledges that both the nurse and the patient introduce to the clinical encounter a cultural background that includes religiosity. The model advises that a nurse's knowledge of differences about religions can help during the actual nurse–patient interaction. The outcome of such interaction should show the nurse's respect for the patient's religiosity—hence, religio-specific nursing practice—and the need to educate nurses regarding religions.

Empirical Evidence

A small number of research studies provide insight regarding how nurse religiosity has an impact on nursing care. This research begins to describe how a nurse's religious affiliation affects attitudes, actual care provided, and how a nurse gives meaning to work. A few studies also describe how religious beliefs help nurses to cope with the stressors of nursing work, as well as how those same beliefs can potentially create dissonance.

Religion Affects Nurses' Attitudes and Care. Religious nurses often view their work as a "calling"—clearly conferring religious meaning upon their work as nurses.[22–24] In Grant's survey of nurses, a quarter of both those identifying themselves as religious and spiritual (i.e., not religious) acknowledged their work was a calling.[25] Indeed, nurses of many other religious traditions likewise view their vocation as a sacred and divinely called—or even as ministry. A Christian nurse participating in a phenomenological study about spiritual care illustrates this point:

> We have so many opportunities to share and to witness. I've always used nursing as a springboard for ministry. I look at nursing as a ministry, not a job. Maybe that's why I've always enjoyed 32 years and still enjoy it. I still have a passion in working for Christ.[26]

Whereas some religious nurses view nursing as the end, some (presumably more evangelically oriented) nurses perceive nursing as a means to an end rather than an end in itself. What the "end" is, will vary and reflect the beliefs of the nurse. For example, the ultimate purpose of nursing for some may be to "glorify God" or be a conduit of Love; for others, it may be converting patients to their religious beliefs. These ends raise a vital question for religious nurses: Is the value of my being a nurse in the nursing I do, or in the witnessing I do in the context of nursing? To put this in moral terms, "Is nursing a good in itself, or simply an instrumental good to other ends?"

While some nurses may perceive their call to ministry via nursing in an understated and general way, others may have an acute awareness of specific circumstances leading them into nursing that they attribute to divine guidance. As another Christian nurse observed:

> I look at my job as a calling and as a mission field . . . I do believe that the [way for the] door to be open, way back, to even go to nursing school, was divinely appointed. I was sitting in church. Single mom, divorced, no home, no car. No means other than the job and just to survive and I've always wanted to go back to school. And it was just not part of what I could swing. And I got a true word that this was the desire of my heart and shortly thereafter the doors began to open and I was able to do that. . . . The calling got louder. And so it's always been in my heart to be a minister, for my hands to be trained. And this is just how God trained my hands to deliver that.[27]

This quote also suggests how when a nurse frames the work of nursing as a response to a divine calling, this meaning inevitably manifests in what the "hands deliver"—that is in how care is given.

Most of the research quantitatively linking a nurses' religiosity with attitudes that influence nursing practice is research exploring spiritual care attitudes and practice. This research fairly consistently suggests that nurse religiosity is linked with positive attitudes toward providing spiritual care, which is directly related to the frequency of giving spiritual care.[28-31] An exception to this trend was found in a study of mostly Israeli Jewish nurses among whom no differences in spiritual care attitudes were found between those who were secular or religious.[32] Furthermore, the religious Jewish nurses tended to have possibly less positive attitudes about giving spiritual care, likely reflecting a belief that spiritual needs are the domain of religious professionals. When measuring religiosity as intrinsic or extrinsic, however, religiosity was found to predict attitude toward spiritual care.[33]

A glimpse of how nurses' private religiosity influences their spiritual caregiving is also seen in data showing how nurses learn about spiritual caregiving. Although basic and continuing education are primary venues for learning, there is evidence that nurses also take what they have learned from their religious leaders, programs, and personal spiritual or religious experiences and apply it to their practice of nursing.[34-36]

Several studies have also examined if nurse religiosity is associated with attitudes regarding euthanasia and physician-assisted suicide. A detailed review of the evidence completed by Gielen and colleagues supported the hypothesis that nurse religiosity and worldview does influence attitudes toward euthanasia and physician-assisted suicide.[37] Religious affiliation and doctrine, observance of religious practices, and the personal importance of religion were found to be factors influencing attitude. These scholars, however, appreciated the diversity of cultures and religious beliefs represented in the collection of reviewed studies made global conclusions inappropriate. They recommend that future research in this area examine how specific theological beliefs (e.g., about the sanctity of life, afterlife, divine intervention, religious authority) influence nurses' attitudes and care.

A couple of studies explore how nurse religiosity has an impact on how nurses converse with patients. Christopher explores nurse religiosity in relation to willingness to release control in conversations with patients about end of life care.[38] It was theorized that when sensitive and morally ambiguous topics, like dying, are discussed with patients, nurses who are personally disconcerted will manage this distress by exerting more control during the conversation. The study involved an online survey of 115 graduate nursing students; religiosity was measured using an intrinsic/extrinsic religiosity scale. It was found that neither type of religiosity correlated with relational control. A direct relationship, however, was observed between intrinsic religiosity and an additional item "I would want a patient to interrupt if I suggested a treatment contrary to his or her religious beliefs." Although these study findings failed to fully support the hypotheses, future research with stronger methods can shed further light on the ways in which nurse religiosity does have an impact on interaction with patients. Pesut and Reimer-Kirkham's ethnographic study describes how nurses sometimes used their religious experience as a connecting point with patients, a way to gain entrée to talk with them about spirituality.[39] Conversely, these researchers also observed that sometimes nurses realized their religiosity was something to hold back. Hence, nurses may juggle whether and when to hide or expose their religion. This is illustrated in Geller and colleagues' survey of genetic nurses.[40] Over a quarter of these 59 nurses responded that they occasionally/commonly felt conflicted about disclosing personal beliefs to colleagues or patients.

Although scanty and weak, this evidence does indeed begin to show how nurses' religiosity influences how they care. The religious beliefs motivating nurses, however, vary. A qualitative study of Iranian Muslim nurses found some nurses viewed the provision of nursing care as an opportunity to worship God.[41] Similarly, nurses of other religious traditions may be motivated by an experience of divine love, and wish to reciprocate this through nursing caring.[42] Many religions espouse a "Golden Rule" and this may form a foundation that motivates a nurse. As one nurse puts it, "I look to Christ as my example and I look at the patient and [consider] how I would want to be treated in the same manner." For others, the presumption of a divine judgment and potential retribution may motivate their good deeds. As the first nurse quoted above stated, "I have to answer to Him at the end of the day."

Religious coping among nurses. A handful of studies about nurses begin to show what has been well-established among patients: Religiosity influences coping. Qualitative studies from Canada, Sweden, and the United States briefly portray how nurses' religious faith help them to maintain hope, find comfort, cope with the stressors of work, and provide a meaningful orientation.[43–46] Bunta explores religious coping among emergency department and intensive care unit nurses and found that both state and trait anxiety were predicted in part by religious coping.[47] That is, negative religious coping (e.g., endorsing items like feeling abandoned or punished by God, questioning the power of God) explained a significant amount of anxiety. Likewise, positive religious coping was linked with lower anxiety among these nurses in stressful work environments. Another study of Hungarian sister nurses (Roman Catholic nuns) demonstrated an inverse correlation between religiosity and burnout, suggesting that religious beliefs and practices can function to protect nurses against burnout.[48]

RECOMMENDATIONS FOR NURSING PRACTICE

> I feel that as a Christian, when the Holy Spirit tells me to pray with that individual even if I'm not supposed to, that the Lord will protect me. And so I don't care; [laughs] so that's always been my attitude.[49]

This nurse's remark raises questions: Under what circumstances is it ethical for religious nurses to introduce their particular religious practices or beliefs to patients? Is it possible that some religious beliefs, such as interpreting promptings as of the Holy Spirit and the omnipotence of God to protect them from ill-conceived nursing care, could sometimes be detrimental to patient care? How can a religious nurse know whether to follow divine promptings that would have an impact on nursing care? These are difficult questions. Some guidelines for helping the religious nurse to address the above questions will be offered following a discussion to increase an awareness of how nurse religiosity can create negative and positive effects in nurse–patient encounters.

The Impact of Nurse Religiosity on Patient Care

Negative Effects
The nurse–patient relationship is inevitably asymmetric in terms of power; a nurse can potentially use his or her religion to harm a patient—albeit unintentionally. Although in theory a patient has the power to refuse a nurse's care, in reality such a refusal is improbable given the resulting challenges it would pose (e.g., "I need nursing help now, and I don't want to have to wait for a different nurse—who might be as bad as this one!" "Might the system hold my refusal against me?"). Thus, the patient is in a vulnerable position as the recipient of nursing care. Given this power imbalance, it can be appreciated how the unwelcomed or inappropriate introduction of religion at the bedside could easily become harmful to the patient or detrimental to the nurse–patient relationship and nursing care.

There are more subtle ways, however, in which religious nurses' beliefs can become hurtful. Taylor identifies ways in which a nurse could speak harmfully, even in an attempt to comfort a patient searching for meaning.[50] For example, a very common misquotation from the Christian New Testament is "God doesn't give you more than you can bear" which may leave the patient confused about a punishing deity and reinforce that they are suffering more than they can bear. Likewise, "Just pray about it" is often unhelpful and may show the patient how the nurse needs to use religion as avoidance coping or for passive decision making. Although a religious nurse likely has the sincerest of intentions, such admonitions can be harmful for patients who are spiritually struggling.

Positive Effects

Whereas the potential negative effects of a nurse introducing personal religious beliefs or practices into nursing care can seem to outweigh the potential positive effects, it is important to remember how religion can benefit—and may outweigh the negatives—in the nurse–patient encounter. Because religions offer individuals ways of understanding suffering, explaining life and death, purpose for living, and guidance in clinical moral decisions, religious nurses have a framework for making sense of the tragedies they continually witness at work.[51,52] Religions characteristically also provide believers with hope, social support, and practices that promote emotional and physical health.[53] If a nurse does find these benefits from a religion, she or he undoubtedly has an important tool for dealing with the stressors of nursing practice.

A common dimensionality applied to religiosity in nursing research is that of intrinsic and extrinsic religiosity. Simply put, intrinsic religiosity is religion that is lived (i.e., religiosity is integrated in all aspects of living), whereas extrinsic religiosity is used to seek an end (e.g., to gain social status, to achieve immortality). The scanty evidence about nurses' religiosity may mirror that observed among patients: that is, a solid intrinsic religiosity is associated with positive outcomes, whereas extrinsic religiosity may not be helpful.[54,55] Furthermore, positive religious beliefs are associated with positive outcomes, and negative religious beliefs are linked to negative outcomes.[56] Thus, it is likely that it is the nurse with high intrinsic religiosity and a paucity of negative religious beliefs who is well equipped for the rigors of nursing. We conjecture that such "armor" should allow nurses to be able to be more peacefully present to a patient and offer more wisdom when the patient asks for it.

When Personal and Professional Beliefs Clash

Occasionally, a nurse's personal religious beliefs contradict professional beliefs. Perhaps the most common instance of such a clash is when nurses whose religious beliefs maintain it is morally wrong to abort a fetus are asked to assist with an abortion procedure or counsel couples about it as a therapeutic option. Winslow and Wehtje-Winslow maintain that nurses should provide care that is consonant with their beliefs.[57] Pellegrino agrees, and suggests that during initial contact with patients, clinicians should inform patients of their religious perspective if it is likely to influence the subsequent care they deliver.[58]

Both the American and Canadian Nurses' Associations codes of ethics contain a "conscientious objection" clause.[59,60] Conscientious objection permits a nurse to refuse to participate in a nursing duty on the grounds of moral or religious objection. Conscientious objection can be invoked for categories of activity (e.g., participation in abortion or sexual reassignment) or for particular interventions for particular patients on the grounds of moral inappropriateness for that patient (e.g., not in the patient's best interests, or the patient did not want it). Both codes state that although patient safety is foremost, the nurse must provide safe, compassionate, and competent care for a patient requiring care the nurse believes to be morally unacceptable until alternative arrangements can be made. The patient is never to be abandoned. Nurses can and should, however, communicate this objection in advance. Conscientious objection to participation in particular treatments ought to be discussed with employers (including patients, if the nurse is in solo practice). For example, a midwife may have a brochure introducing herself, as well as a verbal introduction, that indicates how her religious beliefs could affect her nursing care. A nurse employed by an institution that offers treatments morally objectionable to the nurse should opt out of participation, in writing, at the start of employment. This, of course, would not affect conscientious objection on the grounds that a particular treatment was contrary to the patient's best interests or wishes. Pellegrino suggests that when clinicians refuse to provide care due to religious reasons, they should assist patients to find a replacement.

Proselytizing

Proselytizing, an attempt to convert another to one's own religion, is the most essential concern about religious nurses sharing their religious beliefs or practices with patients. However, proselytizing should not be confused with openness about one's religious faith when a patient asks. Proselytizing, or evangelizing, seeks the end of conversion. It is generally considered to be morally objectionable to proselytize in illness settings where that setting is not explicitly and openly religious. There is a power differential between nurse and patient, and patients are generally made more vulnerable by illness. These factors combine to constrain a patient's freedom in the face of proselytizing.

Thiessen proposes that there is a continuum of persuasion. At a gentle end of this continuum is education.[61] While moving toward a more aggressive end of coercion, one passes through advisement and persuasion. This can be schematically presented as:

$$\text{educate} \rightarrow \text{advise} \rightarrow \text{persuade} \rightarrow \text{coerce}$$

Thiessen posits proselytization can be moral when it is nonaggressive and noncoercive; immoral proselytization, in contrast, is aggressive and coercive. Thiessen argues that proselytizing is ethical or moral when it is done as an expression of care and respect for the other person. It should be done in a way that protects the dignity and worth of the individual. Thus, this philosopher offers a framing for the possibility of an ethical sharing of nurse religiosity with patients.

Fowler disagrees. However soft the attempt at proselytizing, it is intrinsically coercive in a nonreligious setting, and seeks the end of conversion. It also subordinates nursing to evangelization. Fowler would, however, allow that when a patient asks about a nurse's own faith, the nurse is free to share—as a part of a duty to self to maintain wholeness of person—but it is only permissible if that sharing preserves and affirms the patient's freedom and autonomy. In these instances, sharing is at the patient's request, is welcomed by the patient, and aims to support (not convert) the patient. Because such welcome sharing also has the potential to deepen a dialogue with patients that moves them toward greater clarity of the *patients'* own values, or healing, or a relationship that addresses their spiritual needs in the face of illness or trauma, it should not be foreclosed. Sharing one's faith, then, must be done only with an eye to the *health-related concerns,* even health-related spiritual concerns, of the patient, and not disconnected from that for some salvific aim.[62]

Guiding Principles. The ANA and CNA codes of ethics mandate that patients' "religious beliefs" or "unique values, customs and spiritual beliefs" be respected to preserve their dignity.[63,64] The interpretive statements accompanying these codes also provide guidance on this issue of proselytization. The ANA *Code of Ethics with Interpretive Statements* states:

> In situations where the patient requests a personal opinion from the nurse, the nurse is generally free to express an informed personal opinion as long as this preserves the voluntariness of the patient and maintains appropriate professional and moral boundaries. It is essential to be aware of the potential for undue influence attached to the nurse's professional role. Assisting patients to clarify their own values in reaching informed decisions may be helpful in avoiding unintended persuasion.[65]

Similarly, the CNA *Code of Ethics* states:

> Nurses maintain appropriate professional boundaries and ensure their relationships are always for the benefit of the persons they serve. They recognize the potential vulnerability of persons and do not exploit their trust and dependency in a way that might compromise the therapeutic relationship. . . .[66]

These Codes remind nurses of their primary role of supporting patient health (not religious indoctrination) and of the powerful position the nurse holds intrinsically in any nurse–patient relationship. Sharing of a religious "opinion" can threaten this delicate relationship if the patient did not volunteer for it, and if the nurse exploits a patient's request for it.

Greenway's fundamental principles for religious evangelism provide further guidance for the nurse whose patient has asked for a religious perspective.[67] These principles include:

- *Reciprocity.* This means that the nurse sharing religious beliefs and the patient ought to have equal opportunity to share their ideas. Such a stance requires that the nurse is respectful and not defensive. Guidelines for nurse self-disclosure include not only initially asking "whose needs am I meeting by self-disclosing?" but also following up self-disclosures with a question for the patient that allows them the opportunity to respond so the nurse can gauge the therapeutic value of the disclosure.
- *Honesty in both message and methods.* Not only must the message given be truthful, but the means whereby it is delivered is not deceptive. Asking a patient, "Do you mind if I ask you a question?" to gain entrée to share religious beliefs is misleading and coercive. Another subtle way some religious nurses may coerce their beliefs is by preaching—sharing beliefs—during a prayer, when a patient has only asked for prayer. "Bait and switch" tactics become unethical in the context of caring for vulnerable people (e.g., having nursing students obtain patients' permission to survey them about their spirituality, then ending the "survey" with a conversation where their religious beliefs are shared.) This principle should also encourage heart-searching among missionary nurses about methods for health evangelism (e.g., is material assistance or health care used as bait for evangelism among disadvantaged people?)
- *Humility.* The nurse who shares her or his faith must not be arrogant or condescending, and not self-serving or self-glorifying. The nurse who is sharing religious beliefs must not be doing it for personal gain (e.g., to gain her own salvation, or to get "another jewel in my crown"). Rather, sharing must have an authentic desire for the well-being of the other's health. It is also done to please God, not self or others. Nurses who believe they are responsible for converting others are trusting themselves, not their God.
- *Respect.* The nurse must recognize that patients are not objects to manipulate. Instead of coercion, the religious nurse should respect and support a patient's freedom to make choices. Of course, this includes the freedom to not discuss religious matters.

Again, Fowler would maintain that proselytizing is impermissible in the nonreligious health care context, that it wounds a patient's freedom, that it makes nursing subservient to other ends, and that it disconnects faith from health concerns that are the proper purview of the nurse.[68] However, she would affirm that Greenway's principles should be attributes of all nurse–patient relationships: reciprocity, honesty, humility, and respect.

Although there may be times when a religious nurse is asked by a patient to address religious concerns, it is important for nurses to remember that they are the spiritual care generalists.[69] Spiritual care experts such as trained chaplains, pastoral counselors, spiritual directors, and clergy are the specialists. Sometimes nurse–patient conversations about religious concerns will inform the nurse that a serious issue exists. At such times, the nurse should ask the patient for permission to make a referral and discuss with the patient which expert is preferred.

CONCLUSION

Many nurses are religious. The religious dimension of their personhood cannot be extracted and placed in the nurse's locker while she or he works. Indeed, a small body of evidence indicates nurse religiosity is related to attitudes and practice, especially about spiritual care and end-of-life care. It is important for nurses to reflect on how their personal religiosity does have an impact on their provision of care. Without this bracketing, it is inevitable that the nurse's religiosity will manifest in disrespectful and harmful ways at the bedside. This chapter provides recommendations for how nurses can ethically bring their religion to the bedside. More clinical guidelines are provided in the companion book *Religion: A Clinical Guide for Nurses*.[70]

NOTES

1. Pollard, Tom. "The Place of Religion in Nursing Practice." *British Journal of Nursing* 18.4 (2009): 217.
2. Grant, Donald, Kathleen M. O'Neil and Laura S. Stephens. "Neosecularization and Craft versus Professional Religious Authority in a Nonreligious Organization." *Journal for the Scientific Study of Religion* 42.3 (2003): 479–87.
3. Cavendish, Roberta, Lynda Konecny, Claudia Mitzeliotis, et al. "Spiritual Care Activities of Nurses Using Nursing Interventions Classification (NIC) Labels." *International Journal of Nursing Terminology Classification* 14.4 (2003): 113–24.
4. Taylor, Elizabeth J., Martha Highfield, and Madalon Amenta. "Attitudes and Beliefs Regarding Spiritual Care: A Survey of Cancer Nurses." *Cancer Nursing* 17.6 (1994): 479–87.
5. Scott, Marshall, Marisue Grzybowski, and Sue Webb. "Perceptions and Practices of Registered Nurses Regarding Pastoral Care and the Spiritual Need of Hospital Patients." *Journal of Pastoral Care* 48.2 (1994): 171–79.

6. Christopher, Stephanie A. "The Relationship between Nurses' Religiosity and Willingness to Let Patients Control the Conversation about End-of-life Care." *Patient Education and Counseling* 78 (2010): 250–55.

7. Taylor, Elizabeth J., Martha Highfield, and Madalon Amenta. "Predictors of Oncology and Hospice Nurses Spiritual Care Perspectives and Practices." *Applied Nursing Research* 12.1 (1999): 30–37.

8. Grant, et al., op. cit.

9. Geller, Gail, Ellyn Micco, Rachel J. Silver, et al. "The Role and Impact of Personal Faith and Religion among Genetic Service Providers." *American Journal of Medical Genetics Part C: Seminars in Medical Genetics* 151C.1 (2009): 31–40.

10. Scott, et al., op. cit.

11. Taylor, Elizabeth J., Iris Mamier, Khalid Bahjri, et al. "Efficacy of a Self-Study Programme to Teach Spiritual Care." *Journal of Clinical Nursing* 18.8 (2009): 1131–40.

12. Pesut, Barb, and Sheryl Reimer-Kirkham. "Situated Clinical Encounters in the Negotiation of Religious and Spiritual Plurality: A Critical Ethnography." *International Journal of Nursing Studies* 47.7 (2010): 85–825.

13. Ibid., 8.

14. Gielen, Joris, Stef van den Branden, Trudie van Iersel, et al. "Religion, World View and the Nurse: Results of a Quantitative Survey Among Flemish Palliative Care Nurses." *International Journal of Palliative Nursing* 15.12 (2009): 590–99.

15. Musgrave, Catherine and Elizabeth McFarlane. "Intrinsic and Extrinsic Religiosity, Spiritual Well-Being, and Attitudes toward Spiritual Care: A Comparison of Israeli Jewish Oncology Nurses' Scores." *Oncology Nursing Forum* 31.6 (2004): 1179–83.

16. Cusveller, Bart S. "A View from Somewhere: The Presence and Function of Religious Commitment in Nursing Practice." *Journal of Advanced Nursing* 22.5 (1995): 973–78.

17. Ibid., 977.

18. Fowler, Marsha. Ed. *Guide to the Code of Ethics for Nurses: Interpretation and Application*. Silver Spring, MD: American Nurses Association, 2008.

19. Pellegrino, Edmund D. "Commentary: Value Neutrality, Moral Integrity, and the Physician." *Journal of Law, Medicine, & Ethics* 28.1 (2000): 78–81.

20. Bjarnason, Dana. "Nursing, Religiosity, and End of Life Care: Interconnections and Implications." *Nursing Clinics of North America* 44.4 (2009): 517–25.

21. Meux, Louis, and Linda A. Rooda. (1995). "The Development of a Model for Delivery of Religio-Specific Nursing Care." *Journal of Holistic Nursing* 13.2 (1995): 132–41.

22. Edwards, Adrian, N. Pang, V. Shui, et al. "The Understanding of Spirituality and the Potential Role of Spiritual Care in End of Life and Palliative Care: A Meta-Study of Qualitative Research. *Palliative Medicine* 24.8 (2010): 753–70.

23. Grant, et al., op. cit.

24. Taylor, Elizabeth J. and Mark Carr. "Nursing Ethics in the Seventh-Day Adventist Religious Tradition." *Nursing Ethics* 16.6 (2009): 707–18.

25. Grant, et al., op. cit.

26. Unpublished data from a phenomenological study of Christian nurses identified as spiritual care "experts" being conducted by Taylor, Elizabeth J., Jane Pfeiffer, and Carla Gober. Loma Linda, CA: Loma Linda University School of Nursing.

27. Ibid.

28. Grant, et al., op. cit.

29. O'Shea, Eileen R., M. Wallace, Margaret Q. Griffin, et al. "The Effect of an Educational Session on Pediatric Nurses' Perspectives toward Providing Spiritual Care." *Journal of Pediatric Nursing* 26.1 (2011): 34–43.

30. Taylor, Elizabeth J. "Spiritual Care Nursing Research: The State of the Science." *Journal of Christian Nursing* 22.1 (2005): 22–28.

31. Chan, Moon Fai. "Factors Affecting Nursing Staff in Practicing Spiritual Care." *Journal of Clinical Nursing* 19.15–16 (2010): 2128–36.

32. Musgrave, Catherine and Elizabeth McFarlane. "Israeli Oncology Nurses' Religiosity, Spiritual Well-Being, and Attitudes toward Spiritual Care: A Path Analysis." *Oncology Nursing Forum* 31.2 (2004): 321–27.

33. Musgrave & McFarlane, 2004, op. cit.

34. Sellers, Sandra C. and Barbara Haag. "Spiritual Nursing Interventions." *Journal of Holistic Nursing* 16.3 (1998): 338–54.

35. Highfield, Martha, Elizabeth J. Taylor, and Madalon Amenta. "Preparation to Care: The Spiritual Care Education of Oncology and Hospice Nurses." *Journal of Hospice and Palliative Nursing* 2.2 (2000): 53–63.

36. Taylor, Elizabeth J., Iris Mamier, Khalid Bahjri, Triin Anton, and Floyd Petersen. "Efficacy of a Self-Study Programme to Teach Spiritual Care." *Journal of Clinical Nursing* 18.8 (2009): 1131–40.

37. Gielen, et al., op. cit.

38. Christopher, op. cit.

39. Pesut & Reimer-Kirkham, op. cit.

40. Geller, et al., op. cit.

41. Ravari, Ali, Zohreh Vanaki, Hydarali Houmann, et al. "Spiritual Job Satisfaction in an Iranian Nursing Context." *Nursing Ethics* 16.1 (2009): 19–30.

42. For example, see: Taylor & Carr, op. cit.

43. Duggleby, Wendy, Dan Cooper, and Kelly Penz. "Hope, Self-efficacy, Spiritual Well-being and Job Satisfaction." *Journal of Advanced Nursing* 65.11 (2009): 2376–85.

44. Ekedahl, Marieanne and Yvonne Wengström. Caritas, Spirituality and Religiosity in Nurses' Coping. *European Journal of Cancer Care* 19.4 (2010): 530–37. (2009 epub).

45. Burkhart, Lisa and Nancy Hogan. "An Experiential Theory of Spiritual Care in Nursing Practice." *Qualitative Health Research* 18.7 (2008): 928–38.

46. Geller, et al., op. cit.

47. Bunta, Adrian. "A Study of Anxiety, Religious Coping, and Selected Predictor Variables in Emergency Room and Intensive Care Unit Nurses at a Hospital in Phoenix, Arizona." *Dissertation Abstracts International: Section B: The Sciences and Engineering* 69.12-B (2009): 7841.

48. Kovacs, Bernadett. "The Relationship between Burnout and Religious Belief among Nuns Serving as Nurses." *Psychiatria Hungarica* 24.1 (2009): 74–87.

49. Taylor, Pfeiffer, & Gober, op. cit.

50. Taylor, Elizabeth J. *Spiritual Care: Nursing Theory, Research, and Practice.* Upper Saddle River, NJ: Prentice Hall, 2002.

51. Cavendish, Roberta, Lynda Konecny, B. K. Luise, et al. Nurses Enhance Performance through Prayer. *Holistic Nursing Practice* 18.1 (2004): 26–31.

52. Gerow, Lisa, Patricia Conejo, Amanda Alonzo, et al. "Creating a Curtain of Protection: Nurses' Experiences of Grief Following a Death." *Journal of Nursing Scholarship* 42.2 (2010): 122–29.

53. Levin, Jeff. *God, Faith, and Health: Exploring the Spirituality-Healing Connection.* New York: Wiley, 2001.

54. Christopher, op. cit.

55. Musgrave & McFarlane, 2004, op. cit.

56. Bunta, op. cit.

57. Winslow, Gerald R. and Betty Wehtje-Winslow. Ethical Boundaries of Spiritual Care. *Medical Journal of Australia* 186.10 Supplement (2007): S63–65.

58. Pellegrino, op. cit.

59. American Nurses Association. *Code of Ethics with Interpretative Statements.* Silver Spring, MD: Author, 2008. Web. 20 March 2011, from http://nursingworld. org/MainMenuCategories/ThePracticeofProfessionalNursing/EthicsStandards/ CodeofEthics.aspx.

60. Canadian Nurses Association. *Code of Ethics for Registered Nurses.* Ottawa, Ontario: Author, 2008. Web. 20 March 2011, from http://www.cna-nurses.ca/CNA/ documents/pdf/publications/Cod_of_Ethics_2008_e.pdf.

61. Thiessen, Elmer J. "The Problems and Possibilities of Defining Precise Criteria to Distinguish between Ethical and Unethical Proselytizing/Evangelism." *Cultic Studies Review* 5.3 (2006): 374–87.

62. Perspective of Dr. Marsha D. M. Fowler, noted nurse ethicist and ordained Presbyterian clergy, in personal communication with the author April 7, 2011.

63. American Nurses Association, op. cit.

64. Canadian Nurses Association, op. cit.

65. American Nurses Association, op. cit., Provision 5.3.

66. Canadian Nurses Association, op. cit. ANA Provision D.7.

67. Greenway, Roger S. "The Ethics of Evangelism." *Calvin Theological Journal* 28 (1993): 147–54.

68. Fowler, op. cit.

69. Taylor, Elizabeth J. *"Spiritual Care: Nursing Theory, Research, and Practice."* Upper Saddle River, NJ: Prentice Hall, 2002.

70. Taylor, Elizabeth J. *"Religion: A Clinical Guide for Nurses."* New York: Springer, in press.

18

The Measurement of Religious Concepts in Nursing

Richard Sawatzky and Landa Terblanche

INTRODUCTION

This chapter addresses approaches to the measurement of religious concepts for nursing theory and practice based on individuals' self-reports. Examples of religious concepts encountered in health research include religious affiliation, religious attendance (participation in religious services or activities), religious orientation, private religiousness, religious coping, and religious beliefs, values, and experiences.[1] Nurses have used established instruments and developed new ones for the measurement of religious concepts to address questions such as: To what extent do individuals draw on their religion to cope with health challenges? What is the impact of religious beliefs, experiences, and practices on health? What are the implications of individual differences in religious beliefs, experiences, and practices for nursing care? The results of studies that answer these questions vary and must be interpreted in light of the characteristics of the measurement instruments that were used and the populations and purposes for which they were developed. It is therefore important for nurses who draw on these studies to be knowledgeable about the processes and assumptions underlying the measurement validation of religious concepts and the corresponding inferences that may be warranted, which is the focus of this chapter.

ABOUT MEASUREMENT VALIDATION

A fundamental premise for the measurement of religious concepts is that, although most are inherently latent (i.e., they are not directly observable and hence not directly measurable), their measurements can be inferred from related observations, such as individuals' reports of their religious beliefs, experiences, and practices.[2,3] This is not unique to religious concepts; there are numerous other latent concepts that are not *directly* observable, such as depression, anxiety, coping, and health. The implication is that the measurement of such concepts requires a theory that relates the concept of interest to the observations from which measurements of the concept are inferred. That is, the measurement of latent concepts requires a theory about the relationship between the conceptual (theoretical) and operational (observable) domains.[4] Here, the conceptual domain refers to the latent concepts and the relationships among them that are not directly observable but inferred from related observations. The operational domain refers to observations that, in the context of self-report measurements, consist of individuals' responses to questions or statements (e.g., *items* of a measurement instrument or questionnaire) that function as *measurement indicators* of the latent concept. For example, it has been suggested that a measure of religious well-being (a latent concept) can be inferred from individuals' responses to questions about their relation with "God." This is the case in the Spiritual Well-Being Scale that includes 10 questions for the measurement of religious well-being (e.g., "I feel most fulfilled when I am in close communion with God" and "My relation with God contributes to my sense of well-being") that are rated on a six-point scale ranging from strongly agree to strongly disagree.[5] The theory underlying the measurement of a latent concept should provide an explanation of how the measurement indicators represent (or reflect) the concept and the mechanisms by which they produce a *measure* (i.e., a scaled score) of the degree to which a concept is manifest. The resulting measure is viewed as an "empirical analog" of the concept of interest.[6]

These considerations are foundational to the validation of self-report measures. Within the field of educational testing, Messick[7] offers a comprehensive and influential perspective of measurement validity that he defines as "an overall evaluative judgment of the degree to which empirical evidence and theoretical rationales support the adequacy and appropriateness of interpretations and actions on the basis of test scores or other models of assessment." In this sense, measurement validation is viewed as a theory-laden activity that involves: (a) the use of empirical approaches (statistical as well as qualitative approaches) to investigate the meaning or interpretation of a measured concept and (b) theoretical and pragmatic considerations about the utility of the measurement in terms of its intended purpose(s) and any related social and ethical consequences.[8–11] That is, measurement is not merely a mechanical procedure; it is an *inferential process* "by which an attempt is made to understand the nature of a variable [or concept]."[12] In the context of our discussion, the measurement validation of religious concepts, therefore, refers to the analytical processes (theoretical and empirical) through which we come to understand concepts that pertain to religion, religiosity, religiousness, religious affiliation, and religious beliefs, experiences, and practices. This includes the justification of inferences pertaining to the measurement of these concepts and their relationships with other concepts of relevance to nursing's theoretical and clinical purposes.

These perspectives of measurement validation have important implications for the measurement of religious concepts. At the *operational* level, a religious concept is understood through the question(s) and statement(s) (items) from which a measure of the concept is inferred. This necessitates an examination of individuals' interpretations of the items and whether these are congruent with those of other individuals and the concept that is being measured. The operational level also pertains to the processes by which responses to the items (measurement indicators) are used to produce a measure (scaled score) that is reliable and valid with respect to the intended purpose(s) for which the measure is to be used. At the *conceptual* level, the measurement of a religious concept (i.e., the interpretation of the measurement scores) requires an in-depth understanding of its relationships with other relevant concepts. This has traditionally been called the "nomological network"[13,14] of a concept and includes knowledge about its *antecedents* (i.e., concepts that contribute to a change in the religious concept) and *consequences* (i.e., outcomes or concepts that are affected by the religious concept). An implication of a *philosophical* nature is that the measurement of a religious concept inevitably reflects a frame of reference by which the relationships between the religious concept and the measurement indicators are understood. This frame of reference includes theoretical, philosophical, theological, religious, or spiritual understandings that inform how the concept is measured (e.g., the wording of questions and statements) and how the measure is to be used. In summary, the measurement of a religious concept requires an in-depth examination of the following: (a) the *operational characteristics* that define how the concept is measured (i.e., including its measurement indicators and the operations by which a measure of the religious concept is obtained), (b) the *conceptual relationships* of the religious concept with other concepts of relevance to nursing, and (c) the *philosophical underpinnings* (frame of reference) by which the religious concept is understood and corresponding measurement instruments are constructed. Examples of considerations pertaining to each of these premises are provided in Table 18.1.

In the following sections, we discuss the above premises with the intent of explicating some of the analytical processes by which nurses have pursued the measurement of religious concepts. Our intention is not to provide a taxonomy or evaluation of particular measurement instruments; extensive reviews of instruments for the measurement of religious concepts have already been provided by other authors.[15–18] Nor do we strive to critique particular studies or provide an in-depth account of the analyses and

TABLE 18.1 Considerations for the Measurement of Religious Concepts

	Antecedents	Consequences
Operational characteristics	The "why and how" of individuals' responses to question(s) and statement(s) used to measure the religious concept: • To what extent is the religious concept adequately represented by the questions and statements that are used to measure it? • Are there any factors other than the concept being measured that may influence individuals' responses? • Are the items interpreted by all individuals within the intended target population in the same way?	The processes by which the measurement indicators produce a measure (scaled score): • How are responses to multiple questions and statements combined to produce a measure of the religious concept? • Do the indicators produce a measure that is reliable and sensitive with respect to the desired purposes and usages of the measure?
Conceptual relationships	The concepts that influence or explain the religious concept of interest: • What concepts of relevance to nursing explain or contribute to individual differences (variability) in the religious concept?	Nursing relevant outcomes and other concepts affected by the religious concept: • To what extent does the religious concept influence outcomes or other concepts of relevance to nursing?
Philosophical underpinnings	The underlying theoretical and philosophical frame of reference: • What are the theoretical and philosophical understandings from which the measurement instrument was constructed?	The intended and unintended implications: • What are the intended purposes of measuring the religious concept? • What are the social and ethical consequences of the approach taken for the measurement of the religious concept?

results. Rather, we extracted several examples from published studies to elucidate the types of questions and considerations that guide the interpretation of scores derived from individuals' responses to questions and statements that have been used for the measurement of religious concepts. We have limited our selection of studies to those that have been conducted by nurses or for nurses and that serve to exemplify the measurement of selected religious concepts in terms of their: (a) operational characteristics, (b) conceptual relationships, and (c) philosophical underpinnings.

OPERATIONAL CHARACTERISTICS

The operational domain is about understanding how and why individuals respond the way they do to questions and statements used for the measurement of a religious concept. To what extent is the religious concept adequately represented by the questions and statements that are used to measure it? How are responses to multiple questions and statements combined to produce a measure of the religious concept? Do all individuals within the intended target population interpret each of the questions and statements in the same way? The answers to these questions necessitate careful examination of the wording of the items and the statistical models that are applied to examine individuals' responses to the items. We draw on examples from published studies to illustrate several approaches to answering such questions and highlight particular challenges.

The Wording of Items

The first example is a study by Ng, Fong, Tsui, Au-Yeung, and Law who examine the validation of a translated Chinese version of the 16-item Daily Spiritual Experience Scale (DES) in a sample of 245 Chinese individuals living in Hong Kong.[19] The original English version of the DES was developed by Underwood for use in health studies as a measure of "ordinary experience of the transcendent or sense of the divine" that crosses the boundaries of particular religions or spiritual groups.[20] The original instrument was based on in-depth interviews and focus groups with people from various religious backgrounds. Ng et al. set out to examine whether the DES could be translated and meaningfully applied to a different cultural context, namely that of Chinese people living in Hong Kong. The translation process, which involved a team of Chinese mental health practitioners and the use of forward and backward translation techniques, revealed ambiguity regarding the Chinese translation of the term "God" that was used in several of the questions. Specifically, the researchers found that "God" in Chinese could refer to a "humanized God" (as represented in some of the religious rituals of Confucianism, Buddhism, and Daoism) or to a philosophical higher power as reflected in discourses about spiritual transcendence. Ng et al. therefore added an explanatory statement to the measurement instrument to ensure that the term "God" was interpreted in the manner that was consistent with its intended meaning.

Translation challenges, such as the one described by Ng et al.,[19] are not surprising considering the central of role of language in the social construction of religious concepts. Similar challenges could arise in situations where questions and statements for the measurement of a religious concept might have different meanings for people with different religious or cultural backgrounds or life experiences. For example, Dunn and Horgas explore gender differences in religious coping styles related to the experience of pain in older adults ($N = 200$) as one of their study objectives.[21] The authors used an adaptation of Pargament's Religious Problem-Solving Scales (RPSS) that consists of 18 items for the measurement of three religious coping styles (self-directed, deferring, and collaborating) pertaining to an individual's relationship with God.[22] For instance, the item "When it comes to deciding how to manage my pain, God and I work together as partners," is a measurement indicator of the collaborative religious coping style, which Pargament interprets as reflective of an active partnership between the individual and God that would be particularly representative of some Jewish and Christian traditions.[22] Dunn and Horgas observed that the mean score for the collaborative religious coping style, as well as the other religious coping styles, was greater in women than in men. It appears that women use religious coping strategies more frequently than men for the management of their pain. Although there are many possible explanations for this observation, a question of particular relevance to our discussion is whether these findings point toward *actual* differences in the religious coping styles or whether they are an artifact of the way in which the religious coping styles were measured. The measurement approach that was taken assumes that the measurement indicators represent particular religious coping styles in ways that are equivalent for women and men (i.e., the measurement approach is equivalently applicable to women and men). Although the women had relatively higher average scores for the combined measurement indicators for each coping style, it is not known whether this difference is the same for all of the 18 measurement indicators individually. That is, do the religious coping styles have the same meaning for women and men, and are they manifested (via their measurement indicators) in the same way in both groups?

Similar questions apply when measures of religious concepts are used to compare other groups, such as religious or cultural groups, or when they are applied to a population that is different from the one for which the measurement instrument was developed. For instance, the above example item suggests that the RPSS is specifically representative of monotheistic religious beliefs. The application and use of this instrument for the measurement of religious coping styles in people who have other religious beliefs is likely unwarranted. Like the RPSS, many instruments for the measurement of religious concepts have been developed within particular, often Christian dominant, populations. In such situations, the concept may not be measured in a way that is congruent with other religious, spiritual, or cultural traditions. Researchers who use measures of religious concepts must therefore consider whether the instrument that was used is congruent with the characteristics of the population to which it was applied.

Statistical Approaches

In addition to paying attention to the wording of items used for the measurement of a religious concept, it is important to examine the statistical relationships between the measured concept and its measurement indicators. This is particularly important when multiple items are used as measurement indicators of the same concept. The construction of a scale for the measurement of a religious concept requires that a *measurement model* of the relationships between the measurement indicators and the measured concept to be established and validated. One of the most common approaches is to use factor analysis techniques to determine whether the measurement indicators are reflective of the same concept.[23] The premise of factor analysis is that the measurement indicators and the correlations among them arise from a common source, called a latent factor (i.e., a measure of the concept of interest), plus some degree of error. Specifically, factor analysis addresses the following questions about the relationships between the measurement indicators and the measured concept: (a) Do the measurement indicators reflect a common concept (factor)? and (b) Do the measurement indicators that reflect the same concept do so to the same extent?

An example of a factor analysis is found in a study by Lim and Yi[24] who examine the validity of the six-item Spiritual Well-Being subscale of the Quality of Life-Cancer Survivor instrument,[25] which they translated into Korean. For the original English translation of the instrument, the responses to the six items could purportedly be combined to produce a measure of spiritual well-being. Lim and Yi examine whether this approach of combining the six items into a single measure was warranted in a sample of breast and gynecological cancer survivors among Koreans living in Korea ($N = 110$) and in the United States of America ($N = 51$). The results of their exploratory factor analysis suggested that the six items (measurement indicators) should not be combined in a single measure of spiritual well-being because they reflect two (rather than one) latent factors, which the authors labeled *religiosity* and *spirituality*. The religiosity factor was represented by the following three items: "Importance of participation in religious activity," "Religious or spiritual life change as a result of the cancer diagnosis," and "Importance of other spiritual activity (meditation)." The other three items for the measurement of spirituality were: "Positive change in life because of illness," "Sense of purpose or mission for life or a season for being alive," and "Feeling about uncertainty about the future." The results also revealed that, although five of the items had relatively strong associations with either the religiosity or the spirituality factor (with factor loadings ranging from 0.80 to 0.92), one of the items for the measurement of spirituality, "Feeling about uncertainty about the future," had a factor loading of only 0.43. Statistically, this means that this item was a relatively weak measurement indicator of spirituality in this sample. That is, there were sources, other than the latent factor, that were unaccounted for and that influenced the individuals' responses to this item. These may have included random sources, due to sampling variability, and systematic sources such as cultural or spiritual beliefs that may have influenced individuals' interpretations and responses to the item.[26]

Another statistical approach has been demonstrated in a study by Gielen, van den Branden van Iersel, and Broeckaert who use latent class analysis to classify Flemish palliative care nurses based on their responses to a variety of questions about religious or worldview perspectives, affiliation, and various beliefs and practices.[27] These researchers found that the sample could be divided into the following five groups (called latent classes): atheists/agnostics, doubters, church-going respondents, religious but not church-going respondents, and devout church-going respondents. What is of interest to the discussion here is that the measurement indicators were used to *group* respondents in the sample and to characterize those groups in terms of common patterns of responses to the questions. This is different from the previously discussed factor analysis approach, where measurement indicators were used to obtain scaled measures of religiosity and spirituality in the overall sample. That is, the purpose of latent class analysis is to identify and characterize different sampling groups that are not known *a priori* (it is not known a priori how many groups exist in the sample and to which group an individual belongs). The theoretical premise is that individuals' responses to the items are reflective of group membership (represented as *latent classes*). In contrast, the factor analysis approach that was used in the study by Ng et al. seeks to produce a measure (scaled score) of one or more *latent factors* that is applicable to the overall sample. The theoretical premise of factor analysis is that individuals' responses to the items are determined by their score on the latent factor (i.e., the extent to which the concept is present). The important point for the discussion here is that both of these approaches can be used to examine various explanations for individuals' responses to items, which is what measurement is all about.

These statistical approaches illustrate how items could be used to produce a measure of a religious concept (represented as a latent factor) or to identify subgroups (represented as latent classes) within a sample. Whatever approach is taken, a fundamental premise of all self-report measures is that individuals in the sample are consistent in their interpretations of the questions or statements used to measure the concept of interest. Psychometric approaches, such as factor analysis, have been extensively used to examine the measurement validation of religious concepts. However, the possibility of heterogeneity with respect to the individuals' interpretations of the questions or statements (items) used to measure a religious concept has been much less extensively examined. It is often unclear to what extent people from different backgrounds and with different life experiences and beliefs may variously interpret and respond to questions and statements that are used as measurement indicators. Considering the different populations in which religious concepts are often measured, it is plausible that people may not interpret all of the indicators in the same way (e.g., as may result from the use of the term "God" in measurement instruments such as the DES). Sophisticated statistical techniques, such as differential item functioning and latent variable mixture modeling, should be more extensively used to examine sources of heterogeneity that may help to explain why individuals interpret and respond to questions and statement in different ways.[28,29] Qualitative analysis techniques, such as cognitive interviewing, can provide additional valuable insights for understanding potential differences in individuals' interpretations of the items.[30–32] Regardless of the techniques that are used, compelling evidence must be provided to ensure that the religious concept of interest is accurately reflected in the items that are used to measure it, and that individuals are consistent in their interpretations of the items such that their responses can be meaningfully evaluated and compared.

CONCEPTUAL RELATIONSHIPS

Many studies have examined the associations of religious concepts with various other health-related concepts.[33,34] Of interest, here are the processes by which the meaning of a religious concept is understood through its relationships with other relevant concepts, which include *antecedents* that predict or explain the religious concept and *consequences* that are affected by the religious concept. Related questions include: To what extent is the religious concept associated with other similar or dissimilar concepts? What are possible explanations for individual differences (variability) in the religious concept? To what extent does the religious concept influence outcomes or other concepts of relevance to nursing? A relatively common approach is to examine measures of religious concepts in terms of their correlations with other measures of the same concept and with measures of different concepts (this corresponds to the examination of convergent and discriminant validity).[4] This approach contributes to an understanding of the measured concept in terms of the amount of variance it shares with other measured concepts (or the extent to which the concepts overlap). However, it is important to remember that correlations may be due to the influences of other potentially confounding extraneous variables. Another approach is to examine the extent to which a religious concept uniquely explains (or accounts for) the variance in another concept (often a particular outcome of interest), in the context of other explanatory variables. Conversely, one can examine the extent to which other concepts explain variance in a religious concept (specified as the response variable). This "unique variance approach" is used to adjust for the potentially confounding effects of extraneous variables when examining the association between the religious concept and another concept.[35] A limitation of the unique variance approach is that it does not consider the relationships among the explanatory variables. A third approach is to use structural equation modeling, or path modeling, to further examine the associations among the explanatory variables for the purpose of revealing a network of relationships between the religious concept and other concepts of interest. This approach could, for example, be used to reveal hypothesized mechanisms (or paths) by which a religious concept may be associated with an outcome variable through its associations with other (mediating) variables. Whatever the approach taken, the concern of interest to the discussion here is that a religious concept must be understood in terms of its associations with other concepts within a purposefully constructed theoretical framework so as to avoid erroneous conclusions about its meaning and theoretical relevance. We discuss three examples to illustrate these approaches.

Bivariate Associations

The first example is a study by Rohani, Khanjari, Abedi, Oskouie, and Langius-Eklöf who develope and evaluated Persian translations of established English instruments for the measurement of health, sense of coherence, religious coping, and spiritual perspective.[36] The authors specifically explored the validation of the translated instruments for the measurement of these concepts by examining the associations among them. Translation was facilitated by the use of recommended procedures, including forward and backward translation, expert reviews, and pilot testing. Religious coping was measured using the translated Brief Religious Coping instrument that consists of 14 items for the measurement of the following two forms of religious coping: (a) "positive religious coping" (seven items; high scores indicate positive religious coping), defined as "an expression of a sense of spirituality, a secure relationship with God, a belief that there is meaning to be found in life, and a sense of spiritual connectedness with others" and (b) "negative religious coping" (seven items; high scores indicate negative religious coping), which purportedly reflects "a less secure relationship with God, a tenuous and ominous view of the world, and a religious struggle in search for significance."[37] The reliability of the translated instrument was supported by the examination of internal consistency among the items (Crohnbach's alphas ≥ 0.87 and 0.76 for the positive and negative religious coping scales, respectively) and test–retest reliability estimates (intra-class correlations of 0.80 and 0.74, respectively). The authors used similar procedures to translate the Spiritual Perspective Scale that consists of 10 items addressing a variety of religious and spiritual behaviors and beliefs with higher scores purportedly indicating greater integration of spirituality in one's life.[38]

The following discussion focuses on the results pertaining to the correlations between spiritual perspective and the religious coping variables.[39] The authors hypothesized that positive religious coping would be positively associated with spiritual perspective, which was supported by the findings. However, the hypothesized negative association between negative religious coping and spiritual perspective was not supported; the correlation was found not to be statistically significant. What are some possible explanations for these findings? One possibility suggested by the authors is that spiritual perspective and negative religious coping may indeed be different and unassociated concepts in this particular sample. This explanation raises questions about the conceptualizations of spiritual perspective and religious coping. It is also possible that the meanings of the measured concepts based on the translated instruments are not the same as those of the English versions. Another possibility is that the results were obtained due to chance or random error. It is always important to remember that inaccurate results from individual studies may have been obtained as a result of sampling variability. Further investigation is needed to determine why the hypothesized association between spiritual perspective and negative religious coping was not observed in this sample. Nonetheless, this study exemplifies that the measurement of religious concepts is a theory-laden activity, where the religious concepts are understood in terms of their associations with other concepts.

The Unique Variance Approach

Another commonly used approach is to evaluate the extent to which the variance in an outcome of interest is uniquely explained by a religious concept in the context of other potentially relevant explanatory variables. For example, Newlin, Melkus, Tappen, Chyun, and Koenig examine the relevance of religious and spiritual factors in relation to glycemic control in a sample of 109 "Black" women in the United States of America suffering from diabetes (the term "Black" was used to refer to a group of African American women).[40] The Spiritual Well-Being Scale was used for the measurement of two factors: religious well-being (10 items) and existential well-being (10 items) (higher scores indicate greater well-being).[41] Hemoglobin A1c (HgA1c) was used to assess glycemic control. The authors observed that a relative increase in religious well-being was associated with higher levels of HgA1c, whereas a relative increase in existential well-being was associated with lower levels. What are some possible explanations for these findings? Is it likely that religious and spiritual well-being are predictive of HgA1c? Or can these associations be explained by other variables that were not examined in this study? In correlational analyses, it is important to remember that a relationship between two variables can occur for several reasons. It is possible that the association is due to the impact of confounding variables that were not considered in this study or that the relationships are mediated by other explanatory variables of HgA1c. Another possibility is that the direction of the relationship was misspecified; the positive association between religious well-being and HgA1c may reflect a tendency to rely more intensely on the religious beliefs and practices that are used as indicators for the measurement of religious well-being. The authors used regression modeling to examine several possible explanations, including the possibility that the associations may be mediated by psychosocial factors, such as emotional distress and social support. However, compelling support for these explanations was not achieved. Nonetheless, the study raises important questions regarding the meaning and interpretation of religious and existential well-being scores with respect to a particular clinical outcome. In this case, although a correlation between religious well-being and a clinical outcome was observed, theoretical mechanisms underlying this correlation were not revealed.

Exploration of Relationships Among All Observed Variables

There are other studies that have more explicitly examined the *mechanisms* by which a religious concept may contribute to outcomes of relevance to nursing. For example, Musgrave and McFarlane combine results from several regression models to determine whether the potential effects of intrinsic and extrinsic religiosity on attitudes toward spiritual care in a sample of Israeli oncology nurses was mediated by their spiritual well-being while taking the antecedents of gender, ethnicity, and education into account.[42] Here, intrinsic and extrinsic religiosity referred to the motivation underlying religiosity, where the former (internal) pertained to the use of religiosity for the sake of one's own faith, and the latter (extrinsic) to a "utilitarian approach to religious beliefs." The researchers used translated versions of the Revised Age University I/E Scale[43] and the Spiritual Well-Being Scale[34] for the measurement of intrinsic and extrinsic religiosity and spiritual well-being (higher scores indicate greater religiosity or spiritual well-being). They used the Spiritual Care Perspective Survey[44] to measure nurses' attitudes to spiritual care, with higher scores indicating greater regard for spiritual care in nursing. The results provided support for the authors' propositions that intrinsic and extrinsic religiosity could be viewed as antecedents of nurses' attitudes to spiritual care and that these relationships were partially mediated by nurses' reports of their spiritual well-being. Intrinsic and extrinsic religiosity was positively associated with nurses' reports of their spiritual well-being, which, in turn, was positively associated with their attitudes to spiritual care. However, the negative total effect of extrinsic religiosity on attitudes toward spiritual care suggests that Israeli nurses with higher extrinsic religiosity had relatively poorer attitudes to spiritual care. Although there are many possible explanations for these findings that provide ground for further research, the relevance of this study to the discussion is that the study addresses a hypothesized mechanism that further facilitates the interpretation of religious concepts in terms of their associations with potential antecedents and consequences.

There are many other descriptive studies that have similarly examined the associations between religious concepts and other concepts of relevance to nursing. Some studies contribute valuable insights and most provide ground for new questions about the conceptualization and measurement of religious concepts and their potential value to nursing theory and practice. A general caution applies to all these studies: considering that alternative explanations resulting from measurement bias, confounding, and sampling variability exist for any individual study, some degree of skepticism is called for, at least until an association appears consistently in multiple studies involving samples from different populations.[45] The meaningful interpretation of scores pertaining to the measurement of a religious concept necessitates that the measure is examined in different samples and in relation to various other relevant concepts such that consistencies and inconsistencies in the results across several studies are understood.

PHILOSOPHICAL UNDERPINNINGS

The philosophical underpinnings refer to the theories, values, and beliefs that comprise the frame of reference underlying the conceptualization and measurement of a religious concept. Related questions include: What are the theoretical and philosophical understandings from which the instrument was constructed? What are the intended and unintended social and ethical consequences of measuring a religious concept in a particular way? These questions are particularly relevant when individuals from different cultural or religious backgrounds or with different life experiences might not be equivalently represented by the questions and statements from which a measure of a religious concept is inferred (e.g., questions using terms such as God, sin, and forgiveness may be relevant for some religious traditions but not others). A related unintended consequence is that particular religious or cultural groups might be essentialized of the use of predefined, and sometimes stereotypical, measurement indicators. Conversely, the existence of purportedly universal measures of religious concepts has been questioned by several authors who suggest that religious concepts should be measured in relation to specific theological or religious traditions.[46,47]

Hamilton, Crandell, Carter, and Lynn develope the Perceived Support from God Scale with the specific intention of addressing these types of concerns with respect to the shared religious and cultural backgrounds in a sample of Christian African American cancer survivors.[48] The authors argue that the spiritual and religious perspectives of Christian African Americans have been uniquely shaped by the shared historical and contemporary contexts of racial oppression. Consequently, their religiosity may not be congruent with many of the purportedly universal measures of religious and spiritual concepts used in health research. To address this concern, Hamilton, Powe, Pollard, Lee, and Felton set out to construct a new measurement instrument that specifically reflects the religious and spiritual experiences and beliefs of Christian African Americans. The resulting instrument consists of 15 items that were based on a qualitative study of 28 Christian African American cancer survivors.[49] A factor analysis suggests that these items reflect two factors, one measuring "support from God" (nine items) and the other measuring "God's purpose for me" (six items). The authors conclude that the instrument provides valid measurements of these religious concepts for Christian African American cancer survivors. However, despite the authors' laudable efforts to represent accurately the spiritual and religious perspectives of Christian African Americans, there remain potentially unintended consequences that deserve consideration. For example, there is a risk of essentializing the spiritual and religious perspectives of Christian African Americans through the use of potentially stereotypical measurement indicators such as "God allows to suffer" and "Illness made me a better person." The use of these indicators implies that the Christian African Americans' perceived support from God would, in part, be defined by their affirmative responses to statements about the extent to which God allows suffering and the extent to which illness made them a better person. Is this necessarily the case for all Christian African American cancer survivors? What does it mean if patients do not respond affirmatively to these indicators? What would nurses do with this information? These types of questions apply to all measures of religious concepts and point to the need for careful consideration of the social and ethical consequences of measuring religious concepts in a particular way.

CONCLUSION

Examination of the operational characteristics, conceptual relationships, and philosophical underpinnings pertaining to the measurement of religious concepts often reveals challenges and questions about the interpretation of the measurement scores and their relevance to nursing. At times, it is unclear what the measures actually mean and why they are relevant to nursing. Further more, empirical research, both quantitative and qualitative, is needed to understand the "why and how" of individuals' responses to questions and statements about their religiosity. Are the items and questions used for the measurement of religious concepts interpreted in the same way by all people? We must also understand how the measures of religious concepts relate to other concepts of relevance to nursing. Are the measurement scores relevant with respect to particular nursing outcomes and clinical decisions? Empirical research and philosophical inquiry are needed to evaluate the social and ethical consequences pertaining to the use of religious measures for both theoretical and clinical purposes. What are the implications of using individuals' self-reports to classify them into predefined religious groups or to determine the extent to which a religious concept is manifest? What are the social and ethical consequences of any inadequately represented religious traditions in the measurement of religion for theoretical and clinical purposes? In clinical practice, are patients who have provided information about their religiosity treated differently from patients who have not provided such information, and does this bring about differences in the outcomes and quality of nursing care? Does knowledge about individuals' self-reported religiosity contribute to improved decision making, or does it possibly lead to erroneous assumptions and preconceived notions about individuals' preferences and beliefs? Considering the complexity involved in answering these questions, we recommend a cautionary stance to the measurement of religious concepts to avoid that individuals or groups with particular religious or cultural histories are systematically disadvantaged or advantaged by means of the instruments used for the measurement of religious concepts.

In conclusion, we offer the following considerations that we hope will facilitate the meaningful interpretation and use of measures of religious concepts for nursing's theoretical and clinical purposes:

- A measure of a religious concept must be interpreted with respect to the actual wording of the questions and statements that serve as its measurement indicators. Considering the diversity in conceptual and operational definitions of many religious concepts, there is a significant risk that the results of studies will be misunderstood unless the operational characteristics of instruments for the measurements of religious concepts are explicated and considered in the interpretation of study results.

- A measurement model must be specified and examined to determine whether and how various measurement indicators can be combined to produce a measure that is reliable and valid for its intended purposes. This may include factor analyses, analyses of internal consistency among the measurement indicators (Cronbach's alpha), and other analyses of measurement reliability. These analyses must be performed within the sample that is a representative of the population of interest, and the results must be compared with those of other studies conducted in other samples. There is a significant risk for incorrect inferences based on measurement scores when the statistical properties of the measurement instrument are inadequately examined or poorly understood.

- Understanding a religious concept requires that its associations with other relevant concepts are examined and understood. This necessitates examination of potential antecedents and consequences of the religious concept, and the comparison of results of such analyses across multiple studies.

- The purposes and contexts to which a measure of a religious concept is applied must be congruent with its philosophical, theoretical, religious, and cultural underpinnings. Nurses who use an instrument for the measurement of a religious concept must be familiar with its frame of reference as the basis for evaluating its appropriateness for particular theoretical and clinical purposes and populations.

- The use of an instrument for the measurement of a religious concept must be evaluated in consideration of any intended and potentially unintended social and ethical consequences. Particular attention must be paid to individuals or groups who may be systematically disadvantaged, or advantaged, through the use of a particular measurement instrument.

NOTES

1. Hall, Daniel, Keith Meador, and Harold Koenig. "Measuring Religiousness in Health Research: Review and Critique." *Journal of Religion and Health* 47.2 (2008): 134–63.
2. Berry, Devon. "Methodological Pitfalls in the Study of Religiosity and Spirituality." *Western Journal of Nursing* 27.5 (2005): 628–47.
3. Miller, William, and Carl Thoresen. "Spirituality, Religion, and Health. An Emerging Research Field." *American Psychologist* 58.1 (2003): 24–35.

4. Viswanathan, Madhu. *Measurement Error and Research Design*. Thousand Oaks, CA: Sage, 2005.

5. Paloutzian, Raymond, and Craig Ellison. "Loneliness, Spiritual Well-Being and Quality of Life." *Loneliness: A Sourcebook of Current Theory, Research and Therapy*. Ed. Lititia Peplau and Daniel Perlman. New York: John Wiley, 1982. 224–37.

6. Stine, William. "Meaningful Inference: The Role of Measurement in Statistics." *Psychological Bulletin* 105.1 (1989): 147–55.

7. Messick, Samuel. "Validity of Psychological Assessment: Validation of Inferences from Persons' Responses and Performances as Scientific Inquiry into Score Meaning." *American Psychologist* 50.9 (1995): 741–49.

8. Zumbo, Bruno. "Validity as Contextualized and Pragmatic Explanation, and Its Implications for Validation Practice." *The Concept of Validity: Revisions, New Directions and Applications*. Ed. Robert Lissitz. Charlotte, NC: Information Age Publishing, 2009. 65–82.

9. Messick, Samuel. "Test Validity: A Matter of Consequence." *Social Indicators Research* 45.1–3 (1998): 35–44.

10. Zumbo, Bruno. "Validity: Foundational Issues and Statistical Methodology." *Handbook of Statistics*. Ed. C. Radhakrishna Rao and Sandip Sinharay. Vol. 26. Psychometrics, Amsterdam: Elsevier Science, 2007. 45–79.

11. Hubley, Anita, and Bruno Zumbo. "A Dialectic on Validity: Where We have Been and Where We are Going." *Journal of General Psychology* 123.3 (1996): 207–15.

12. De Ayala, Rafael. *The Theory and Practice of Item Response Theory*. Methodology in the Social Sciences. New York: Guilford Press, 2009.

13. Cronbach, Lee, and Paul Meehl. "Construct Validity in Psychological Tests." *Psychological Bulletin* 52.4 (1955): 281–302.

14. Hubley, op. cit.

15. Hall, Daniel, Keith Meador, and Harold Koenig. "Measuring Religiousness in Health Research: Review and Critique." *Journal of Religion and Health* 47.2 (2008): 134–63.

16. Kilpatrick, Shelley, Andrew Weaver, and Michael McCullough, et al. "A Review of Spiritual and Religious Measures in Nursing Research Journals: 1995–1999." *Journal of Religion and Health* 44.1 (2005): 55–66.

17. Egbert, Nichole, Jacquelyn Mickley, and Harriet Coeling. "A Review and Application of Social Scientific Measures of Religiosity and Spirituality: Assessing a Missing Component in Health Communication Research." *Health Communication* 16.1 (2004): 7–27.

18. Hill, Peter, and Ralph Hood. *Measures of Religiosity*. Birmingham, AL: Religious Education Press, 1999.

19. Ng, Siu-Man, Ted Fong, Elaine Tsui, et al. "Validation of the Chinese Version of Underwood's Daily Spiritual Experience Scale: Transcending Cultural Boundaries?" *International Journal of Behavioral Medicine* 16.2 (2009): 91–7.

20. Underwood, Lynn, and Jeanne Teresi. "The Daily Spiritual Experience Scale: Development, Theoretical Description, Reliability, Exploratory Factor Analysis, and Preliminary Construct Validity Using Health-Related Data." *Annals of Behavioral Medicine* 24.1 (2002): 22–33.

21. Dunn, Karen, and Ann Horgas. "Religious and Nonreligious Coping in Older Adults Experiencing Chronic Pain." *Pain Management Nursing* 5.1 (2004): 19–28.

22. Pargament, Kenneth, Joseph Kennell, William Hathaway, et al. "Religion and the Problem-Solving Process: Three Styles of Coping." *Journal for the Scientific Study of Religion* 27.1 (1988): 90–104.

23. Gorsuch, Richard. *Factor Analysis*. 2nd ed. Hillsdale, NJ: L. Erlbaum Associates, 1983.
24. Lim, Jung-won, and Jaehee Yi. "The Effects of Religiosity, Spirituality, and Social Support on Quality of Life: A Comparison between Korean American and Korean Breast and Gynecologic Cancer Survivors." *Oncology Nursing Forum* 36.6 (2009): 699–708.
25. Ferrell, Betty, Karen Hassey Dow, and Marcia Grant. "Measurement of the Quality of Life in Cancer Survivors." *Quality of Life Research* 4.6 (1995): 523–31.
26. Viswanathan, Madhu. *Measurement Error and Research Design*. Thousand Oaks, CA: Sage, 2005.
27. Gielen, Joris, Trudie van Iersel, and Bert Broeckaert. "Religion, World View and the Nurse: Results of a Quantitative Survey among Flemish Palliative Care Nurses." *International Journal of Palliative Nursing* 15.12 (2009): 590–600.
28. Hancock, Gregory, and Karen Samuelsen. *Advances in Latent Variable Mixture Models*. The CILVR Series on Latent Variable Methodology. Charlotte, NC: Information Age Pub., 2008.
29. Zumbo, Bruno. "Three Generations of DIF Analyses: Considering Where It Has Been, Where It Is Now, and Where It Is Going." *Language Assessment Quarterly* 4 (2007): 223–33.
30. Drennan, Jonathan. "Cognitive Interviewing: Verbal Data in the Design and Pretesting of Questionnaires." *Journal of Advanced Nursing* 42 (2003): 57–63.
31. Morell, Linda, and Rachel Jin Bee Tan. "Validating for Use and Interpretation: A Mixed Methods Contribution Illustrated." *Journal of Mixed Methods Research* 3.3 (2009): 242–64.
32. Willis, Gordon. *Cognitive Interviewing: A Tool for Improving Questionnaire Design*. Thousand Oaks, CA: Sage Publications, 2005.
33. Miller, op. cit.
34. Williams, David, and Michelle Sternthal. "Spirituality, Religion and Health: Evidence and Research Directions." *Medical Journal of Australia* 186.10 Suppl (2007): S47–50.
35. Miller, op. cit.
36. Rohani, Camelia, Sedigheh Khanjari, Heidar-Ali Abedi, et al. "Health Index, Sense of Coherence Scale, Brief Religious Coping Scale and Spiritual Perspective Scale: Psychometric Properties." *Journal of Advanced Nursing* 66.12 (2010): 2796–2806.
37. Pargament, Kenneth, Bruce Smith, Harold Koenig, et. al. "Patterns of Positive and Negative Religious Coping with Major Life Stressors." *Journal for the Scientific Study of Religion* 37.4 (1998): 710–724.
38. Reed, Pamela. "Religiousness among Terminally Ill and Healthy Adults." *Research in Nursing and Health* 9.1 (1986): 35–41.
39. Rohani, op. cit.
40. Newlin, Kelley, Gail Melkus, Ruth Tappen, et al. "Relationships of Religion and Spirituality to Glycemic Control in Black Women with Type 2 Diabetes." *Nursing Research* 57.5 (2008): 331–9.
41. Paloutzian, op. cit.
42. Musgrave, Catherine, and Elizabeth McFarlane. "Israeli Oncology Nurses' Religiosity, Spiritual Well-Being, and Attitudes toward Spiritual Care: A Path Analysis." *Oncology Nursing Forum* 31.2 (2004): 321–7.
43. Gorsuch, Richard, and Susan McPherson. "Intrinsic/Extrinsic Measurement: I/E-Revised and Single-Item Scales." *Journal for the Scientific Study of Religion* 28.3 (1989): 348–54.

44. Johnston Taylor, Elizabeth, Martha Highfield, and Madalon Amenta. "Predictors of Oncology and Hospice Nurses' Spiritual Care Perspectives and Practices." *Applied Nursing Research* 12.1 (1999): 30–7.
45. Taveggia, Thomas. "Resolving Research Controversy through Empirical Cumulation: Toward Reliable Sociological Knowledge." *Sociological Methods Research* 2.4 (1974): 395–407.
46. Hall, Daniel, Keith Meador, and Harold Koenig. "Measuring Religiousness in Health Research: Review and Critique." *Journal of Religion and Health* 47.2 (2008): 134–63.
47. Moberg, David. "Assessing and Measuring Spirituality: Confronting Dilemmas of Universal and Particular Evaluative Criteria." *Journal of Adult Development* 9.1 (2002): 47–60.
48. Hamilton, Jill, Jamie Crandell, J. Kameron Carter, et al. "Reliability and Validity of the Perspectives of Support from God Scale." *Nursing Research* 59.2 (2010): 102–9.
49. Hamilton, Jill, et al. "Spirituality among African American Cancer Survivors: Having a Personal Relationship with God." *Cancer Nursing* 30.4 (2007): 309–16.

19

Looking Back and Looking Ahead: A Concluding Postscript

Marsha D. Fowler, Sheryl Reimer-Kirkham, Richard Sawatzky,
Elizabeth Johnston Taylor, and Barbara Pesut

Dating from as early as the third millennium BCE, Ancient Near Eastern religious texts display a substantial body of prophetic literature. Ugaritic, Phoenician, Aramaic, Urukan, Marian, Assyrian, Ischchalian, and Egyptian prophets all spoke to the people in words of social and religious criticism, of announcements of things to come, and as charismatically authorized messengers from God to the people. Depending on the sociopolitical and religious context of the prophet, in any given example their words may not have reflected all three functions of prophets. In the Jewish Biblical tradition, at times they would speak a word of warning (e.g., pre-exilic prophets), at times a word of hope (exilic prophets), and at times an announcement of a world to come (post-exilic prophets). It seems fitting in a book on religion and nursing to end with a prophetic word—words of warning, hope, encouragement, critique, and of that which may lie ahead.

RELIGION, NURSING IDENTITY, AND ASPIRATION

Nursing's current neglect of religion as it affects patient care extends to a neglect of religion as it has contributed to modern nursing's development of nursing schools, education, research, and practice. Both directly and indirectly, religion has played an historical role in shaping modern nursing and in internationalizing nursing in underserved regions, a role that remains largely

379

unexplored though eminently worthy of research. Shunning religion in the service of nursing's ambition toward social recognition as a science and a profession has not served nursing well in at least two ways. First, patients have not benefited from religiously competent nursing care. Such care could have drawn upon religious understandings of duties toward health and wellness, and in caring for others, and comfort in grief or at the end of life. Our intent is not to erase the ways in which nursing's focus on spirituality in the last three decades has benefited nursing care, but rather to underscore the incompleteness of approaches that overlook religious understandings. Second, nursing's long-standing social ethics has never been systematically developed. Some of the health-related social policies developed by religious denominations are of exceptional breadth, depth, coherence, and comprehensiveness as models for how nursing might do health policy and social ethics. Contemporary religious policies regarding health and health care often address health disparities and the social determinants of disease. As policies, they demonstrate how the value structure and metaphysics of a tradition might coherently inform and articulate with a social policy. Nursing has much that it could learn if it would permit itself to be informed by the extensive and mature body of social–ethical literature developed over centuries by many religious traditions.

Nursing's attempt to work in isolation, as it has with *spirituality*, poses a risk to its study of religion. On the one hand, it runs the risk of essentializing religion, as has been done in any number of *Introduction to Nursing* textbooks, or reducing it to a set of attributes that reify religion into a static, and largely lifeless entity. On the other hand, religion can be understood so broadly that it fails to provide anything to work with in terms of informing actual patient care. We must not forget that the concern of nursing is religion as it interacts with health; nursing need not define religion per se as much as identify the boundaries of its domain of concern.

RELIGION AND THE BOUNDARIES OF NURSING PRACTICE

A careful reading will indicate that this work is not simply another pro-religion source that gives nurses license to discuss religious beliefs with patients or to introduce religious practices into nursing care. Nurses who practice outside of religious hospitals or agencies are not often given ethical guidelines for discussing religion with patients, even though accrediting bodies mandate nurses be taught to assess and care for the spiritual dimension. As integrated, whole persons, nurses inevitably bring their personal religious faith or philosophy to the bedside. As nursing begins to explore the import of religion on nursing and nursing care, attention will need to be given to appropriate moral boundaries for discussing religion in the clinical context. This will also have curricular implications for basic as well as graduate education in nursing.

There is little research data to guide nurses regarding how they might support patients spiritually or religiously. While evidence indicates that religion can create both positive and negative outcomes for patients, nurses are not prepared to assess or intervene appropriately in either case. And while there is some research that incorporates religion, most of it is on religion as a coping strategy or as one of several factors in coping. Yet there is substantially more to religion than coping that is relevant to nursing practice. Additional research is needed to explore the ways in which the metaphysics of a religious tradition influences bioethical and clinical decision making, whether by patients or by nurses. There are, thus, implications for nursing research, instrument development, education, and practice.

Nursing urgently needs to wrestle with the implications of including religion in nursing education, research, and practice. More specifically, nursing needs to grapple with what is or is not within its purview with regard to religion and health/illness and to delimit its involvement to religion vis-à-vis health. Even so, there are levels of involvement that may be appropriate to advanced nursing practice that are not appropriate to basic nursing practice that remain to be discussed. In addition, future study and translational research are needed to create processes for improved, effective, and ethical collaboration between nurses and non-nursing experts who can support adaptive patient religiosity.

CONSTRAINTS AND PRACTICE ENVIRONMENTS

While the point can be well-argued that the profession of nursing needs to tend to the influence of religion in the lives of their patients and that religious ethics provides guidance to nurses who care for patients affiliated with particular religious traditions, or who are themselves adherents, we would be amiss not to acknowledge the contextual or social constraints that may make this integration difficult. With the development of nursing ethics as distinct from bioethics or medical ethics, attention has been put on the moral climate of the practice environments of nurses. The priorities of the modern health care system of efficiency and cure do not align easily with tending to the sacred. Quality practice environments, such as those found in magnet hospitals, provide the resources, support, and climate required for nurses to enact their moral agency to operationalize ethical principles and values. A question that requires examination is whether the leadership and organizational culture that facilitates quality practice environments would equally support the enactment of religious ethics. It could be anticipated that nurses working in faith-based organizations, or in organizations loosely or historically affiliated with faith traditions (such as hospitals administered by the Catholic Health Association or the Salvation Army) might have more support for the integration of religious ethics. Spiritual care providers (also referred to as chaplains) typically cite spiritual support to staff as an integral aspect of their role, suggesting that spiritual care services in hospitals open dialogic space for tending to matters of the spirit, and departments legitimate the role of religion and spirituality more generally in relation to the illness experience. Health care administrators likewise play a key role in creating a climate where religion and spirituality might be incorporated into care, for all faith perspectives. Undoubtedly, the contextual influences that must be negotiated for the inclusion of religious ethics vary considerably from unit to unit, organization to organization, and society to society. Our work on this volume with contributors from several continents has reminded us of these variations, with the clear message that although numerous health care services, especially those providing public health and community development services, are provided by religious organizations, in many places religion is not always welcomed into the public sphere of health care.

RELIGION IN PUBLIC LIFE

No discussion of the intersections between religions, nursing, and ethics could be complete without acknowledging the contested role of religion in public life, and more specifically in the case of this volume, the role religions should play in the development of public policies and practices in the realm of health care. This question becomes more urgent in pluralistic societies where it is not one religious perspective that is accommodated, but rather multiple voices that may not always agree. Assumptions that secularism provides a neutral space in which to provide health care without the messy interruptions of religion are increasingly challenged, not as obviously in nursing literature to date, but increasingly in the social sciences and humanities. With globalization, religions that do not distinguish between public and private, secular and sacred, are being established in western secular nations to compel an examination of the role of religion in public life.

At the least, nurses and other health care professionals must seek to recognize the influence of religion in patients' lives and not demean patients on this account. Nursing codes of ethics underscore nurses' duty to provide safe, competent, compassionate, and ethical care extending to an accommodation of religious, spiritual, and cultural values and practices. Any tendency to relegate religiously informed values and beliefs to the domain of the private and thus as not relevant to health care services and the experience of health and illness risks imposition of the dominant Western cultural worldview (a hegemonic centre) that holds to secular/sacred, public/private binaries. But more than respect for individual values and beliefs, the question of the role of religion in public life extends to the contributions of religious discourse to ethical theories.

The role of religion in public life at the level of the state continues to engage scholars, politicians, and policy makers, and citizens alike in debate, and produces complicated political effects. Sacralization, with the widespread diffusion of the sacred across society, also to what is deemed secular, adds further complexity by its more implicit influences. The challenge is one of achieving a form of responsible pluralism, where multiple religious, spiritual, and nonreligious views are welcomed equally, without relativizing, syncretizing, or homogenizing the underlying belief systems, and without succumbing to the dynamics of power that inevitably shape which of multiple perspectives are foregrounded. Hence, pluralism is qualified with *responsible*, a term that underlines the need for inclusive dialogic space, but also agreement that there is judgment and negotiation in how one's own views are enacted in the public realm. At its basis, a responsible pluralism seeks common ground by balancing unity and plurality, recognizing the universality of human experience with detailed engagement with the particularities of various traditions. The challenge—and the opportunity—is that of bringing many perspectives into the realm of professional ethical discourses, including those of religious traditions, rather than confining them to the private realm, and thus enlisting the support of all reliable moral discourses in support of respect, dignity, and equity.

RELIGIOUS IDENTITY, INCLUSION, AND EXCLUSION

Religion has played, and will continue to play, a significant role in the lives of nurses and hence in the profession of nursing. Religion can have numerous benefits for individuals including social support, a sense of significance, and answers for those questions in life that, while common to the human condition, are notoriously hard to answer—what is my purpose, why does suffering exist, and what comes after? Indeed, religion can provide a profound sense of identity whereby one belongs to a special group, with a special purpose, that contributes something good and meaningful to the world.

This sense of identity may be one of the reasons that religion has been so enduringly significant for nursing. The history of nursing appears at times to be one long identity crisis, as the profession has struggled to carve out its niche alongside medicine. Carving out this identity has been attempted through many ideals. Nursing models, the adoption of concepts such as caring to uniquely define nursing, and, more recently, calls for social justice and equity grounded in theoretical perspectives such as feminism, poststructuralism, and postcolonialism have arisen out of a desire to find common ground for a nursing identity. This common ground is moral ground. Within these ideals, nursing is striving to implement change for the betterment of society. Religion too makes an important contribution to nursing as a moral and meaningful practice. What we have sought to reveal in this book is a deeper understanding of how those contributions occur for nurses and patients alike. In contrast to a caricature of religion that superficially deals with belief and ritual, we have sought to illustrate how religions can provide thoughtful and nuanced answers to the complexities of life. Or in some cases, not answers but rather mystery that, while defying answers, may nevertheless contribute profoundly to meaning.

However, inevitably, those things that are most powerful also carry the most risk and such is the case with religion in nursing. As religion becomes more globalized, and the discourse of spirituality becomes more accepted in nursing, there are inherent risks. Professional nursing organizations are consistent in prohibiting proselytizing by nurses. Caution is in order. One of the highest risks is that the same religious identity that provides such a powerful sense of belonging and purpose will ultimately become exclusionary. Paradoxically, the strongest group identities are often built around a sense of owning something special that necessitates the presence of an "other" that does not bear the same privileges. It is this risk that becomes ours as we embrace the idea of religion in nursing. The task then becomes creating a space within which individuals are free to create and enact their sense of religious identity while holding equal space for the religious or nonreligious identities of "others."

This exclusionary sense is rarely intentional. Rather, it tends to arise when we are passionate about some truth and have the most altruistic sense of wanting to do something right and just with that truth. This happens not only within religion in nursing but in all of those ideals (e.g., caring, equity, social justice) that have informed nursing theory and epistemology over the past decades. They perhaps become most problematic when they are positioned as *the* lens rather than *a* lens by which to inform the profession. Spaces for diverse ideals are perhaps better made by anchoring the common ground in the more pragmatic tangibles of practice than in the metaphysical and social claims that by necessity are so complex that they inform one aspect of a more complete picture. We need to be cautious about creating any type of globalizing nursing theory, model, or concept (even that of spirituality) that attempts to reconcile the inherent diversities of religion.

And yet, we can envision a time when nursing must do the difficult task of reconciling diverse religious perspectives. Religions, as this book illustrates, contain sacred and powerful ideas of what is good, and how one should live rightly in relation to that goodness. That is, religion is about morality, but that morality takes on different forms both within religions and across religions. A debate within nursing is where the moral authority comes from that undergirds nursing ethics. Religious nurses have argued that it should be derived from religion. If that is so, in the face of religious diversity, is there a common morality that crosses religions? Others have argued that morality can and should be constructed and negotiated within our shared humanity. In that case, religion is just one aspect that informs that humanity. These approaches may indeed lead to quite different places. As society continues to struggle to accommodate emerging forms of religious and spiritual diversity, we anticipate that these questions will generate significant debate.

RELIGION, NURSING THEORY, AND THE HUMAN CONDITION

Nursing theories define the foundational concepts of nursing—nursing, person, health, and environment—in ways that identify what nursing is, its phenomena of concern, and its ends. Nurses' understanding of *health*, defined in vitro, risk running afoul of patients' in vivo religiously informed understanding of health and the attendant duties regarding health. It is less likely that there is an outright conflict than that the religious understanding of health in a given tradition is more expansive than that of nursing, set as it is within the broader context of a particular religious worldview. There are, thus, two avenues that nursing might pursue to its own benefit and the benefit of patients. First, nursing might become informed about and by the comprehensive worldview and ethical systems of religious traditions in which *health* is defined. Beyond health, nursing needs to know more about how these traditions approach concepts such as suffering, compassion, wholeness, striving, equanimity, well-being, justice, illness, and care of the stranger—and the attendant moral issues that arise from them such as quality and value of life, euthanasia, reproductive issues, homosexuality, marriage and family, family breakdown, domestic violence, abortion, vegetarianism, leisure and rest, drug use, the place of elderly persons, conflict, and more. Second, nursing might examine its own theoretical conceptualizations in the light of what religion might offer to enrich, clarify, or critique those conceptualizations. Every day nurses are confronted by human strength and human frailty, wholeness and brokenness, goodness and evilness. These are part and parcel of the human condition and our consanguinity as humans, and the substance of millennia of religious reflection, wisdom, and concern. Nursing's understanding of itself and of humanity can only be enriched by breaking the taboo against engaging with religion.

For nursing ethics, a renewed attention to religion could mean opening an entire universe of discourse that is as rich and diverse as humanity itself—and from which nursing has largely excluded itself. Religious traditions have much to teach us about how ethical matters are lived out individually and communally in the day-to-day, not necessarily by the application of elegant ethical decision-making frameworks or studied ethical principles, but by reliance on virtues, sacred teachings, and communitarian mores. Examples from religions such as Judaism and Engaged Buddhism can teach us how to apply social justice at once at individual and social levels for human flourishing. Were nursing to open itself to the reflection and wisdom on the human condition, responsibility, and community offered by religious traditions, it would find itself able to think in new and more capacious ways about its identity, theory, practice, and ethics.

LIVED RELIGION, LIVED ETHICS

Finally, traditional ethics, particularly bioethics, has increasingly been critiqued as "armchair" ethics, debating formal systems of theory (such as the merits of deontological and utilitarian approaches) and prescribing principled solutions and decision-making algorithms for those ethical quandaries that stand out as extraordinary. In contrast, the recent move to "lived ethics" puts forward not a system of formal theory, but rather an approach to ethics that attends to moral assumptions and ideals that shape how individuals and groups live their lives. Lived ethics resonates for nurses who understand the mutual shaping of ideas and real life, where all of one's professional practice becomes an ethical way of being. Religions too must be understood as lived, not as codified, discrete systems of beliefs and practices. As amply illustrated in this volume, individuals take up religious affiliation, practices, and beliefs in various ways. Other social classifications and phenomena intersect with religion, so that the study of religion in isolation from other social considerations risks reification, conflation, and/or essentialisms. Recurrent in the preparation of this volume is the challenge of teasing out and articulating ethical systems of thought from everyday lived religion. Religious ethics, in particular, are lived in the everyday as an integrative way of life, as individuals and communities take direction from various sources of moral authority that may simultaneously emphasize virtuous living and communal responsibilities for all members of society. Religious ethics—whether indigenous, emergent, Hindu, Jewish, or Sikh—for this reason alone, serves as a remarkable resource for nurses, for it represents a completely different integrative approach to ethics than the bioethical models that dominate Western health care. Too often, nurses align with a particular school of ethics, such as feminist ethics, relational ethics, virtue ethics, contextual ethics, Kantian ethics, or principle based ethics, all of which have their strengths, but which alone do not provide sufficient resource for the complexity of moral practice in today's diverse societies. Religious ethics, with injunctions for everyday life embedded in strong social networks, can offer many lessons for nursing ethics on the everyday mutual shaping of ideas and practice.

Glossary

Adhyatma: Spiritual, principle of self.

Amidah: Also called *Shmoneh Esreh* (meaning 18), the central prayer of Jewish liturgy found in the prayer book, and recited in prayer services, originally containing 18 constituent blessings.

Amoraim (plural, meaning "those who tell over" or "those who say"): Refers to the scholars who follow the Tannaim, whose debate and reflection upon the oral law is eventually codified as the Gemara. This period covers approximately 200–500 CE in Babylonia and Israel.

Ashkenazim (plural): Originally Jews from Germany, later also applied to Jews from Western and Central Europe.

Atman: Individual self or the eternal soul, which is identical to Brahman in essence.

Ayurveda: A traditional system of medicine, regarded as the Hindu science of healing that originated in India during the Vedic age.

Bhagavad Gita: Literally translated as the song of God, the "Gita" is a sacred Hindu text considered to be a concise guide to Hindu theology and a practical guide to life. The text of the Gita is written as a conversation between Lord Krishna and Arjuna who is experiencing confusion and moral dilemmas on the battlefield about fighting his own cousins. Lord Krishna explains to Arjuna his duties as a warrior and prince and elaborates on the Hindu philosophies with examples and analogies that are considered life lessons from the divine.

Bhagya: Fate or destiny. It is the fruit of all karma (past and present) and is not in the hands of human beings.

Brahman: Absolute God who is beyond the thinking power of human beings. Brahman is great and infinite. Brahman transcends matter, time, space, energy, being, and everything beyond.

Buddhi: The rational and logical capacity or thinking of the brain. It is the instrument of intellect, knowledge, discernment, and decision and thus is considered a high mental faculty.

Carak (or Charak) Samhita: An ancient, comprehensive, and authoritative work of Ayurveda. This is the earliest literature on Indian medicine and health. The book is written in the form of the teachings of Atreya imparted to his pupil Agnivesa. It is central to modern day Ayurvedic medicine. Unique scientific contributions credited to the *Caraka Samhita* include a rational approach to the causation and cure of disease, and an introduction of objective methods of clinical examination.

Church: The body of Christians of which Jesus Christ is the head. It can also mean a subgroup of Christians, such as the Roman Catholic Church or the Protestant Church. It can also mean the building in which Christians worship.

Dharma: Signifies the divine law or divine path.

Fardh kifaya: A societal duty, specifically knowledge, that is required by the Muslim community; requires that the community have a scholar or expert in Islamic religious obligations to the community.

Fatwa: A formal religious legal opinion.

Fidiah: A payment.

Fiqh: Islamic jurisprudence (literally: understanding and acquisition of knowledge); the knowledge of practical Islamic rulings as deduced from detailed statements and religious texts.

Gita: See Bhagavad Gita.

Gospel: A writing that relates the life and teachings of Jesus Christ.

Gunas: Attributes. In Hindu philosophy, every worldly thing has three attributes: sattva, rajas, or tamas. Sattva is characterized by goodness, purity, illumination, order, stability, permanence, happiness, spirituality, cleanliness, and health. Rajas is characterized by passion, action, creation, desire, lust, attachment, movement, and striving. Tamas is characterized by darkness, destruction, madness, disease, dissolution, ignorance, intoxication, heaviness, and sleep.

Hadith: Saying(s) or action(s) ascribed to the Prophet or act(s) approved by the Prophet.

Halacha: The collective body of Jewish law, including Biblical, Talmudic, and rabbinic law.

Halal: The word *Halal*, as used by Arabs and Muslims, refers to anything that is considered permissible and lawful under religion. The word is derived from the verb *Halla*, to be or become lawful, legal, licit, legitimate, permissible, permitted, allowable, allowed, admissible, unprohibited, and unforbidden.

Haram: What is forbidden and punishable according to Islamic law. Prohibited, banned, illegal, and impermissible from a religious standpoint.

Haredim, Charedim: The most conservative form of Orthodox Judaism, sometimes referred to as Ultra-conservative.

Hijra: The emigration of the Prophet Muhammad from Mecca to Medina in 622 CE.

Holy Communion: Also called the Eucharist, this is the ritual whereby Christians commemorate the last supper when Christ shared bread and wine with his disciples and commanded them to continue to remember him in this way. The Eucharist is viewed in different ways in different churches. To some the bread and wine are actually mysteriously changed to Christ's flesh and blood, to others the change is more symbolic. Where it is celebrated, it is usually the most important sacrament of the church.

Ihsan: Perfection or excellence; requires that one takes faith into deed and action.

Ishwar: God.

Islam: The Qur'an defines Islam as the natural course of life that God has bestowed on humanity.

Ithm: Harm.

Kabbala: A school of rabbinic Judaism concerned with the mystical tradition of the faith that uses a set of primary texts that exist apart from the Jewish canon. These works include mystical ascent literature, exegetical literature, mystical Biblical commentaries, and philosophical works.

Karma: Literally means "actions or deeds." In Hinduism, karma refers to the law of causality where actions or deeds (whether voluntary or involuntary) lead to beneficial or harmful effects. The effects may not be immediate but are accumulative and may be experienced later in one's current life or in subsequent lives.

Kavanah: "Intention" or "direction of the heart."

Midrash: A homiletic (public preaching) method of Biblical exegesis or a collection of homiletic teachings.

Moksha: Release from the cycle of birth and death. In moksha, there is ultimate peace, ultimate knowledge, and ultimate enlightenment.

Monk: A person who has chosen to live a life of discipline and asceticism devoted to God. Monks either live alone or in communities with other monks.

New Testament: The second major part of the Christian Bible consisting of works written from about 50 CE to the mid-2nd century and telling of the life and teachings of Jesus Christ. While there is some disagreement among churches about which books should be included, most Christians agree on 27.

Old Testament: The first major part of the Christian bible consisting of works written from circa 13th century BCE to circa 2nd century BCE. There are between 39 and 51 books in the Old Testament, depending on the usage of a specific Christian Church. Much of what Christians call the Old Testament is known in Judaism as the *Tanach* or Hebrew Bible.

Parable: A story that teaches a moral or religious lesson.

Paramatman: Great Soul, God.

Perichoresis: This Greek word expresses the intimate fellowship between the three persons of the Trinity; as if they dwell in each other or interpenetrate each other.

Prakriti: Nature.

Prophet: The Prophet Muhammad, the Messenger of God. Any reference to the Prophet is usually followed by the symbol صلى الله عليه وسلم meaning "Peace be upon him."

Qur'an: The Holy Book of Islam; the highest and most authentic authority in Islam. Quotations from the Qur'an are normally followed by a reference to the chapter number (Sura).

Ramayana: A Hindu scripture that describes the life of Lord Rama. It depicts the duties and relationships, portraying ideal characters like the ideal servant, the ideal brother, the ideal wife and the ideal king, and serves as a guide for righteous conduct in daily life.

Responsa literature: A body of written legal decisions given by scholars to questions brought to them. Responsa address ordinary life situations. They are a unique category of rabbinic literature.

Sacraments: These are visible signs of the invisible grace of God. Usually they are in the form of church rituals such as baptism and Holy Communion. An act can be called a sacramental if it is thought to have a sacramental quality or be like a sacrament even if it is not a recognized sacrament.

Sanatan Dharma: Eternal religion that exists in God and is revealed by God.

Sansara or Samsara: The world where the cycle of birth, life, death, and rebirth (reincarnation) occurs.

Sat-Chit-Anand: A metaphor for God. Sat is existence, Chit is consciousness, and Ananda is bliss. Sat-Chit-Anand is existence–consciousness–bliss that can be experienced by human beings through self-realization. It also means God.

Schools of Fiqh: The schools of Islamic thought or jurisprudence; the four most important of which were founded by Malik, Abu Hanifa, Al-Shafie, and Ahmad Ibn Hanbal.

Segulot (plural; segulah, singular): Symbols created or actions performed for mystical, sometimes supernatural, purposes.

Sephardim (plural): Refers to Jews from the Iberian peninsula (Spain) who use a Sephardic liturgy; can also sometimes used to refer to all Jews who are not Ashkenazic.

Seva: Service.

Shari'a: The body of Islamic law based on the Qur'an and the Sunna.

Shulchan Aruch: Known as the code of Jewish Law. Written by Yosef Karo in 1563 and published in Venice in 1565. It is the most widely accepted compilation of the Jewish Law.

Sunna: Practices undertaken or approved by the Prophet Muhammad and established as legally binding precedents.

Synoptic gospels: The first three books of the New Testament: Matthew, Mark, and Luke.

Talmud: Includes the Mishneh (c. 200 CE), a collection and codification of oral law compiled by Rabbi Judah Ha-Nasi (the Prince) and his school in Palestine, c. 160–200 CE. Also includes the Jerusalem Gemara, a compilation of the commentary on the Mishnah by the Amora'im in Palestine c. the end of the 4th century. Together with the Mishnah this comprises the Jerusalem Talmud. Also includes the Babylonian Gemara (c. 500 CE), a compilation of the commentary on the Mishnah by scholars of the Babylonian academies, c. the end of the 5th century. This is a much more substantial and significant work than the Jerusalem Gemara. Together with the Mishnah this comprises the Babylonian Talmud.

Tanach: The Jewish scriptures. Tanach is an acrostic for Torah, Nevi'im, and Ketuvim. Also known as the Hebrew Bible and (by Christians) as The Old Testament.

Tannaim (plural): Refers to the Rabbinic sages, after the destruction of the Temple in Jerusalem (70 CE to 200 CE), whose exegesis is recorded in the *Mishnah*. The 130-year period of the Tannaim is referred to as the Mishnaic period. These sages directly transmitted the oral tradition, in uncodified form.

Therapeusis: A noble profession, which God honored by making it the miracle of Jesus, son of Mary. Abraham enumerating his Lord's gifts upon him, including "and if I fall ill He cures me."

Vedic Age: The time period during which Hindu religion evolved and the four *Vedas* (Rigveda, Yajurveda, Samveda, and Atharveda) were composed. It is thought to have been written between 3500 and 1500 BCE. This period is considered as an immortal era of the Indian civilization.

Index